PSYCHIATRIC PRESENTATIONS OF MEDICAL ILLNESS

Somatopsychic Disorders

PSYCHIATRIC PRESENTATIONS OF MEDICAL ILLNESS

Somatopsychic Disorders

Edited by

Richard C.W. Hall, M.D.
Professor of Psychiatry and Medicine
Medical College of Wisconsin
Milwaukee, Wisconsin

SP MEDICAL & SCIENTIFIC BOOKS

New York • London

Softcover reprint of the hardcover 1st edition 1980

SPECTRUM PUBLICATIONS, INC.
175–20 Wexford Terrace, Jamaica, N.Y. 11432

Library of Congress Cataloging in Publication Data
Main entry under title:

Psychiatric presentation of medical illness.

Includes index.

1. Psychological manifestations of general diseases. I. Hall, Richard C. W. [DNLM: 1. Mental disorders— Etiology. 2. Diagnosis. WM100.3 P9745]

RC71.3.P79 616.89 80-10344

ISBN-13: 978-94-011-7679-8 e-ISBN-13: 978-94-011-7677-4
DOI: 10.1007/ 978-94-011-7677-4

Second Printing, 1981

DEDICATED TO
Ryan C. W. Hall
and
The Children of His Generation

ACKNOWLEDGMENTS

I would like to thank Mrs. Dorothy Manley, for her painstaking and careful work in managing the collection, proofing, and preparation of the chapters of this volume, as well as for her equanimitas and helpful advice. I am grateful to Dr. Earl R. Gardner and Mrs. Sondra K. Stickney, for their thoughtful comments and advice while editing this volume.

Contributors

RICHARD A. DeVAUL, M.D.
Associate Professor of Psychiatry
Department of Psychiatry
The University of Texas
Medical School at Houston
Houston, Texas

NEIL EDWARDS, M.D.
Associate Professor of Psychiatry
Department of Psychiatry
University of Tennessee Center for the Health Sciences
Memphis, Tennessee

LOUIS A. FAILLACE, M.D.
Professor and Chairman
Department of Psychiatry
The University of Texas
Medical School at Houston
Houston, Texas

ARTHUR M. FREEMAN, III, M.D.
Professor of Psychiatry
Department of Psychiatry
University of Alabama in Birmingham
Birmingham, Alabama

EARL R. GARDNER, Ph.D.
Assistant Professor of Psychiatry
Department of Psychiatry
The University of Texas
Medical School at Houston
Houston, Texas

MOHAN GEHI, M.D.
Assistant Professor of Psychiatry
Center for the Health Sciences
University of Tennessee
Memphis, Tennessee

ROBERT W. GUYNN, M.D.
Associate Professor of Psychiatry
Department of Psychiatry
The University of Texas
Medical School at Houston
Houston, Texas

RICHARD C. W. HALL, M.D.
Professor of Psychiatry and Medicine
Department of Psychiatry
Medical College of Wisconsin
Milwaukee, Wisconsin

THOMAS H. HOLMES, M.D.
Professor of Psychiatry and Behavioral Medicine
Department of Psychiatry
University of Washington
Seattle, Washington

BRIAN KIRKPATRICK, M.D.
Department of Psychiatry
University of North Carolina
Chapel Hill, North Carolina

WILLIAM W. LUKENSMEYER, M.D.
Associate Professor of Psychiatry
Department of Psychiatry
University of Alabama in Birmingham
Birmingham, Alabama

T.B. MACKENZIE, M.D.
Assistant Professor of Psychiatry and Medicine
University of Minnesota Medical School
Department of Psychiatry
Minneapolis, Minnesota

GUSTAVE NEWMAN, M.D.
Associate Professor of Psychiatry
Department of Psychiatry
University of Florida
Gainesville, Florida

MARK PERL, M.B.B.S.
Assistant Professor of Psychiatry
Department of Psychiatry
The University of Texas
Medical School at Houston
Houston, Texas

JOHN PETRICH, M.D.
Assistant Professor of Psychiatry
Department of Psychiatry
and Behavioral Sciences
University of Washington
Seattle, Washington

MICHAEL K. POPKIN, M.D.
Associate Professor of Psychiatry and Medicine
Department of Psychiatry
University of Minnesota Medical School
Minneapolis, Minnesota

MARVIN M. SCHUSTER, M.D.
Professor of Medicine
Assistant Professor of Psychiatry
Departments of Medicine and Psychiatry
Johns Hopkins University
School of Medicine
Baltimore, Maryland

JOHN J. SCHWAB, M.D.
Professor and Chairman
Department of Psychiatry
and Behavioral Sciences
University of Louisville
Louisville, Kentucky

SONDRA K. STICKNEY, R.N., C.
Psychiatric Liaison Nurse
Department of Psychiatry
Hermann Hospital
Houston, Texas

WILLIAM L. WEBB, JR., M.D.
Professor and Chairman
Department of Psychiatry
University of Tennessee
Memphis Mental Health Institute
Memphis, Tennessee

Introduction

When my colleagues and I began the task of assembling this volume, several difficult questions arose: For whom were we writing? Was the purpose to elucidate psychiatric or medical presentation? Should references reflect specific topical areas, or lead the reader to a more general view of a particular topic? Would a symptom or system approach best serve the reader? Should the volume cover a few areas in detail, or attempt to survey a larger area of knowledge?

The present text reflects an attempt to answer these questions. It is designed for the student of medicine who desires a broader understanding of those medical illnesses that produce psychiatric aberration. We hope it will be of assistance to the medical student or house officer studying medicine, neurology, family practice, pediatrics, or psychiatry; as well as to the practicing clinician who wishes a refresher on this subject or a reference for his library. The text is intended to strike a useful balance between medicine and psychiatry by providing a list of differentials for specific symptoms or conditions, as well as suggestions for medical evaluation.

References have been chosen which we hope will assist the reader in further study. We have attempted to diversify them and list a spectrum of articles that deal with both academic and practical treatment considerations.

The initial volume is divided into four sections that address both a symptom and system approach. Section I provides an overview defining the scope of the problem of medical illnesses producing psychiatric illness. Section II presents a differential approach to specific psychiatric symptoms, or conditions, with a review of pertinent literature and suggestions for further workup of the specific problem. Section III provides an approach by system, permitting the clinician who has a patient with a specific medical disorder to review its psychiatric presentation. These chapters are designed to provide the reader with an academic as well as a clinical understanding of psychiatric symptoms that may precede or occur simultaneously with other medical indicators of disease. Section IV defines drug-induced and drug-related psychiatric disorders.

In each section, an attempt has been made to define clinically useful information rather than that of a purely theoretical nature. We have purposely striven to encompass as large an area as possible within the pages allotted. Subsequent volumes will deal at greater length with more diverse topics.

Finally, one must address the question of why, and why now? It is the hope of all contributors to this volume that medicine and psychiatry form a closer union with a better understanding of their interface so that patients, both medical and psychiatric, are able to obtain the most direct and humane care. If this text contributes to the proper diagnosis of any of the 5 to 10 percent of psychiatric patients with medically produced symptoms, or to the better understanding of the 35 percent of medical patients with psychiatric symptoms, we will consider our endeavor worthwhile.

Richard C. W. Hall, M.D.

Foreword

The founding fathers of psychiatry always envisioned psychiatry as an extension of medicine. However, during the period of the 1950s and 1960s, as social psychiatry, humanistic psychiatry, existential psychiatry, and community psychiatry were undergoing a period of rapid progress, the field as a whole loosened its ties with the traditional medical arts. A minority in the field warned of future adverse consequences if we continued our non-medical drift.

New journals abounded and the public's imagination was captured by theorems designed to: prevent war, facilitate nuclear disarmament, save cities from ruin, eliminate criminality from society, develop alternate life styles, eliminate mental illness through "prevention," and produce inner happiness and growth through self-help. Although noble, these goals remained for the most part unattainable.

The new egalitarianism of psychiatry, predicated on concepts of the indigenous worker, psychiatric technicians, crisis intervention by non-professionals, community mobilization, and citizen involvement, further removed psychiatry from its medical foundations. Many espoused a new doctrine of separatism, which stated that a medical workup or intervention was unnecessary and, with the possible exception of psychosis, relief could be obtained through talking or behavioral therapies. A flood of articles appeared that proposed routes to modify intrapsychic distress.

The encounter movement burgeoned and was commercially fed by advertisements in local newspapers such as: "Get your head straight. Forty-eight-hour nude marathon encounter offered by experienced psychotherapist at attractive hillside home. Meet with others; explore yourself and attain new mental comfort. Fee for entire weekend, including food, $500."

In a land where the dollar is king, it is no surprise that these movements did well. As has been the tradition of psychiatry from its onset, a polarization of the new disciplines followed. Many of these groups began to exercise, in the best American tradition, their political, social, and economic power. The conservative and traditional values held by medically oriented psychiatrists seemed out of place, and began to appear archaic. Biologically oriented psychiatrists were characterized as insensitive or simply misinformed in their attempts to treat mental illness with medication, or to find biological causes for its occurrence. Non-psychiatric physicians viewed these developments in psychiatry with remote and distant amusement.

Once the premise that the mind and body could be treated independently was accepted, proponents of the new techniques argued that traditional medical approaches had no place in the treatment of emotional disorders. The government substantiated this hypothesis when it failed to mandate medical evaluation for patients seen at community mental health centers.

Freedom of choice was encouraged. This doctrine suggested that it was no longer important for a practitioner of the psychiatric art to be schooled in medicine. Psychologists argued, as did social workers, family counselors, ministers, and nurses, that a medical degree was not important in counseling situations. For awhile, psychiatry concurred with this view. Internships in the traditional medical disciplines of internal medicine, general medicine, and pediatrics were felt to be superfluous, and many argued that psychiatrists need not suffer such additional training in order to practice their art.

During the 1960s and early 1970s, at the urging of the then leaders in psychiatry, the government committed billions of dollars to the Community Mental Health Movement, predicated on the promise that mental illness would be drastically reduced and treatment would be available to all. The failure and unrealistic promises of the Community Mental Health Movement disillusioned both the populace and the politicians. The government began to expound a need to intervene. Psychiatry felt special pressure, since debate on early bills suggested that the government could not be responsible for paying practitioners of empathy, or social trainers—roles traditionally reserved for the ministry. There again rose voices within organized psychiatry that reminded the profession of its legitimate place in medicine and of the tradition of the "alienist" as one who cares for the sick. In my opinion, healthy changes occurred. Universities took a leadership role in exploring new avenues of medical, biological, and cognitive intervention. Liaison services reshaped their operational styles, and residency programs once again began the Socratic teaching of psychiatric medicine. Rotation on medical services was again made mandatory during the first year of training. It is within this framework that we arrive at the present tumultuous period of psychiatry.

Psychiatry finds itself at a crossroad. We have to decide what kind of discipline we are going to be. Are we to stay in medicine, or are we to gravitate in many diverse areas and become primarily a collection of social sciences? To many of us, it is very clear that we are physicians first and then psychiatrists. Psychiatrists have tended to neglect their roles as physicians, which has isolated the psychiatrists from the rest of their medical colleagues. Recently, because of increased government regulation regarding the payment for treatment, many psychiatrists are suddenly becoming aware that in order to be reimbursed, they must be physicians. It is unfortunate that it has taken the impairment of financial gain to force many psychiatrists to remember that they are physicians.

Because one espouses the idea that he or she is a physician does not mean the abandonment of one's social and community responsibilities, nor of the commitment to improve the care of the disadvantaged. However, the concept that anyone can take care of psychiatric patients is a fallacy and a disservice to the patient.

Dr. Hall and his colleagues clearly demonstrate in this book that there are many psychiatric illnesses with primary physical etiologies. The unrealistic and unattainable promises of the 1960s have given way to the more realistic and rewarding goals of physicians diagnosing and treating psychiatric illnesses, and when appropriate, the underlying physical illnesses.

Knowledge of the physical causes of psychiatric symptoms is essential if the psychiatrist is to fulfill his role as physician, and in so doing to offer his patient the best medical and psychiatric care. It is this knowledge that distinguishes the psychiatrist from the psychologist, nurse, and social worker and defines his primary care role in the management of the psychiatrically ill.

This volume provides, in a single source, the most complete and comprehensive presentation of this subject currently available. The annual volumes to follow will review and reference current important work in the area and will permit the clinician to keep abreast of the field and sharpen his diagnostic and treatment skills.

Louis A. Faillace, M.D.

Contents

PSYCHIATRIC PRESENTATIONS OF MEDICAL ILLNESS

Somatopsychic Disorders

Section I
AN OVERVIEW

CHAPTER 1

Medically Induced Psychiatric Disease– An Overview

RICHARD C. W. HALL, M.D.

It is our hope that this text will serve as a guide in assisting the physician to recognize at least some of those medical illnesses that present as psychiatric disorders. Few doctors have difficulty in recognizing or evaluating a full-blown organic brain syndrome. They do, however, often have difficulty with psychiatric symptoms not characteristic of the organic brain syndrome, but which mimic those of the major psychoses or psychoneuroses. Physicians must regard the mind—its functions and aberrations—in a manner similar to other organ systems, realizing that psychiatric symptoms are non-specific and may occur as the result of medical as well as psychiatric disorders. Cognitive and behavioral disorders represent a final common pathway resulting from central nervous system insult of any etiology.

It has long been known that psychiatric patients are at higher risk for concurrent medical illness than are their age- and sex-matched counterparts in the general population. Comroe (1936) evaluated 100 patients who were diagnosed as suffering from psychoneurotic disorders and found that 24 percent of these patients developed significant organic disease within 8 months of their initial psychiatric evaluation. He suggested that psychiatric and behavioral symptoms are often the harbingers of an unrecognized medical illness, and pleaded for medical evaluation of such patients. Marshall (1949) confirmed these studies by demonstrating a physical morbidity of 44 percent in patients admitted to psychiatric hospitals.

Many articles subsequently appeared in the literature, suggesting systems to differentiate these patients based upon their psychological profiles. Meyer (1958), while investigating the relationship of surgical illness to psychiatric disorders, cautioned against assigning functional causes to elusive symptoms simply because they arose in the midst of emotional crises. His report was timely since several cluster studies had appeared and provided lists of characteristics by which to differentiate the medically ill patient from those with functional complaints. There is little question that these lists have a utilitarian value in surveying large numbers of patients. The danger in their use lies in the fact that they provide a significant number of falsely positive patients who, in fact, suffer from underlying medical illnesses. Such patients, once having a psychiatric label applied, are unlikely to receive a full medical evaluation until their physical symptoms become so compelling and clear that workup is mandated.

Let us examine some of the dilemmas inherent in the use of such a profile. (See Table 1.)

TABLE 1. REPORTED CHARACTERISTICS OF PSYCHIATRIC PATIENTS WITH FUNCTIONAL MEDICAL COMPLAINTS

- A history of anxiety or unusual behavior present since childhood or adolescence.
- The patient evidences a multiplicity of symptoms that involve several organ systems.
- The patient evidences unusual symptoms that are difficult for the physician to deal with.
- A history of atypical response or failure to respond to treatment.
- A history of doctor shopping.
- A failure to carry out the physician's recommendations.
- The absence of concern in the face of serious complaints.
- Symptom onset concomitant with, or exacerbated by, particular people or stressful life events.
- Apparent secondary gain resulting from physical symptomatology.

1. *A history of anxiety or unusual behavior present since childhood or adolescence.*

Medical illness is no respecter of social adjustment; psychiatric patients also become medically ill. Many insidious or debilitating diseases, such as nutritional disorders, parasitic infestations, epilepsy, chronic anemia, post-rubella syndrome, and endocrine disorders, may produce anxiety or unusual behavior during childhood or adolescence.

2. *The patient evidences a multiplicity of symptoms that involve several organ systems.*

Although this statement follows Osler's caveat that a physician should attempt to explain symptoms on the basis of a single disease, it begs the issue since many of the illnesses presenting with psychiatric symptoms are polysystem diseases. Collagen vascular and endocrine disorders frequently affect multiple organ systems, as do chronic infectious diseases and poisoning.

3. *The patient evidences unusual symptoms that are difficult for the physician to deal with.*

One need only think of the exacerbation, remissions, and fleeting symptoms seen with chronic demyelinative diseases, such as multiple sclerosis, and disorders such as pernicious anemia and chronic metal poisonings to realize that simply because a symptom is unusual, does not in and of itself suggest a psychogenic origin.

4. *A history of atypical response or failure to respond to treatment.*

What this statement really means is that the patient has not responded because he has not been appropriately diagnosed or treated. For the majority of medically ill patients with psychiatric symptoms, the above caveat represents a problem of physician recognition rather than patient compliance.

5. *A history of doctor shopping.*

Although of value in recognizing dependent patients who are somatizing, the overapplication of this principle can be dangerous. Consider for a moment the situation of a patient with "real" symptoms, unrelieved by long-term treatment offered by a physician who is unable to make a definite diagnosis. Fear of dependency, helplessness, or insanity may prompt this patient to seek another physician. Doctor shopping in this case may represent prudent judgment.

6. *A failure to carry out the physician's recommendations.*

Medical compliance for any patient may be limited at best. Non-compliance is not confined to the patient with psychiatric or emotional problems. Lasagna (1954, 1958, 1962, 1963) has demonstrated that compliance with physicians' orders diminished as diagnostic uncertainty increased and the number of therapeutics used for symptomatic relief increased. In cases where medications prove ineffective in relieving symptoms, their elimination by the patient may represent "the better part of valor."

7. *The absence of concern in the face of serious complaints.*

Of all the items on this list, this is perhaps the most useful, yet the least applicable to a large number of patients. True "la belle indifference" is useful in establishing the diagnosis of conversion hysteria when it is coupled with symptoms of inexplicable pain or sensory loss; however, indifference also occurs with illnesses producing deterioration of the frontal cortex or generalized cerebral atrophy.

8. *Symptom onset concomitant with, or exacerbated by, particular people or stressful life events.*

This guideline is useful when carefully defined, but it is too frequently employed to justify dismissal of an underlying physical disorder when such dismissal is not based upon medical fact. Consider for a moment, the relationship between psychiatric and metabolic stress and the exacerbation of diabetes mellitus—with increased stress prompting an increased demand for insulin, or emotional stress precipitating atrial flutter in a patient with paroxysmal atrial tachycardia. Holmes and Rahe (1967) have shown that stress beyond a finite limit is associated with an increased vulnerability for the development of subsequent medical illness. To obtain a history of stress and then to dismiss the patient's medical complaints on the basis that stress preceded their development, would be parabolic folly in the extreme.

9. *Apparent secondary gain resulting from physical symptomatology.*

Secondary gain is a major factor in patients who malinger, in the passive dependent, and in the hysterical. However, it too provides enough false positives to make its value in dismissing further medical workup useless. In a study conducted by the author, of 150 patients about to undergo their second surgery for chronic lumbar pain, my associates and I were unable to predict, with any statistical certainty, the operative findings, based upon an analysis of any combination of the above factors. It has long been recognized that when people are frightened, placed in a position of enforced dependency, or adapting to a more limited life because of physical symptoms, they tend to regress and become more dependent. Physicians should bear this in mind before dismissing their symptoms on the basis of the patient's increased dependency, which may be interpreted as secondary gain.

INCIDENCE OF MEDICAL ILLNESS PRODUCING PSYCHIATRIC DISORDERS

What is the incidence of previously unrecognized medical disorders in a general psychiatric population? One of the first etiological classification studies was conducted by Herridge (1960). He found a 50 percent physical morbidity in 209 consecutive psychiatric patients, in spite of previous medical examination. After careful evaluation, he believed that there was a 5 percent incidence of medical disorders that were causative of psychiatric symptoms. Twenty-one percent of his patients had a significant medical illness, which he considered "concomitant" and apparently contributing to the onset of psychological symptoms. Eight percent of his population developed "consecutive" physical disorders, which "apparently" resulted from the psychological illness or its treatment. Of the remaining patients, 34 percent had physical illnesses that required attention but were not related to their psychiatric symptoms. Davis (1965), while evaluating psychiatric outpatients, found a 42 percent incidence of physical disease that he considered causative of psychiatric complaints. Fifty-eight percent of all patients attending his psychiatric clinic were found to suffer from some physical illness that required medical attention. Johnson (1968) conducted detailed physical examinations on 250 consecutive admissions to a psychiatric inpatient service and found a 12 percent incidence of cases where physical illness represented an important etiological factor in the patients presenting psychiatric symptoms. Eighty percent of the illnesses were "missed" by the physicians who examined these patients prior to admission. In 6.6 percent of the cases, the underlying cause of medical illness was not initially recognized during the patients' psychiatric hospitalization. Sixty percent of the patients in this study demonstrated positive physical findings. Maguire and Granville-Grossman (1968) demonstrated a 33.5 percent incidence of medical illness in 200 consecutive psychiatric inpatients, 70 percent of which were considered severe. Forty-nine percent of these patients had illnesses that were previously unknown to either them or their family physician.

Hall et al. (1978), in a study of 658 consecutive psychiatric outpatients, demonstrated a 9.1 percent incidence of medical disorders that were felt to be the definite or probable cause of the patients' psychiatric symptoms. Cardiovascular and endocrine disorders were the most frequent causes of psychiatric symptomatology, followed by infections, pulmonary disease, gastrointestinal and hematologic disorders, central nervous system diseases and malignancies. They demonstrated that psychoneurotic depression and anxiety neurosis were the most frequent psychiatric diagnoses made in patients with medical illnesses producing psychiatric symptoms. It was noteworthy that 28 percent of the group was diagnosed as being functionally psychotic. The majority of these patients did not present with organic brain syndromes, but rather with symptoms of depression, anxiety, sleep disturbance, appetite disorder, diminished concentration, speech difficulty or change in speech pattern, hyperacusis, auditory or visual hallucinations, recent personality change, or the sudden intensification of premorbid personality in previously stable patients. Twenty percent of those patients with medically induced psychiatric symptoms experienced visual hallucinations, distortions, or pronounced visual illusions. Similar symptoms were seen in less than 0.5 percent of non-medically impaired patients. Thus, the presence of visual hallucinations, distortions, or illusions should be considered pathognomonic of an underlying medical disorder until carefully proven otherwise. This study also demonstrated that a detailed medical review of systems, in combination with a careful physical examination and a SMA-34 biochemical screen, would define the probable medical cause of psychiatric symptoms in 80 percent of cases where such disorders existed. It was noteworthy that only 25 percent of the medically ill patients, or their physicians, were aware of the specific underlying medical illness that affected them. No differences were found between the medically and psychiatrically ill patients concerning the availability of a family physician or the frequency with which they visited that doctor. One striking finding was that, although approximately 70 percent of all patients considered themselves to have a family physician, 72 percent had not been physically examined during the preceding year.

In studying the medical practice of psychiatrists, McIntyre and Ramano (1977), found that 66 percent did not perform physical examinations. Only 32 percent of the psychiatrists questioned felt competent to perform such an examination. In looking at the practice of psychiatric residents in an emergency room situation, 59 percent failed to perform physicals. When physical examinations were performed, they yielded useful information in 92 percent of the cases. Koranyi (1977) draws the medical alienation dilemma into sharp focus in his report of 28 deaths occurring in a psychiatric outpatient population. Of these

28, 13 were caused by significant underlying medical illnesses, 6 of which were unrecognized because of failure to medically evaluate the patient. Four additional deaths could have been prevented had a diagnosis been made. This dilemma is further highlighted by the report from a Texas psychiatric hospital: Of 9 deaths that occurred in that hospital in 1977, 3 were the result of previously undiagnosed carcinoma of the pancreas (Symposium on Organic Diseases and Psychiatry, 1977).

In conclusion, the evidence is overwhelming that psychiatric symptoms frequently belie underlying medical illness. The incidence of such diseases producing psychiatric symptoms ranges from 5 to 42 percent, reflecting the population and selection variables employed. The incidence of unrecognized medical disease producing psychiatric symptoms is in the range of 10 percent for psychiatric outpatients. These disorders are only detected when a careful medical history, physical examination, and laboratory workup are initiated. The presence of a physician of record, or a family doctor following the patient, does not protect either the patient or the treating psychiatrist from the presence of an unrecognized medical disorder. Demographic variables, in and of themselves, do not in any meaningful way predict risk. Visual hallucinations, illusions, or distortions are perhaps the most specific signs indicating underlying medical illness, and when present, should be considered as indications of medically induced symptoms until proven otherwise. Although the majority of patients present with psychoneurotic symptoms, it is crucial that the physician bear in mind that approximately 30 percent of patients with underlying medical illnesses have symptoms of functional psychoses. Prompt recognition of an underlying medical disorder lessens the probability that the illness will progress, or that the patient will develop irreversible damage. It mitigates against long-term treatment with psychotropic drugs, changes in the patient's legal status, and the possibility of long-term psychiatric hospitalization. The misdiagnosis of psychiatric disease and the application of psychiatric labels to medically ill patients significantly reduces their chances for improvement and often results in a worsening of both their physical and psychiatric condition. Adequate medical investigation, on the other hand, assures safety for both the patient and his doctor.

REFERENCES

Comroe, B. I. Follow-up studies of one-hundred patients diagnosed as neurotic. *J. Nerv. Dis.* 83:679–684 (1936).

Davis, D. W. Physical illness in psychiatric outpatients. *Brit. J. Psychiat.* 111:27–33 (1965).

Hall, R. C. W., Popkin, M. K., DeVaul, R., Faillace, L. A., and Stickney, S. K. Physical illness presenting as psychiatric disease. *Arch. Gen. Psychiat.* 35:11:1315–1320 (1978).

Herridge, C. F. Physical disorders in psychiatric illness: A study of 209 consecutive admissions. *Lancet.* 2:949–951 (1960).

Holmes, T. H. and Rahe, R.H. The social readjustment rating scale. *J. Psychosom. Rsch.* 11:213–218 (1967).

Johnson, D. A. W. The evaluation of routine physical examination in psychiatric cases. *Practitioner.* 200:686–691 (1968).
Koranyi, E.K. Fatalities in 2,070 psychiatric outpatients. *Arch. Gen. Psychiat.* 34:1137–1142 (1977).
Lasagna, L. The investigator's responsibility to the patients. *J. Chron. Dis.* 16:955–959 (1963).
Lasagna, L. Psychological effects of medication (abridged). *Proc. Royal Soc. Med.* 55:773–776 (1962).
Lasagna, L., Laties, V. G., and Dohan, J. L. Further studies on the "pharmacology" of placebo administration. *J. Clin. Invest.* 37:533–537 (1958).
Lasagna, L., Mosteller, F., von Felsinger, J. M., and Beecher, H. K. A study of the placebo response. *Am. J. Med.* 16:770–779 (1954).
Maguire, G. P., and Granville-Grossman, K. L. Physical illness in psychiatric patients. *Brit. J. Psychiat.* 114: 1365-1369 (1968).
Marshall, H. Incidence of physical disorders among psychiatric inpatients. *Brit. Med. J.* 2:468–470 (1949).
McIntyre, J. S., and Ramano, J. Is there a stethoscope in the house (and is it used?). *Arch. Gen. Psychiat.* 34:1147–1151 (1977).
Meyer, B. C. Some psychiatric aspects of surgical practice. *Psychosom. Med.* 20:203–214 (1958).
Symposium on Organic Diseases and Psychiatry (verbal presentation). Texas Research Institute of Mental Sciences, Houston, Texas (October 1977).

Section II

THE MEDICAL DIFFERENTIAL OF PSYCHIATRIC SYMPTOMS

CHAPTER 2

Anxiety

RICHARD C. W. HALL, M.D.

Freud (1936) termed anxiety "the hallmark of neurosis" and rightly defined it as a major constituent of psychiatric disorders. With the possible exception of depression, no psychiatric symptom is more well known, for all of us have experienced periods of anxiety or depression. Low levels of anxiety facilitate adjustment, adaptation, and personal progress. Higher levels disorganize—concentration becomes impaired; autonomic symptoms develop; sleep is disturbed; and sensations of dysphoria, fatigue, and exhaustion become prominent.

It has been variously estimated that up to 50 percent of patients seen in general practitioners' offices complain of anxiety or anxiety-related symptoms. Most physicians recognize the anxiety states, but few proceed with full medical workup when such symptoms are unaccompanied by clearcut indicators of other medical disease. Yet, anxiety may be a symptom of either a medical or psychiatric disorder (Bailey and Murray, 1928; Berson, 1956; Bingley, 1958; Cohen et al, 1948; Ferrer, 1968; Frostig and Spies, 1940). The complex nature and variability of somatic complaints reported by anxious patients may encourage the physician to dismiss symptoms which, if evaluated, could define an underlying physiologic disorder.

FORMS OF ANXIETY

Anxiety may de defined as a state of fear, where the cause of the fear is unknown. Psychiatrically, it is an unpleasant feeling associated with psychophysiological changes that occur in response to unknown intrapsychic conflict. In contrast to fear, the danger or threat is unreal, yet the patient has a feeling of being overwhelmed. Exhaustion results from prolonged hypervigilance. Similar symptoms occur in patients experiencing metabolically induced anxiety. In these cases, the anxiety is not related to intrapsychic conflict, but rather to a derangement of physiologic homeostasis (Cohen et al., 1948).

In an analytic context, *neurotic anxiety* arises from a threat that deeply repressed and dangerous impulses may enter consciousness and disrupt ego function. Conscious recognition of these impulses would produce unacceptable consequences for the individual. Anxiety mobilizes other defense mechanisms, which keep this material out of awareness (More and Fine, 1967).

The term *normal anxiety* is used to define those situations where anxious feelings are logically connected to some current or impending test of the individual, such as in the case of the student about to take an examination. Anxiety may spring from his lack of preparedness, his competitive strivings, or his need to do well to obtain a seat in graduate school. In such cases, there is reasonable ground for apprehension.

When anxiety arises suddenly, is severe, and is unattached to any ideational content, it is termed *free floating*. If anxiety is not subjectively experienced by the individual, but manifests itself only through somatic symptoms, it is termed *covert*. Where anxiety is the dominant symptom in an individual who evidences the recruitment of various other defensive mechanisms, an *anxiety neurosis* is said to exist.

If anxiety becomes so severe as to disrupt a patient's ego functioning and is accompanied by severe and overwhelming somatic manifestations, a state of *panic* occurs. Periods of panic may be accompanied by short-lived episodes of psychosis with hallucinations, delusions, derealization, and depersonalization. Misinterpretations followed by projection are felt by many to represent the mechanism by which hallucinations occur. When present, such hallucinations usually have a threatening or accusatory quality and may be further structured into delusions of persecution. During these states, the patient may either become agitated and aggressive—running about aimlessly or evidencing other flight mechanisms—or become immobilized by his somatic symptoms. Should the latter occur, the patient will appear overwhelmed and bewildered. Suicide during states of panic is not uncommon (Ackner, 1954; Cattell and Scheier, 1958).

More and Fine (1967) define the typical intrapsychic fears and dangers seen in patients with anxiety as follows:

1. *Object loss:* Separation or actual loss of person (real or symbolic) on whom the person depends for care or love.
2. *Loss of love:* Anger or disapproval on the part of a person upon whom one depends.
3. *Castration anxiety:* Fear of injury to genital or other bodily parts; threats to body integrity.
4. *Bad conscience:* Guilt because one's own moral standards have been violated, in reality or fantasy.
5. *Loss of self esteem:* The result of inability to live up to one's own ideals.

SYMPTOMS OF ANXIETY

Anxiety, whether due to physical or psychological causes, can present with disruption of practically any bodily system. (Ackner, 1954; Allan, 1944; Bartley, 1957; Cattell and Scheier, 1958; Cohen et al., 1948; Dill, 1939; Garmany, 1955; Lader and Satorius, 1968; Noreik, 1970; Roth, 1959; Thompson, 1965; Wheeler et al., 1950; Winokur and Holemon, 1963). Symptoms may be aggregated into clusters or appear selectively. (Cattell and Scheier, 1958) There is currently no rational explanation as to why a given individual manifests symptoms involving specific organ systems.

The manifestations of anxiety may be divided into 3 subgroups:

Psychological Manifestations

These represent the inner feelings of terror, tension, apprehension, and dread, as well as the more extreme manifestations that occur with panic, such as derealization, depersonalization, hallucinations, fear of impending insanity, impulsivity, aggressiveness, psychomotor immobilization, and suicidal ideation.

Intellectual Disturbances

Such disturbances are evidenced by diminution of the patient's basic intellectual strengths and manifested primarily by diminished concentration, disruption of logically associated thought patterns, inability to perceptually organize and integrate the life space, cyclical thinking, and sensory flooding (i.e., a sensation of being overwhelmed by input stimuli).

Somatic Manifestations

These are autonomic and visceral symptoms, which include: palpitations; precordial pain or pressure; lightheadedness; tachycardia; elevated blood pressure; easy fatigability; increased perspiration, particularly of the face and hands; vasomotor changes, such as, coldness of hands or feet, flushing, blushing, pallor, numbness, and tingling of the extremities; sensations of vertigo, dyspnea, and air hunger; chest pain; headache; blurred vision; tinnitus; interference with sexual function; anorexia; diarrhea; weight loss or gain; fine tremor of the extremities; brisk tendon reflexes; pupillary dilatation; abdominal pain or cramping; syncopal episodes; non-specific muscular weakness; and urinary urgency, hesitancy, or frequency.

SPECIFIC ANXIETY CONSTELLATIONS

Some authors feel that specific anxiety constellations may be seen in certain defined situations (Winokur and Holemon, 1963; Cameron, 1963; Klein, 1964; Beebe, 1955; Bettelheim, 1953; Hall and Simmons, 1972). For example, sudden panic episodes are felt to be related to increased sympathetic and adrenal medullary output, and are thus associated with tremor, tachycardia, hypertension, diaphoresis, pupillary dilatation, and diminished salivation and gastric acid secretion.

Chronic stress, such as occurs in combat situations and in people living in countries under siege, produces a condition known as *battle fatigue*. Here, tension, nervousness, and a tendency to be easily startled are noted. Physical complications of headache, anorexia, and diarrhea dominate the clinical picture (Beebe, 1955; Bettelheim, 1953; Hall and Simmons, 1972; Chodoff, 1963; Eitinger and Strom, 1972; Grinker and Spiegel, 1945; Hocking, 1970).

Acute anxiety attacks are most likely to present with palpitations, difficulty in falling asleep, sensations of constriction in the chest, or a feeling that the lungs are not adequately filled. Deep sighing respirations and an increased respiratory rate lead to respiratory alkalosis, producing giddiness, visual field constriction, and tachycardia, as well as circumoral and peripheral paresthesias which may progress to tetany with carpopedal spasm and syncope *(the hyperventilation syndrome)* (Garmany, 1955; Lader and Sartorius, 1968; Roth, 1959).

Chronic anxiety states, which may or may not be punctuated by acute anxiety episodes, are characterized by steady, prolonged, and distressing disturbances of mood (Wheeler et al., 1950). These symptoms are less intense, though not necessarily qualitatively different from those seen in patients with acute anxiety. Patients having chronic anxiety symptoms frequently report depression, hopelessness, and feelings of sadness, as well as diminished concentration, intellectual performance, and thought disruption. Intelligence testing may show deficits similar to those seen in patients with early dementia i.e., diminished concentration, diminished short-term memory, and diminished serial task performance). Somatic complaints accompanying chronic anxiety most frequently include: dyspnea, palpitations, chest pain, dizziness, dysmenorrhea, fatigue, difficulty falling asleep, nausea, vomiting, frontal and occipital headache, anorexia, diarrhea, and weight loss (Winokur and Holemon, 1963). Physical examination may reveal signs of constant tension, such as a fine tremor of the extended arms, brisk tendon reflexes, rapid heart rate, increased blood pressure, and pupillary dilatation. Laboratory studies show reduced gastric acid secretion and increased adrenal cortical activity (Perkoff et al., 1954; Rioch, 1956; Venning et al., 1957).

DIAGNOSIS OF PSYCHOGENIC ANXIETY

As stated in the preceding chapter, in the absence of full medical evaluation, no specific symptom or historical item can differentiate psychogenic from medically produced anxiety. Certain factors, however, are useful in suggesting its etiology.

Psychogenically produced anxiety rarely makes its appearance before the age of 18, or after the age of 35, with the age of peak incidence being 25; females predominate 3:2, with most patients having a positive family history (Cohen et al., 1948). When initially seen, the patient's chief complaint usually centers on emotional distress. More than 60 percent of patients with psychogenic anxiety have other psychiatric symptoms, such as phobias, conversion syndromes, or psychoneurotic depressions, present or elicitable at the time of examination (Cohen et al., 1948; Winokur and Holemon, 1963). Psychogenic anxiety states are most likely to occur in individuals with compulsive, hysterical, or passive dependent personalities. In over 80 percent of cases, some immediate ego threat such as job loss, impending divorce, fear of loss or separation from a loved one, etc., can be elicited. Contrary to popular thought, the presence of *angor animi* (a sense of imminent danger, where the patient feels that he will suddenly lose his mind, or die) does not differentiate psychogenic from medically produced anxiety.

A physical etiology should be sought in individuals younger than 18, or older than 35, who suddenly develop anxiety which disrupts their normal activity, and who have an otherwise negative psychiatric history. Those patients with illnesses known to be associated with the production of anxiety states should be considered at high risk and carefully evaluated.

TABLE 1. MEDICAL CAUSES OF ANXIETY

NEUROLOGICAL – 25%

1. Cerebral vascular disorders
2. Sequelae to head injury
3. Postencephalitic disorders
4. Cerebral syphilis
5. Multiple sclerosis
6. Brain tumor (general)
7. Tumors of third ventricle (specifically)
8. Diencephalic autonomic epilepsy
9. Posterolateral sclerosis
10. Postconcussive syndrome
11. Wilson's disease
12. Huntington's chorea
13. Combined systemic disease
14. Polyneuritis
15. Myesthenia gravis

ENDOCRINE – 25%

1. Thyroid disorders
    a. Hyperthyroidism
    b. Hypothyroidism

TABLE 1. MEDICAL CAUSES OF ANXIETY (Cont.)

2. Pituitary disorders
   a. Hypopituitarism
   b. Hyperpituitarism
3. Parathyroidism
   a. Hypoparathyroidism
   b. Hyperparathyroidism
4. Ovarian dysfunction
5. Testicular deficiency
6. Pancreatic disorders
   a. Hypoglycemia
   b. Diabetes mellitus
   c. Pancreatic carcinoma
7. Adrenal cortical disorders
   a. Adrenal cortical insufficiency (Addison's Disease)
   b. Adrenal cortical hyperplasia (Cushing's)
   c. Adrenal tumors

CHRONIC INFECTIONS – 12%

1. Tuberculosis
2. Brucellosis
3. Malaria
4. Atypical viral pneumonia
5. Viral hepatitis
6. Mononucleosis

RHEUMATIC – COLLAGEN VASCULAR DISORDERS – 12%

1. Rheumatoid arthritis
2. Lupus (systemic lupus erythematosus)
3. Polyarteritis nodosa
4. Temporal arteritis

CIRCULATORY DISORDERS – 12%

1. Anemia (various causes)
2. Cerebral anoxia
3. Cerebral insufficiency
4. Paroxysmal atrial tachycardia
5. Coronary insufficiency

OTHER – 14%

1. Nephritis
2. Other malignancies (e.g. oat-cell carcinoma of the lung)
3. Nutritional disorders
4. Drug-induced, particularly in the elderly
5. Meniere's disease (early)
6. Drug abuse

MODEL FOR MEDICALLY INDUCED ANXIETY

Medical illnesses producing anxiety states can be etiologically subdivided into 3 classes:

1. Those interfering with stimulus discrimination.
2. Those producing sympathetic nervous system disruption.
3. Those producing direct end organ changes.

The classical discrimination model first proven by Pavlov has long provided a basis for many attractive psychological theories of anxiety. I believe that it is equally important in explaining anxiety of medical origin. This model helps one understand how life events can trigger episodes of anxiety that are determined by an underlying physical disease.

Pavlov trained his dogs to respond to the picture of a circle by rewarding correct responses with food. He alternated presentation of the circle with that of an ellipse which, when responded to, failed to produce a reward. He then reduced the discriminatory value of the rewarding and non-rewarding symbols by compressing the ellipse so that it gradually approximated the shape of a circle, thus progressively making discrimination between the rewarding and non-rewarding symbols more difficult. The emotional response this change elicited in his dogs was quite remarkable. His personable laboratory animals became ferocious and violent. They tore at their harnesses, barked and snapped uncontrollably, appeared chronically nervous, startled easily, and evidenced autonomic symptoms similar to those seen in anxious patients.

Stimulus discrimination that is impaired by such illnesses as, degenerative diseases, metabolic and endocrine disorders, toxic states, or brain tumors, may produce anxiety as their first and only manifestation. Mild organic brain syndromes reduce the organism's ability to discriminate. Consequently, sudden environmental changes that demand an immediate response, based on a discriminating analysis of variables, may produce a rapidly developing anxiety state.

In other situations, specific metabolic or biochemical imbalances, such as anoxia (Adams, 1957), hypoglycemia, or thyroid disorders (Schwab, 1969), directly produce anxiety by effecting end organ change.

TENSION, NERVOUSNESS AND FATIGUE

Although some patients present specifically with a complaint of anxiety, the majority report symptoms of tension, nervousness, or fatigue (Allan, 1944; Bartley, 1957; Dill, 1939; Sayers, 1942; Shands et al., 1949; Shaw et al., 1962). *Nervousness* implies a state of mental or physical restlessness, where the patient's capacity for performing purposeful activity is impaired. He complains of uneasiness and indecisiveness, which makes him apprehensive. By *fatigue,* the patient usually means that he is no longer able to work at full capacity because of a loss of interest or ambition, as well as the feeling of being tired.

These symptoms are perhaps the most common complaints heard by physicians who must be cognizant that, although such sensations can be caused by psychic tension, they may also be caused by physical conditions affecting those hypothalamic centers that regulate drive, level of consciousness, and energy balance. Nervousness arises as a result of any condition that disrupts the complex neural integration necessary for the maintenance of normal behavior. It is particularly likely to occur when the source of disturbance is unknown to the patient, such as during the prodrome of a chronic disease, like cancer (Avery, 1971; Blumer, 1970; Blustein and Seeman, 1972; Fras et al., 1967) or tuberculosis (Schwab, 1969). These complaints may also constitute the initial symptoms of an impending psychosis, such as schizophrenia or mania. Neurologically, they occur following encephalitis (Azar et al., 1966; Schwab, 1969; Himmelhoch, et al., 1970), epilepsy (Bingley, 1958), and the degenerative disorders (McAlpine, 1964), or as the sequelae of head trauma (Thompson, 1965; Modlin, 1967). Endocrine (Treadway, 1969; Hossain, 1970; Hall and Joffe, 1972), collagen vascular (Ford and Siekert, 1965; O'Connor and Musher, 1966), and nutritional disorders (Frostig and Spies, 1940; Hall and Joffe, 1973; Bram, 1969) commonly produce such symptoms as do chronic infections (Hall and Popkin, 1977; Hall et al., 1978a; Schwab, 1969), toxic conditions resulting from the ingestion of drugs or poisons (Hall and Kirkpatrick, 1978; Bram, 1969; Shader, 1972; Hall and Popkin, 1977; Hall et al., 1978b; Hall and Joffe, 1972; Preu, 1956), and self-poisonings such as those that occur with alcoholism and drug abuse (Hall et al., 1978a) (Hall et al., 1978b).

To evaluate the cause of anxiety, it is necessary to ascertain when the nervousness began, as well as its pattern of occurrence. Does it occur when the patient is alone, or is it related to a specific person or situation? What is its duration? What increases or decreases its intensity? Are there specific physical complaints with which it is associated? Are there recent changes in the patient's dietary habits or patterns of drug or alcohol use?

It is diagnostically useful for the physician to determine whether nervousness or fatigue was the patient's initial symptom. Fatigue resulting from organic disease may produce fear or frustration expressed as nervousness (Allan, 1944; Sayers, 1942; Shands et al., 1949). If nervousness antedated the appearance of fatigue, there is a higher probability that the source of difficulty is psychological. If fatigue predated nervousness, a somatic cause is more likely. Another useful generalization is: Those cases of anxiety that have been present for periods in excess of 2 years, with little fluctuation in their intensity, are most likely related to psychological factors. Organically produced anxiety characteristically fluctuates in both its severity and duration. Careful medical evaluation will define the underlying medical etiology of anxiety in about 90 percent of cases (Hall et al., 1978a).

In a study at the Lahey Clinic conducted by Allan (1944), 20 percent of 300 consecutive admissions with a chief complaint of nervousness, weakness, or fatigue, were found to suffer from a previously unrecognized medical disorder.

Of these patients, 4.3 percent suffered from chronic infections, 4 percent had metabolic disorders, 5.5 percent had neurological disorders, 2.7 percent had heart disease, 1.7 percent had anemia, and 1 percent had nephritis. The remaining patients suffered from such conditions as unrecognized lung tumor, vitamin deficiency, Hodgkin's disease, or lymphoma.

The majority of these patients complained of *pathological fatigue* (fatigue that was unrelieved, and in most cases, made worse by sleep), which was felt to be an important diagnostic feature suggestive of organically produced anxiety. Pathological fatigue frequently occurs following head injury, and is associated with diabetes mellitus, nutritional disorders, chronic infections, toxic states and poisonings; or with conditions that deprive the brain of oxygen and/or glucose, such as congenital heart defect, anemia, and disturbances of carbohydrate metabolism. It is produced by disturbances of hydrogen ion concentration and alterations in the concentration of serum calcium, sodium, and potassium. The hypoproteinemia of chronic renal and hepatic disease, and the accumulation of metabolic waste seen in these conditions also produce it. It is a striking symptom of thyroid disease, ovarian malfunction, pancreatic insufficiency states, pituitary disorders, and adrenal hypofunction (Allan, 1944; Sayers, 1942; Shands, 1949; Ferrer, 1968; Howland et al., 1929; Adams, 1957; Dalessio, 1965; Read et al., 1967; Stenbäck and Haapanen, 1967; Tyler, 1968; Shands et al., 1949).

DIFFERENTIAL DIAGNOSIS OF ANXIETY STATES

Psychiatric Disorders

Although it is beyond the scope of this chapter to specifically delineate the psychiatric disorders related to anxiety, a few points may be of use to the clinician. Any mental disorder may begin with, or evidence during its course, symptoms of anxiety. Such symptoms are non-specific. Of the major psychotic disorders associated with anxiety, manic depressive psychosis (depressed phase) is perhaps the most frequently overlooked. Anxiety may occur in acute reactive psychoses and as an early or mid-course symptom of acute schizophrenia. It is common in patients suffering from hysteria, obsessive compulsive, or other neuroses and hypochondriasis (Andresen, 1963; Bennett, 1963; Berger, 1962).

Anxiety is also a prominent feature of *neurocirculatory asthenia*. Patients with such manifestations give a history of having been extremely susceptible to fatigue from early childhood. They evidence defects of vasomotor regulatory mechanisms with moderate stress, or exercise, producing symptoms of breathlessness, palpitations, anxiety, sweating, and fatigue. These patients develop excess levels of lactic acid under conditions of moderate exertion (Cohen et al., 1948; Wheeler et al., 1950).

Medical Differential of Anxiety

A partial list of medical conditions responsible for anxiety states is shown in Table 1. Neurological disorders are the primary cause of anxiety in approximately 25 percent of cases with specific medical etiology. Endocrine disorders cause 25 percent; chronic infections, 12 percent; rheumatic and collagen vascular disease, 12 percent; circulatory disease, 12 percent; with the remaining 14 percent caused by various other conditions. It may be worthwhile at this time to look at a few of the more prominent causes.

NEUROLOGICAL DISEASES

Among the neurological disorders, *cerebral vascular insufficiency* is the most common cause of anxiety. *Cerebral vascular accidents* are generally associated with other symptoms, and therefore do not create diagnostic difficulty (Baker, 1965). The *cerebral insufficiency* associated with *transient cerebral ischemia* may be difficult to define (Scheinberg and Rice-Simons, 1964). Often, there are premonitory recurrent focal ischemic attacks lasting from 10 to 15 seconds to as long as an hour, with most persisting from 2 to 10 minutes. Anxiety frequently accompanies these episodes and may precede other signs by weeks or months. The condition is frequently associated with narrowing of the extracranial arteries, particularly the internal carotid at its origin in the neck, by arteriosclerotic plaques (Bradshaw and Casey, 1967). When internal carotid involvement becomes significant, the patient may develop contralateral weakness, numbness, or dysphasia. Anxiety progresses to a more global confusional state, and memory becomes poor (Fazekas, 1964).

Another condition creating diagnostic confusion occurs with partial occlusion of the subclavian or innominate arteries, causing the *subclavian steal syndrome* (episodes of anxiety associated with dizziness and intermittent confusion) (Santschi et al., 1966).

Relative cerebral vascular insufficiency may also occur secondary to extracranial causes, such as chronic anemia, cardiac arrythmias, or conditions producing intermittent or sustained hypotension. Regardless of the etiology of the cerebral vascular insufficiency, the early symptoms are the same and include significant anxiety (Fazekas, 1964; International Conference on Vascular Disease, 1961).

Anxiety states associated with personality change are a frequent sequelae of *head injury* (Merskey and Woodforde, 1972). A transient loss of consciousness following injury, persisting for a few seconds or minutes, is indicative of concussion (Denny-Brown, 1945). The duration of unconsciousness following such trauma is related to both the site and extent of injury (Evans, 1966a). Following mild concussion, the patient may show normal alertness within a few minutes. If laceration or contusion of the brain occurs, more severe symptoms develop, with anxiety becoming prominent (Miller and Stern, 1965). In these cases, anxiety is associated with other specific signs, such as motor weakness, aphasia, or cranial nerve palsies (Evans, 1966a; Evans, 1966b). Ipsolateral pupillary dilatation indicates dural hemorrhage. It is important to note that during the recovery phase and for months thereafter, the patient may experience episodes of overwhelming anxiety; dizziness; lability of mood; personality change; headache; the *post-concussive syndrome,* or *post-traumatic cerebral syndrome,* which is characteristically made worse by changes in posture, exposure to heat or sunlight, alcohol ingestion, and strenuous exercise (Miller and Stern, 1965; Merskey and Woodforde, 1972).

Anxiety states frequently follow *encephalitis. Subclinical encephalitis* produces profound psychiatric disturbance. Such patients give a history of psychiatric symptoms with onset 6–12 weeks following an upper respiratory infection associated with headache, fever, nuchal rigidity, or photophobia. Lumbar puncture, with chemistries, cell count, and viral titers demonstrating a fall from acute phase levels, facilitates diagnosis (Azar et al., 1966; Blumer, 1970; Himmelhoch et al., 1970; Schwab, 1969).

Multiple sclerosis (disseminated sclerosis) is another central nervous system disease, which early in its course, is frequently thought to be psychogenic (Blumer, 1970; McAlpine, 1964; Dalessio et al., 1965; Ross and Reitan, 1955). It usually presents with sudden, transient motor and sensory disturbances; periods of impaired vision; and diffuse, fleeting neurological signs that characteristically exacerbate and remit. Early symptoms are associated with a dysphoric mood state and episodic anxiety (Symposium on Disseminated Sclerosis and Allied Conditions, 1961). As the illness progresses, significant depression may occur, followed by a state of euphoria during which the patient has little insight into his condition (Ross and Reitan, 1955; Ivers and Goldstein, 1963). Manic episodes may also occur (See *Chapter 3, Depression.*)

Wilson's disease, or *hepatolenticular degeneration,* is a familial disorder that may occur in the "asymptomatic" or "carrier" form, manifested by psychiatric symptoms alone, or as the full blown disorder, with basal ganglion degeneration, cirrhosis, greenish-brown corneal pigmentation (Kayser-Fleicher ring), and psychiatric symptoms (Goldstein et al., 1971). The onset is insidious, usually occurring between the ages of 11 and 25. Early symptoms are psychiatric in nature and usually consist of severe anxiety or episodes of frank psychosis. As the disease progresses, basilar symptoms become apparent; the patient develops tremor, rigidity, and gait disturbances. Tremors are of the intention or alternating type. "Wing beating" tremors of the upper extremities, accentuated by extension of the arms, are thought by some to be characteristic. Laboratory findings include elevations of: liver function tests, urinary copper, and amino acid levels; accompanied by decreased serum copper and ceruloplasmin (Sternlieb and Scheinberg, 1968; Walshe, 1969).

Chronic progressive, or *Huntington's chorea,* is a hereditary disorder involving the basal ganglion and cerebral cortex, having its onset in adult life. Severe anxiety, lability, rage, and personality change, progressing to labile psychosis with mental deterioration and chorea, are characteristic. When present, choreiform movements tend to be abrupt and jerky, but less rapid or lightening-like than those seen with Sydenham's chorea. The disease is chronically progressive and leads to death within 15 years (James et al., 1969; McCaughey, 1961).

Posterolateral sclerosis (combined system disease) is frequently misdiagnosed as a psychiatric disorder during its early stages. Patients with such symptoms present with unusual histories and moderate to severe anxiety. The vagueness and unusual nature of their complaints suggests a diagnosis of hysteria. Complaints of anxiety, numbness, "pins and needles," weakness, tenderness, and feelings of heaviness in the limbs and digits are frequent. The patient may evidence stocking- or glove-sensory loss. Later in the course, hyperreflexia and flexor spasm, followed by hyporeflexia and flaccid paralysis, occur. Posture and vibratory senses are lost during the mid-course of the disease. Mental changes begin with episodes of fatigue and diffuse anxiety. As the disease progresses, memory becomes impaired, and a frank psychosis may develop. Laboratory evaluation may show the associated blood and gastric findings of pernicious anemia. The clinician must remember that all of these symptoms may occur in the absence of clear-cut hematologic findings. If the patient evidences a macrocytic anemia, achlorhydria, and a positive Schilling's test, the diagnosis is certain.

The primary pathology involves progressive degeneration of the posterior and lateral columns of the spinal cord, as well as occasional degeneration of peripheral nerves. The disease is most likely to affect people in the middle and older age groups. The severity of spinal cord changes does not parallel the degree of severity of anemia, and as stated previously, psychiatric symptoms and spinal-cord degeneration may develop without manifest anemia (Shulman, 1967).

Polyneuritis (peripheral neuritis) is frequently initially misdiagnosed as conversion hysteria or anxiety neurosis (Mulder, 1964). Patients with such symptoms evidence slowly progressive muscular weakness, parasthesias, tenderness and pain in distal portions of their extremities, and frequently give a history of stocking or glove hyperesthesia or anesthesia. During the mid-course of the disease, hyporeflexia or areflexia may occur, accompanied by muscular wasting of the extremities. The condition may appear at any age, but is most common in young and middle-aged males. It may be caused by a series of chronic intoxications with substances, such as: carbon disulfide, alcohol, benzene, sulfonamides, arsenic, or phosphorus. It is seen following infections, particularly diphtheria, syphilis, tuberculosis, pneumonia, mumps, viral meningitis, and as a component of the Guillain-Barré syndrome (Heller and DeJong, 1963). Nutritional causes such as cachectic states, beri-beri, and chronic vitamin deficiencies have also been implicated. The presence of trophic changes over the skin of the extremities (thinned, reddened, glossy), with impaired ability to sweat, are useful in making the diagnosis, as is the presence of muscular tenderness and hypersensitivity.

Inexplicable and severe anxiety states also occur in association with *convulsive disorders* and *tumors of the nervous system*. These are addressed in subsequent chapters (Bailey and Murray, 1928; Bartley, 1957; Berson, 1956; Bingley, 1958; Blumer, 1970; Blustein and Seeman, 1972; Avery, 1971, Daly, 1958; Horton, 1976; Mulder et al., 1957; Patton and Sheppard, 1966; Soniat, 1951). Suffice it to say at this point that anxiety is, according to Penfield and Jasper (1954), a predominant feature of tumors involving the third ventricle, and of diencephalic epilepsy. Acute anxiety episodes, or panic attacks, may occur as part of the aura of grand mal epilepsy or following a convulsion during the post ictal period.

Cerebral syphilis and early myasthenia gravis are other disorders frequently associated with severe anxiety states (Zimmerman, 1964; Humphrey, 1965; Simpson et al., 1966).

ENDOCRINE DISORDERS

Endocrine disorders account for approximately 25 percent of medically produced anxiety states.

Hypopituitarism, although a relatively rare condition, may mimic many functional neuroses and/or psychoses, as well as anorexia nervosa (Bauer, 1954; Friesen and Astwood, 1965; O'Dell, 1966). Routine endocrine workup in such cases reveals diminished T_3, T_4, and T_7; FSH, urinary 17 ketosteroids, and corticoids. Skull x-rays may define stellar erosion. On physical examination, visual field defects and loss of axillary and pubic hair are seen. The fasting blood sugar is usually low, with a flat glucose tolerance curve, while insulin-tolerance testing shows increased insulin sensitivity.

Cachectic malnutrition, such as occurs in anorexia nervosa, may produce functional hypopituitarism. Growth hormone assays, which are increased in anorexia nervosa, are usually reduced in patients with true hypopituitarism (Williams, 1958; Mecklenburg et al., 1974; Lucas et al., 1976; Liebman et al., 1974; Dally, 1969).

Hypopituitarism may present as a nephrosis or "pernicious anemia" accompanied by psychiatric symptoms, and should be considered in the differential diagnosis of these disorders. The severe hypoglycemia that occurs after fasting may suggest a diagnosis of primary hyperinsulinism. The associated mental changes are frequently misdiagnosed as a primary psychosis (Bauer, 1954; Friesen and Astwood, 1965).

Although rare, *hyperpituitarism,* which is secondary to eosinophilic adenoma of the anterior pituitary, often presents with symptoms of overwhelming anxiety and sympathetic discharge. The diagnosis of *acromegaly* is not difficult when the patient presents with classical findings of excessive growth of the hands and feet, increased shoe and glove size, and protrusion of the lower jaw. The patient may, however, present with more discrete symptoms, such as mental change (particularly overwhelming anxiety), intermittent headache, fatigue, anergia, weakness, diaphoresis and visual disorders. Laboratory findings may confuse the picture, since glycosuria and phosphaturia may be prominent, suggesting diabetes mellitus. The patient may evidence insulin-resistent diabetes, or hypermetabolic goiter, and be unresponsive to antithyroid drugs. Pituitary adenomas are frequently associated with adenomas elsewhere in the body, particularly in the parathyroids and pancreas (Young et al., 1965). The incidence of carcinoid tumors is also increased in such patients.

The findings of headache, bitemporal hemiopia, diplopia, lethargy, and anxiety strongly suggest hyperpituitarism. As mentioned, long-standing cases may develop secondary hormonal changes, including diabetes mellitus, hypermetabolic goiter, and abnormal lactation. Excessive sweating is the most reliable sign of activity and progression of the disease. X-rays may show enlargement of the sella with destruction of the clinoids; however, a normal sella does not rule out the diagnosis. Other radiographic findings may include: enlargement of the frontal sinuses, thickening of the skull and long bones, bony overgrowth of the vertebral bodies with spur formation, dorsal kyphosis and "tufting" of the terminal phlanges of the fingers and toes (Hamwi, 1960).

Thyroid disorders are the most common endocrine causes of severe episodic anxiety (Berson, 1956; Hall and Popkin, 1977; Treadway, 1969; Flagg et al., 1965). These conditions will be discussed in detail elsewhere in this volume, but a few words are in order.

Simple goiters usually present with few or no specific psychiatric symptoms. Symptoms, if any, are produced by glandular compression of structures in the neck. Basal metabolic rate, PBI, T_3, T_4, T_7, and serum cholesterol are all normal; radioiodine uptake may be either elevated or normal (Astwood et al., 1960).

Adult hypothyroidism frequently presents with symptoms of anxiety, depression, and fatigue. These patients specifically complain of muscular weakness, increased fatigability, intolerance to cold, constipation, menorrhagia, and/or hoarseness. Physical findings include: dry, cold, yellow, and puffy skin, scant eyebrows, thickened tongue, "water bottle heart," bradycardia, and delayed return of deep tendon reflexes. Anemia may be present. Hypothyroidism may also present as a macrocytic anemia requiring differentiation from pernicious anemia, as a menstrual disorder requiring differentiation from various pelvic diseases, or as a frank psychosis (myxedema madness). Myxedema should always be considered in the differential of a patient with neurasthenia, or one who evidences the psychiatric triad of anxiety, fatigue, and intermittent depression. As the illness progresses, a frank organic psychosis with paranoid delusions may occur (Watanakunakorn et al., 1965).

The physician must remember, when treating agitated myxedema patients, that they are unusually sensitive to opiates and other central nervous system depressants, and that reports have emerged of patients dying from the administration of average doses of these medications (Catz and Russell, 1961). It is strongly urged that thyroid function studies be obtained as part of the routine workup for any patient with anxiety.

Hyperthyroidism may present as a classic anxiety neurosis, particularly in women during the menopause. It is one of the most common endocrine disorders and has a peak incidence in women between the ages of 20 and 40 (Treadway, 1969).

Little diagnostic challenge exists when the exopthalmia and diffuse goiter characteristic of *Graves' disease* are present. However, diffuse goiter is absent in many cases, being replaced by a toxic nodular goiter or no goiter at all. In these instances, all of the metabolic features of thyrotoxicosis may be present (Ingbar, 1966). Signs indicative of a hypermetabolic state may be conspicuously absent, particularly in elderly patients: *apathetic Graves' disease* (Greer, 1964).

Over 95 percent of patients with undiagnosed Graves' disease have nervousness or episodic anxiety as their primary complaint. Over 70 percent of these patients also complain of hyperhydrosis, palpitations, fatigue, tachycardia, dyspnea, or weakness. Characteristically, the psychiatric picture changes rapidly (Flagg et al., 1965). Initial fatigue and anxiety give way to episodes of mild exhilaration, which progress to full-blown dementiform organic brain syndromes. Manic-like episodes, with agitation, precognition, paranoia, and delusions, or conditions resembling severe endogenous depression, may occur.

The most reliable physical signs include goiter, tremor, bruit over the thyroid, eye signs, atrial fibrillation, splenomegaly, gynocomastia, and liver palms. Reflexes are increased; hair is thin and of silky texture; skin is smooth and oily; hyperpigmentation and/or vitiligo may be seen. Spider angioma are common (Greer, 1964; Gilliland, 1975; Vagenakis et al., 1976).

Psychiatrically, these patients may give a history of sleep disruptive anxiety episodes associated with tachycardia and a fear of death. The symptoms may be so severe as to suggest a diagnosis of pavor nocturnus; however, the absence of nightmares preceding the awakening provides insight into the correct diagnosis.

The laboratory diagnosis of Graves' disease is made on the basis of: thyroid function studies, increased radioiodine and radio T_3 red cell uptake, low serum cholesterol, postprandial glycosuria, increased urinary creatinine, and lymphocytosis. Urinary and serum calcium, thyroid-stimulating hormone, and long-acting thyroid-stimulating hormone may also be elevated (Cassidy, 1962).

Thyroiditis, which occurs from several causes, is perhaps the most misunderstood endocrine disorder producing psychiatric symptoms. These conditions may be insidious or fulminant in their onset and course. They are characterized by sudden fluctuations in the level of circulating thyroid hormone, which disrupt the patient's emotional balance. The sudden alterations from a relatively hypothyroid to hyperthyroid state may produce severe anxiety, rapid mood swings, sensory flooding, delusions, paranoia, impaired cognition and attention, and a sense of unreality (Doniach et al., 1960; Steinberg, 1960; Thomas et al., 1965).

The expected characteristic picture of a painfully swollen thyroid gland, productive of pressure symptoms in the acute and subacute forms, and the painlessly enlarged thyroid of the chronic form occur in only 50 to 60 percent of cases. Diagnosis is confirmed by high antithyroid or microsomal antibody titers.

Thyroiditis may be caused by specific agents, such as pyogenic infection, tuberculosis, or syphilis; or be due to a non-specific autoimmune process. Autoimmune thyroiditis is subdivided into three major groupings: *DeQuervain's thyroiditis, Hashimoto's thyroiditis,* and *Riedell's thyroiditis.*

DeQuervain's thyroiditis, or *giant-cell thyroiditis,* occurs most often in middle-aged women, and is thought to follow viral infections, particularly exposure to mumps. These patients develop an acutely painful enlargement of the thyroid gland with dysphasia.

Hashimoto's thyroiditis, or *chronic lymphocytic thyroiditis,* on the other hand, may be more insidious in onset and global in symptom presentation, making diagnosis difficult. It is the most common form of thyroiditis and occurs principally in middle-aged women. Because of its insidious onset and progression, it produces few pressure symptoms. Psychiatrically, patients experience periods of overwhelming anxiety, tension, restlessness, and sleep continuity disturbance, coupled with significant depression and marked emotional lability. In rapidly progressing cases, hallucinations, delusions, paranoid projective symptoms, derealization, time distortion, and anxiety to the point of panic, occur. Elevated thyroid autoantibodies are most commonly demonstrated in this type of thyroiditis, but may also occur in other forms of the disease.

Riedell's thyroiditis, or *chronic fibrous thyroiditis,* is the rarest form of the condition and is said to occur only in middle-aged women. These patients fortunately have few associated psychiatric findings.

Hypoparathyroidism frequently presents with symptoms of overwhelming anxiety (Hossain, 1970; Fonseca and Calverley, 1967; Nusynowitz et al., 1976; Schneider and Sherwood, 1975). In fully advanced states, these patients complain of: tetany, carpal-pedal spasm, stridor, wheezing, muscular and abdominal cramps, and urinary frequency. The family characteristically reports marked personality change. Episodes of mental slowing alternate with periods of overwhelming anxiety that may border on panic (Denko and Kaelbling, 1964). Idiopathic hypoparathyroidism occurs in association with candidiasis and Addison's disease (Tyler, 1968).

A picture simulating hypoparathyroidism occurs in patients with chronic renal failure and those with pseudohypoparathyroidism, a genetic defect occurring in obese, round-faced, short-statured individuals with short metacarpals, atopic bone formation and hypertension. In the latter, the parathyroids are often hyperplastic and the renal tubules unresponsive to hormonal regulation. The above conditions are associated with lethergy, personality change, and the presence of intermittent, severe anxiety. In fully developed cases, Chvostek's (facial contraction on tapping the facial nerve near the angle of the jaw) and Trousseau's (carpal-pedal spasm after application of a blood pressure cuff) signs are positive. Cataracts may occur. The skin is dry and scaly, and there is a loss of eyebrow hair. Deep tendon reflexes are hyperactive. Alkaline phosphatase is usually elevated in pseudohypoparathyroidism, but normal in hypoparathyroidism (Bronsky et al., 1958).

While primary hyperparathyroidism is relatively rare, it is associated with symptoms of severe anxiety in over 90 percent of cases (Denko and Kaelbling, 1964; Reilly and Wilson, 1965). Other symptoms that develop during the course of the disease include: renal calculi, nephrocalcinosis, hypertension, gastrointestinal symptoms, intractable peptic ulcer, constipation, polyuria, polydipsia, and bone pain. Cystic bone lesions and pathological fractures may occur. Serum and urine calcium are elevated; urine phosphorus is high; serum phosphorus is low or normal. Alkaline phosphatase is usually normal. Other conditions that present with similar physical and biochemical findings and must be differentiated include: carcinoma of the lung, kidney, ovary, and multiple myeloma (Krane, 1961; Bronsky et al., 1958).

Diseases of the *adrenal cortex* frequently present with psychiatric symptoms (Besser and Jeffcoate, 1976; Thorn, 1972). Patients with *Addison's disease* complain of anxiety; depression; weakness; easy fatigability; anorexia; and frequent episodes of nausea, vomiting, and/or diarrhea. The presence of these symptoms may suggest the diagnosis of anxiety neurosis.

Physical examination usually reveals these patients to have sparse axillary hair and increased pigmentation of the intertriginous zones and about the nipple. They are generally hypotensive and have a small heart.

Patients with *Addison's disease* report that anxiety and lability progressing to panic occur if they miss a meal. The anxiety is rapidly relieved following the consumption of glucose. Fasting blood sugars are low. Other laboratory findings useful for the definition of Addison's disease include: hyponatremia, hypokalemia, decreased 17 hydroxy and ketosteroids, moderate neutropenia (white blood cell count 4000–5000), lymphocytosis of 35–50 percent, and eosinophilia, with a total eosinophil count in excess of 300 c/ml. Such patients are usually hemoconcentrated. Serum cortisol levels of less than 8 mcg/100 ml are practically diagnostic (Smilo and Forsham, 1969; Irvine and Barnes, 1972).

Cushing's syndrome is a disorder of multiple etiologies (adrenal cortical hyperplasia, adrenal adenoma or carcinoma, or secondary to basophilic pituitary adenoma), all of which produce similar psychiatric findings (Besser and Jeffcoate, 1976; Ganong et al., 1974; Smilo and Forsham, 1969). Five percent of these cases are associated with adrenal carcinoma, which is usually unilateral and metastasizes late, making prompt diagnosis crucial. The syndrome may also be produced by ovarian adrenal rest tumors, which are also productive of a virilizing syndrome. Cushing's syndrome may rarely be caused by extra-adrenal malignant tumors, such as oat-cell carcinoma of the lung, in which case it is associated with hyperkalemia and marked hyperpigmentation (Friedman et al., 1966).

The psychiatric symptoms of Cushing's syndrome are legend and usually begin with chronic agitation and intermittent anxiety that becomes constant, progressing to the point of panic. Emotional lability, hallucinations, delusions, and frank paranoid psychosis occur (Liddle and Shute, 1969; Herrera et al., 1964).

Physical examination reveals: buffalo hump; hirsutism; moon face; purple stria of the thighs, breast, and abdomen; ecchymoses; a plethoric appearance; and trunkal obesity. A history of diminished menstruation or amenorrhea in females and impotence in males, associated with complaints of weakness, backache, acne, superficial skin infections and headache, are common. Laboratory examination may show evidence of osteoporosis, glycosuria, and 17 hydroxycorticosteroid elevation associated with low serum potassium and chloride. The total eosinophil count is low. A lymphopenia is usually present (Thorn, 1972).

The *virilization* syndromes of adult females are also associated with anxiety. Such patients present histories of menstrual disorder, hirsutism, regression or reversal of secondary sexual characteristics, deepening or hoarseness of voice, acne, clitoral enlargement, and on occasion, balding. A sudden change in the amount of hair, other than at the times of puberty, pregnancy, or menopause, is of greater diagnostic significance than a history of hirsutism being present throughout life (Behrman, 1960).

Virilization syndromes may be caused by such diverse conditions as adrenal hyperplasia; adrenal tumors; ovarian disorders, such as arrhenoblastoma, Stein-Leventhal syndrome, Theca luteinization syndrome, hilar cell tumor, or hyperplasia; ovarian hyperplasia; dysgerminoma; and ovarian adrenal rest tumors. They may also occur following disruption of the hypothalamic-pituitary axis, such as occurs with acromegaly (eosinophilic adenoma) and hyperostosis frontalis internia (*Steward-Morgagni-Morel syndrome*). These syndromes may also be associated with pregnancy, chorioepithelioma, hermaphroiditism, and thymic tumor. If 17 ketosteroid levels are high, the diagnosis of adrenal disorder is likely. Extremely high levels suggest adrenal tumor. In arrhenoblastoma or Stein-Leventhal syndrome, 17 ketosteroids are usually normal or only moderately elevated. The ACTH stimulation test and cortisone suppression test are useful in distinguishing between adrenal tumors, adrenal hyperplasia, and ovarian lesions. Elevations of pregnanediol suggest adrenal abnormality (Behrman, 1960; Segre et al., 1964).

CONCLUSION

As one can see from the preceding pages, anxiety can be a protean initial symptom of a myriad of diseases. Its occurrence as one of the first symptoms of medical disorder may increase the likelihood that a clinician will consider its presence indicative of a psychogenic illness, and thereby dismiss other nonspecific physical findings and arrive at a diagnosis of conversion hysteria, labile personality, or anxiety neurosis.

REFERENCES

Ackner, B. Depersonalization II: Clinical syndromes. *J. Ment. Sci.* 100:854–872 (1954).

Adams, R. D. Neurological manifestations of chronic pulmonary insufficiency. *N. Eng. J. Med.* 257:579–590 (1957).

Allan, F. N. Differential diagnosis of weakness and fatigue. *N. Eng. J. Med.* 231:414–418 (1944).

Andresen, A.F.R., Jr. A practical approach to anxiety reactions. *N. Y. J. Med.* 63:1144–1147 (1963).

Astwood, E. B., Cassidy, C. E., and Aurbach, G. D. Treatment of goiter and thyroid nodules with thyroid. *J.A.M.A.* 174:459–464 (1960).

Avery, T. L., Seven cases of frontal tumor with psychiatric presentation. *Brit. J. Psychiat.* 119:19–23 (1971).

Azar, G. J., Bond, J. O., and Lawton, A. H. St. Louis encephalitis: Aspects of 1962 epidemic in Pinellas County, Florida. *J. Amer. Geriat. Soc.* 14:326–333 (1966).

Bailey, P., and Murray, H. A. A case of pinealoma with symptoms suggestive of compulsive neurosis. Clinical Report. *Arch. Neurol.* 19:932–945 (1928).

Baker, A. B. Common stroke syndromes and their management. *Postgrad. Med.* 37:268–272 (1965).

Bartley, S. H. Fatigue and inadequacy. *Psychol. Rev.* 37:301–324 (1957).

Bauer, H. G. Endocrine and other clinical manifestations of hypothalamic disease. *J. Clin. Endocrinol.* 14:13–31 (1954).

Beebe, G. W. Follow-up studies of World War II and Korean War prisoners II. Morbidity, disabiltiy, and maladjustments. National Research Council, Washington, D. C. (1955).

Behrman, H. T. Diagnosis and management of hirsutism. *J.A.M.A.* 172:1924–1931 (1960).

Bennett, A. E. Anxiety as a symptom of mental illness. *Gen. Pract.* 27:101–106 (1963).

Berger, F. M. The treatment of anxiety. A critical review. *J. Neuropsychiat.* 4:98–103 (1962).

Berson, S. A. Symposium on pathologic physiology of thyroid diseases: Pathways of iodine metabolism. *Am. J. Med.* 20:653–669 (1956).

Besser, G. M., and Jeffcoate, W. J. Endocrine and metabolic diseases: Adrenal diseases. *Brit. Med. J.* 1:448–451 (1976).

Bettelheim, B. Individual and mass behavior in extreme situations. *J. Abn. Soc. Psychol.* 38:417–452 (1953).

Bingley, T. Mental symptoms in temporal lobe epilepsy. *ACTA Psychiat. and Neurol. Supp. 120,* 33:1–151 (1958).

Blumer, D. Neurological states masquerading as psychoses. *Md. St. Med. J.* 19:55–60 (1970).

Blustein, J. E., and Seeman, M. V. Brain tumors presenting as functional psychiatric disturbances. *Canad. Psychiat. Assn. J.* 17:55–59–ss–63 (1972).

Bradshaw, P., and Casey, E. Outcome of medically treated stroke associated with stenosis or occlusion of the internal carotid artery. *Brit. Med. J.* 1:201–204 (1967).

Bram, M. Miscellaneous advances: Neurological manifestations of folate deficiency in recent advances in neurology and neuropsychiatry. L. Bram, and M. Wilkinson eds. Churchill, London, (1969), pp. 129–146.

Bronsky, D., Kushner, D. S., and Dubin, A. Idiopathic hypoparathyroidism and pseudohypoparathyroidism: Case reports and review of the literature. *Med.* 37:317–352 (1958).

Cameron, N. *Personality Development and Psychopathology: A Dynamic Approach.* Houghton Mifflin, Boston, Massachusetts (1963).

Cassidy, C. E. The treatment for hyperthyroidism. *Med. Clin. N. Am.* 46:1201–1221 (1962).

Cattell, R. B., and Scheier, I. H. Nature of anxiety: A review of thirteen multivariate analysis comprising 814 variables. *Psychol. Rep.* 4. So. Univ. Press Monog. Supp. 5, pp. 351–388 (1958).

Catz, B., and Russell, S. Myxedema, shock, and coma. *Arch. Int. Med.* 108:407–417 (1961).

Chodoff, P. C. Late effects of the concentration camp syndrome. *Arch. Gen. Psychiat.* 8:323–333 (1963).

Cohen, M. E., White, P. D., and Johnson, R. A. Symposium on recent advances in medicine; neurocirculatory asthenia (anxiety neurosis, neurasthenia, effect syndrome cardia neurosis). *Arch. Int. Med.* 81:260–281 (1948).

Dalessio, D. J., Benchimol, A., and Dimond, E.G. Chronic encephalopathy related to heart block. *Neurol.* 15:499–503 (1965).

Dally, P. *Anorexia Nervosa.* Grune and Stratton, New York (1969).

Daly, D. Ictal affect. *Am. J. Psychiat.* 115:97–108 (1958).

Denko, J. D., and Kaelbling, R. The psychiatric aspects of hypoparathyroidism. *ACTA Psychiat. Scand.* Supp. 164:40 (1964).

Denny-Brown, D. Disability arising from closed head injuries. *J.A.M.A.* 127:429–436 (1945).

Dill, D. B. Industrial fatigue and physiology of man at work. *Indust. Med.* 8:315–318 (1939).

Doniach, D., Hudson, R. V., and Roitt, I. M. Human auto-immune thyroiditis: Clinical studies. *Brit. Med. J.* 1:365–373 (1960).

Eitinger, L., and Strom, A., eds. *Mortality and Morbidity After Excessive Stress.* Humanities Press, New York (1972).

Evans, J. P. Advances in the understanding and treatment of head injury. *Canad. Med. Assn. J.* 95:1337–1348 (1966a).

Evans, J. P. Acute trauma to the head, fundamentals of management. *Postgrad. Med.* 39:27–30 (1966b).

Fazekas, J. K. Medical management of cerebral vascular insufficiency. *Gen. Pract.* 29:78–83 (1964).

Ferrer, M. I. Mistaken psychiatric referral of occult serious cardiac disease. *Arch. Gen. Psychiat.* 18:112–113 (1968).

Flagg, G. W., Clemens, T. L., Michael, E. A., Alexander, F., and Wark, J. A psychophysiological investigation of hyperthyroidism. *Psychosom. Med.* 27:497–507 (1965).

Fonseca, O. A., and Calverley, J. R. Neurological manifestations of hypoparathyroidism. *Arch. Int. Med.* 120:202–206 (1967).

Ford, R. G., and Siekert, R. G. Central nervous system manifestations of periarteritis nodosa. *Neurol.* 15:114–122 (1965).

Fras, I., Litin, E. M., and Pearson, J. S. Comparison of psychiatric symptoms of carcinoma of the pancreas with those in some other intra-abdominal neoplasms. *Am. J. Psychiat.* 123:1553–1562 (1967).

Freud, S. *The problem of anxiety.* W. W. Norton and Co., New York (1936).

Friedman, M., Marshal-Jones, P., and Ross, E. J. Cushing's syndrome: Adrenocortical hyperactivity secondary to neoplasms arising outside the pituitary-adrenal system. *Quart. J. Med.* 35:193–214 (1966).

Friesen, H., and Astwood, E. B. Hormones of the anterior pituitary body. *N. Eng. J. Med.* 272:1216–1223, 1272–1277, 1325, 1328–1335 (1965).

Frostig, J. P., and Spies, T. D. Initial nervous syndrome of pelagra and associated deficiency diseases. *Am. J. Med. Sci.* 199:268–274 (1940).

Ganong, W. F., Alpert, L. C., and Lee, T. C. ACTH and the regulation of adrenocortical secretion. *N. Eng. J. Med.* 290:1006–1011 (1974).

Garmany, G. Emergencies in general practice. Acute anxiety and hysteria. *Brit. Med. J.* 2:115–117 (1955).

Gilliland, P. F. Myxedema: Recognition and treatment. *Postgrad. Med.* 57:61–65 (1975).

Goldstein, N. P., Tauxe, W. N., McCall, J. T., Randall, R. V., and Gross, J. B. Wilson's disease (hepatolenticular degeneration). *Arch. Neurol.* 24:391–400 (1971).

Greer, M. A. Graves' disease. *Ann. Rev. Med.* 15:65–78 (1964).

Grinker, R. R., and Spiegel, J. P. *Men Under Stress.* Blackeston, New York (1945).

Hall, R.C.W., and Joffe, J. R. Aberrant response to diazepam: A new syndrome. *Am. J. Psychiat.* 129:114–118 (1972).
Hall, R.C.W., and Joffe, J. R. Hypomagnesemia. *J.A.M.A.* 224:1749–1751 (1973).
Hall. R.C.W., and Kirkpatrick, B. The benzodiazepines. *Am. Fam. Phys.* 17:131–134 (1978).
Hall, R.C.W., and Popkin, M. K. Psychological symptoms of physical origin. *Fem. Patient.* 2:43–47 (1977).
Hall, R.C.W. and Simmons, W. C. The POW wife. *Arch. Gen. Psychiat.* 29:690–694 (1972).
Hall, R.C.W., Popkin, M. K., Devaul, R., Faillace, L. A., and Stickney, S. K. Physical illness presenting as psychiatric disease. *Arch. Gen. Psychiat.* 35:11:1315–1320 (1978).
Hall, R.C.W., Popkin, M. K., Devaul, R., Stickney, S. K. The effect of unrecognized drug abuse on diagnosis and therapeutic outcome. *Am. J. Alc. and Drug Abuse.* 4:4:455–465 (1977).
Hall, R.C.W., Popkin, M. K., Stickney, S. K., Gardner, E. R. Covert outpatient drug abuse: Incidence and therapist recognition. *J. Nerv. Ment. Dis.* 166:343–348 (1978).
Hamwi, G. J., Skillman, T. G., and Tufts, K.C. Acromegaly, *Am. J. Med.* 29:690–699 (1960).
Heller, G. L., and DeJong, R. N. Treatment of Guillain-Barré syndrome. *Arch. Neurol.* 8:179–193 (1963).
Herrera, M. G., Cahill, G. F. Jr., and Thorn, G. W. Cushing's syndrome. Diagnosis and treatment. *Am. J. Surg.* 107:144–152 (1964).
Himmelhoch, J., Pincus, J., Tucker, G., and Detre, T. Subacute encephalitis: Behavioral and neurological aspects. *Brit. J. Psychiat.* 116:531–538 (1970).
Hocking, F. Psychiatric aspects of extreme environmental stress. *Dis. Nerv. Syst.* 31:542–545 (1970).
Horton, P. C. Personality disorder and parietal lobe dysfunction. *Am. J. Psychiat.* 133:782–785 (1976).
Hossain, M. Neurological and psychiatric manifestations in idiopathic hypoparathyroidism: Response to treatment. *J. Neurol. Neurosurg. Psychiat.* 33:153–156 (1970).
Howland, G., Campbell, W. R., Maltby, E. J., and Robertson, W. L. Deinsulinism. *J.A.M.A.* 93:674–679 (1929).
Humphrey, J. G. Prognosis and therapy of myasthenia gravis. *Postgrad. Med.* 38:64–71 (1965).
Ingbar, S. H. Management of emergencies. IX thyrotoxic storm. *N. Eng. J. Med.* 274:1252–1254 (1966).
International Conference on Vascular Disease of the Brain. Neurology 11, No. 4, Part 2 (1961).
Irvine, W. J. and Barnes, E. W. Adrenocortical insufficiency. *Clin. Endocrinol. Metabol.* 1:549–594 (1972).
Ivers, R. R. and Goldstein, H. P. Multiple sclerosis: A current appraisal of symptoms and signs. *Proc. Staff Meet. Mayo Clin.* 38:457–466 (1963).
James, W. E., Mefferd, R. B., and Kimball, I. Early signs of Huntington's chorea. *Dis. Nerv. Syst.* 30:556–559 (1969).
Klein, D. F. Delineation of two drug responsive anxiety syndromes. *Psychopharmacologia* (Berlin). 5:397–408, (1964)..
Krane, S. M. Selected features of the clinical course of hypoparathyroidism. *J.A.M.A.* 178:472–475 (1961).
Krupp, M. A., Chatton, M. J., eds. *Current Diagnosis and Treatment.* Lang. Pub., Los Altos, California (1973). (See applicable sections for each medical disorder.)
Lader, M., and Sartorius N. Anxiety in patients with hysterical conversion symptoms. *J. Neurol. Neurosurg. Psychiat.* 31:490–495 (1968).
Liddle, G. W., and Shute, A. M. The evolution of Cushing's syndrome. *Adv. Int. Med.* 15:155–175 (1969).
Liebman, R., Minuchin, S., and Baker, L. An integrated treatment program for anorexia nervosa. *Am. J. Psychiat.* 131:432–436 (1974).
Lucas, A. R., Duncan, J. W., and Piens, V. The treatment of anorexia nervosa. *Am. J. Psychiat.* 133:1034–1038 (1976).
McAlpine, D. The benign form of multiple sclerosis. Results of long-term study. *Brit. Med. J.* 2:1029–1032 (1964).
McCaughey, W.T.C. The pathologic spectrum of Huntington's chorea. *J. Nerv. Ment. Dis.* 133:91–107 (1961).

Mecklenburg, R. S., Loriaux, D. L., and Thompson, R. H. Hypothalamic dysfunction in patients with anorexia nervosa. *Med.* 53:147–159 (1974).

Merskey, H., and Woodforde, J. M. Psychiatric sequalae of minor head injury. *Brain.* 95:521–528 (1972).

Miller, H., and Stern, G. The long-term prognosis of severe head injury. *Lancet.* 1:225–228 (1965).

Modlin, H. C. Post accident anxiety syndrome: Psychosocial aspects. *Am. J. Psychiat.* 123:1008–1012 (1967).

More, B. E., and Fine, B. D. *A Glossary of Psychoanalytic Terms and Concepts.* The American Psychoanalytic Assn., N.Y. (1967).

Mulder, D. W. Diagnosis and management of mononeuropathies. *Postgrad. Med.* 36:321–329 (1964).

Mulder, D. W., Bickford, R. G., and Dodge, H. W., Jr. Hallucinatory epilepsy: Complex hallucinations as focal seizures. *Am. J. Psychiat.* 113:1100–1102 (1957).

Noreik, K. A followup examination of neurosis. *ACTA Psychiat. Scan.* 46:81–95 (1970).

Nusynowitz, M. L., Frame, B., and Kolb, F. O. The spectrum of the hypoparathyroid states: A classification based on physiological principles. *Med.* 55:105–119 (1976).

O'Connor, J. F., and Musher, D. M. Central nervous involvement in systemic lupus erythematosis. *Arch. Neurol.* 14:157–164 (1966).

Odell, W. D. Isolated deficiencies of anterior pituitary hormones. Symptoms and diagnosis. *J.A.M.A.* 197:1006–1016 (1966).

Patton, R. B., and Sheppard, J. A. Intracranial tumors found at autopsy in mental patients. *Am. J. Psychiat.* 113:319—324 (1956).

Penfield, W., and Jasper, H. Functional localization in the cerebral cortex, in *Epipepsy and the Functional Anatomy of the Human Brain.* W. Penfield and H. Jasper, eds. Little, Brown and Co., Boston, Massachusetts (1954), Chap. 3, pp. 41–155.

Perkoff, G. T., Sandberg, A. A., Nelson, D. H., and Tyler, F. H. Clinical usefulness determination of circulating 17-hydroxycorticosteroid levels. *Arch. Int. Med.* 93:1–8 (1054).

Preu, D. Experimental aspects of anxiety. *Am. J. Psychol.* 113:435–442 (1956).

Read, A. E., Sherlock, S., Laidlaw, J., and Walker, J. G. Neuropsychiatric syndromes associated with chronic liver disease and an extensive portal systemic collateral circulation. *Quart. J. Med.* 36:135–150 (1967).

Reilly, E. L., and Wilson, W. P. Mental symptoms in hyperparathyroidism. *Dis. Nerv. Syst.* 26:361–363 (1965).

Rioch, D. Experimental aspects of anxiety. *Am. J. Psychiat.* 113:435–442 (1956).

Ross, A. T., and Reitan, R. M. Intellectual and affective functions in multiple sclerosis. *Arch. Neurol. Psychiat.* 73:663–677 (1955).

Roth, M. The phobic anxiety-depersonalization syndrome. *Proc. Roy. Soc. Med.* 52:587–595 (1959).

Santschi, D. R., Frahm, C. J., and Pascale, L. R. The subclavical steal syndrome: Clinical and angiographic considerations in 74 cases in adults. *J. Thorac. and Cardiovas. Surg.* 51:103–112 (1966).

Sayers, R. R. *Findings From Major Studies of Fatigue..* The Bureau of Mines Information, Circ. 7209. U.S. Dept. Inst., Washington, D.C. (1942).

Scheinberg, P., and Rice-Simons, R. A. The treatment of recurring cerebral ischemic phenomena. *Geriat.* 19:887–893 (1964).

Schneider, A. B., and Sherwood, L. M. Pathogenesis and management of hypoparathyroidism and other hypocalcemic disorders. *Metabol.* 24:871–898 (1975).

Schwab, J. J. Psychiatric illnesses produced by infection. *Hosp. Med.* 5:98–108 (1969).

Segre, E. J., Klaiber, E. L., and Labotsky, J. Hirsutism and virilizing syndromes. *Ann. Rev. Med.* 15:315–334 (1964).

Shader, R. I., ed. *Psychiatric Complications of Medical Drugs.* Raven Press, New York (1976).

Shands, H. C., Finesinger, J. E., and Watkins, A. L. Clinical studies on fatigue. *Arch. Neurol. Psychiat.* 60:210—217 (1948).

Shaw, D. L., Chesney, M. A., Tullis, I. F., and Agersborg, H.P.K. Management of fatigue. *Am. J. Med. Sci.* 243:758–769 (1962).
Shulman, R. Psychiatric aspects of pernicious anemia: A prospective study. *Brit. Med. J.* 3:266–269 (1967).
Simpson, J. F., Westerberg, M. R., and Magee, K. R. Myasthenia gravis, an analysis of 295 cases, *ACTA Neurol. Scand.* Supp. 23, 42:1–27 (1966).
Smilo, R. R., and Forsham, P. H. Diagnostic approach to hypofunction and hyperfunction of the adrenal cortex. *Postgrad. Med.* 46:146–152 (1969).
Soniat, T.L.L. Psychiatric symptoms associated with intracranial neoplasms. *Am. J. Psychiat.* 108:19–22 (1951).
Steinberg, F. U. Subacute granulomatous thyroiditis: A review. *Ann. Int. Med.* 52:1014–1025 (1960).
Stenbäck, A., and Haapanen, E. Azotemia and people. *ACTA Psychiat. Scand.* 43:9–65 (1967).
Sternlieb, U., and Scheinberg, I. H. Prevention of Wilson's disease in asymptomatic patients. *N. Eng. J. Med.* 278:352–359 (1968).
Symposium on Disseminated Sclerosis and Allied Conditions. *Proc. Roy. Soc. Med.* 54:1–42 (1961).
Thomas, W. C., Jr., Anderson, R. M., and Jurkiewicz, M. J. Clinical studies in thyroiditis. *Ann. Int. Med.* 63:808–818 (1965).
Thompson, G. N. Posttraumatic psychoneurosis: A statistical survey. *Am. J. Psychiat.* 121:1043–1048 (1965).
Thorn, G. W., ed. Symposium on the adrenal cortex. *Am. J. Med.* 53:529–532 (1972).
Treadway, C. R. Mental changes accompanying thyroid gland dysfunction. *Arch. Gen. Psychiat.* 20:48–63 (1969).
Tyler, H. R. Neurological disorders in renal failure. *Am. J. Med.* 44:734–748 (1968).
Vagenakis, A. G., Dole, K., and Braverman, L. E. Pituitary enlargement, pituitary failure, and primary hypothyroidism. *Ann. Int. Med.* 85:195–198 (1976).
Venning, E. H., Dyrenfurth, I., and Beck, J. C. Effect of anxiety aldosterone excretion in man. *J. Clin. Endocrinol. Metabol.* 17:1005–1008 (1957).
Walshe, J. M. Wilson's disease. *Biochem. J.* 111:8p–9p (1969).
Watanakunakorn, C., Hodges, R. E., and Evans, T. C. Myxedema. *Arch. Int. Med.* 116:183–190 (1965).
Wheeler, E. O., White, P. D., Reed, E. W., and Cohen, M. E. Neurocirculatory asthenia (anxiety neurosis, effort syndrome, neurasthenia); 20 year follow-up study of one-hundred seventy three patients. *J.A.M.A.* 142:878–889 (1950).
Williams, E. Anorexia nervosa: A somatic disorder. *Brit. Med. J.* 2:190–195 (1958).
Winokur, G., and Holemon, E. Chronic anxiety neurosis. *ACTA Scand.* 39:384–412 (1963).
Young, D. G., Bahn, R. C., and Randall, R. V. Pituitary tumors associated with acromegaly. *J. Clin. Endocrinol.* 25:249–259 (1965).
Zimmerman, H. M., ed. *Infections of the Nervous System.* Proceedings of the Association for Research in the Nervous and Mental Diseases, v. 44. Williams & Wilkins, Baltimore, Maryland (1964).

Psychiatric Presentations of Medical Illness

CHAPTER 3

Depression

RICHARD C. W. HALL, M.D.

Depression is a mood state, a psychiatric symptom and a series of psychiatric diseases. As an emotion, or mood state, it is known to us all. It is the most frequent psychiatric illness treated in America today. Unfortunately, its causation by physical disorders has been largely neglected in the psychiatric and medical literature. Depression and the anxiety states are the psychiatric reactions most likely to be associated with concurrent physical disease, or to be produced by a yet undetected medical illness (see Table 1).

Progress in psychiatric research and psychopharmacology has provided the physician with a two-edged sword when it comes to the management of the depressed patient. Rapid breakthroughs in the understanding of the biochemistry of depression have led to the commonplace use of antidepressant drugs. It has become a simple and routine matter during the last 20 years for a physician to "do something" for his depressed patient—prescribe an antidepressant. Such prescription, unless preceded by careful medical evaluation, may do the patient a great disservice by providing a false sense of security to both he and his physician. Antidepressants may be effective in controlling the depressive symptoms produced by an as yet, unrecognized physical illness, thus aborting medical evaluation and worsening the prognosis; or they may prove ineffective, suggesting a diagnosis of characterological or psychoneurotic depression which is then thought to be amenable only to psychotherapy, once again permitting progression of the underlying medical illness (Blumer, 1970; Hall and Popkin, 1977; Hall et al., 1978a; Nicol, 1968; Korolenko et al., 1969; Colbert and Harrow, 1966).

In evaluating depressive symptoms from a psychiatric point of view, the primary physician must wade through a confusing array of terminology and

TABLE 1. MEDICAL ILLNESSES THAT FREQUENTLY INDUCE DEPRESSION

Pernicious anemia
Folic acid deficiency
Multiple sclerosis
Influenza
Viral hepatitis
Cirrhosis
Uremia
Disseminate carcinomatosis
Oat-Cell carcinoma of the lung
Lymphomas
Chronic myelogenous leukemia
Carcinoma of the pancreas
Cushing's disease
Hyperaldosteronism
Addison's disease
Hyperparathyroidism
Hypoparathyroidism
Hyperthyroidism
Hypothyroidism
Acromegaly
Systemic lupus erythematosus
Ulcerative colitis
Regional enteritis
Whipple's disease
Amyloidosis

theorems which, although useful in characterizing depressed patients for research purposes, may not stand the test of clinical utility. For the purpose of this chapter, it is hoped that the following, more simplified approach will be of use.

CLASSIFICATION OF DEPRESSIVE DISORDERS

The physician in his office practice must differentiate between certain major categories of depression. Each of these will now be examined.

Endogenous (Psychotic) Depression

The patient with an endogenous depression has experienced the relatively sudden onset (i.e., over 2–8 weeks) of a progressive series of depressive symptoms that are qualitatively different from those alterations of mood that he has experienced during the course of his everyday life. These symptoms have become so severe as to totally incapacitate him and imbue him with a sense of helplessness and hopelessness. Such a patient is unable to respond to social support within his environment or to experience periods of pleasure. He generally presents a history of adequate premorbid social and work adjustment. When recovery occurs, it is usually complete, with both the patient and his family being able to separate clearly in their minds the premorbid and postmorbid intervals from the actual depressed state. Although depressed mood is present in an overwhelming number of cases (i.e., feelings of sadness, unhappiness), it is noteworthy that it is not necessary for the diagnosis of endogenous depression. The syndrome is characterized by *psychomotor retardation*, manifested by a slowing or paucity of movement, thought, and speech with prolonged speech latencies; impaired ability to concentrate; indecisiveness; diminished vitality; loss of energy, sexual drive, ambition, and initiative; the inability to experience pleasurable feelings (anhedonia); and apathy manifested by an inability to maintain usual interest levels or emotional involvement. Characteristically, the patient reports a diurnal variation of symptoms, feeling worse in the morning and progressively better as the day goes on. The diurnal changes are associated with early morning awakening, where the patient awakens at 3 to 4 A.M. in an agitated, hopeless, despondent state and is unable to return to sleep. Endogenous depression becomes autonomous once established and is unaltered by changes in the patient's social environment. It may or may not have been initially precipitated by a stressful life event or loss.

Constitutional symptoms of anorexia, constipation, weight loss, and sleep disturbance manifested by insomnia, hypersomnia, sleep continuity disorder, and/or early morning awakening are frequently seen, as are feelings of hopelessness, helplessness, guilt, worthlessness, rumination, demoralization, and suicidal ideation. Hallucinations and delusions of a depressive character (e.g., voices condemning the patient for past failures or notions that his body is rotting or diseased) may occur.

In contrast to the patient with profound psychomotor retardation, some patients present with *agitation*. They appear in a state of turmoil, and manifest increased gross motor movements of an expressive nature, such as hand-wringing or pacing. Often, they are paralyzed by their inability to make even inconsequential decisions, such as which article of clothing to wear. They appear to be suffering intense psychic pain. Some authorities feel that this agitated behavior is associated with involutional depressive syndromes, while others feel it should be considered a core characteristic of endogenous depression. In terms of clinical practice, it is perhaps best to look at the agitated and involutional depressive syndromes as subcategories of unipolar depression. The most important signs include the aforementioned agitation with hand-wringing and pacing, accompanied by delusions of guilt, illness, or body decay; and paranoid ideation. The majority of such patients are over 45, hence the term *involutional depression*. True agitated depression may occur in younger individuals as well.

Depression of psychotic proportion may occur as the result of the administration of such drugs as reserpine (Goodwin et al., 1972); alpha methyl dopa; indomethacin; propanol (Waal, 1967); corticosteroids; (Hall and Reading,

1971; Hall et al., 1978b); clonidine; oral contraceptives (Grant and Pryse-Davis, 1968; Herzberg and Coppen, 1970); diazepam, particularly in patients with renal disorders and in the elderly (Hall and Joffe, 1972); phenylbutazone; chloroquine; and hydroxychloroquine (Rockwell, 1968). They may also be induced by physical illnesses, such as carcinoma of the pancreas (Fras et al., 1968), hypothyroidism (Treadway, 1969); mononucleosis (Schnell et al., 1966; Schwab, 1969), encephalitis (Azar, et al., 1966; Guze and Cantwell, 1964), hypoparathyroidism (Hossain, 1970; Petersen, 1968), renal failure (Stenbäck and Haapanen, 1967), viral hepatitis (Schwab, 1969), influenza (Schwab, 1969), stroke (Ullman and Gruen, 1961), pernicious anemia (Strachan and Henderson, 1965; Lewin, 1959; Wiener, 1959), cirrhosis (Read et al, 1967), and lymphomas.

Exogenous Depressions (Psychoneurotic, Situational, Reactive)

These disorders occur as the result of situational stress, such as the loss of a loved one, a job, a possession, or physical health, which temporarily overwhelms the individual and reduces his ability to cope. *Exogenous depressions*

TABLE 2. MEDICAL CONDITIONS ASSOCIATED WITH REACTIVE DEPRESSIONS

Myocardial infarction
Angina pectoris
Transient cerebral ischemia
Congestive heart failure
Associated loss or distortion of special senses producing blindness, deafness, loss of tactile senses
Spinal cord lesions or injury
Degenerative intervertebral disc disease
Cerebral vascular accident
Paraplegia
Rheumatoid arthritis
Osteoarthritis
Felty's syndrome
Sjogren's syndrome
Marie Strumpell spondylitis
Juvenile rheumatoid arthritis
Psoriasis
Gout
Collagen vascular disorder
Malignancy
Tuberculosis
Sarcoidosis
Epilepsy
Diabetes mellitus

are less severe than the endogenous depressions, and the affective state is not fixed (i.e., changes in life circumstances produce a prompt, although temporary, remission of symptoms). Their course, although variable, is self limited with symptoms generally remitting within a few months. Occasionally, symptoms progress to those of an endogenous depression, at which time they change in character and intensity and become autonomous. In such cases, the patient should be treated for endogenous depression.

The most frequent symptoms seen in patients with exogenous depression are: preoccupation with loss, tension and rumination focused on the current loss, diminished or increased appetite, easy fatigability, difficulty in falling asleep or sleep continuity disorder, spontaneous tearfulness, and a brooding appearance. The patient is able to enjoy pleasurable experiences, which may distract him from his preoccupation with the depressing event. The clinical picture of exogenous depression may be produced by such illnesses as chronic anemia of any cause, influenza, hypothyroidism (Treadway, 1969), and early pernicious anemia. (Strachan and Henderson, 1965) (see Table 2). It may also be induced by such drugs as oral contraceptives, and as an idiosyncratic response to the benzodiazepines, particularly Valium.

Depressive Personality (Chronic Characterological Depression)

This syndrome typically occurs in patients with a life-long history of personality disorder, who react to minor stress or life change with the rapid development of depressive symptoms. Characteristically, these patients describe themselves as impaired in their interpersonal and social adjustment and distant from others. The major symptom constellation seen in such individuals includes: emotional lability, preoccupation with stress or loss, spontaneous intermittent weeping, generalized long-term unhappiness, and dissatisfaction with their lot in life, often feeling that they have been short-changed in their career goals or social standing. They frequently have histories of dramatic, histrionic, attention-seeking behavior and fix blame on other individuals or situations for their failure. They tend to have a clinging, almost consuming dependency with a pessimistic, complaining, and demanding attitude. Dependency needs are often expressed through hypochondriasis. Anxiety episodes punctuate the patient's life. Minor frustrations produce irritability and anger followed by self-pity. These patients are likely to have a history of suicidal threats or gestures and frequently abuse stimulants, alcohol, or sedatives. The secondary gain of their depressive symptoms comes from their ability to manipulate or control others.

These patients are particularly difficult for the practitioner to deal with since their personality attributes, and depressive symptoms are markedly exacerbated by even minor physical ills. Their need to elicit pity and to use symptoms for secondary gain make them frequent visitors to the physician's office. Resentment of their clinging, demanding behavior may lead to disruption of the normal physician-patient relationship and may prompt the physician to dismiss their complaints rather than investigate them carefully.

Demoralization

Although not frequently thought of as a specific psychiatric symptom, Frank (1975) and others have cogently pointed out that the relief of demoralization is essential for successful psychotherapy. Demoralization is perhaps the most common symptom of psychiatric patients. It occurs with high frequency as well in medical patients, where it may be readily mistaken for a primary depressive disorder.

Demoralization represents an alteration of self-image, with the patient believing that he is no longer effective in managing his life. He feels increasingly helpless and dependent on others. Each new catastrophe further adds to his feeling of self-denigration. The syndrome is a frequent feature of depression where patients verbalize their helplessness and hopelessness. As demoralization progresses, the patient becomes unable to engage spontaneously in even the simplest tasks. Activities become restricted, and the capacity for enjoyment diminishes. The patient reports being able to enjoy himself only momentarily and then only in situations which make no external demands upon him. The demoralized patient characteristically maintains a normal appetite and sleep pattern and is able to respond to encouragement. His despair is typically unrelieved by antidepressants or other medications. If demoralization progresses, classical symptoms of exogenous depression may appear.

Demoralization is particularly likely to occur as a consequence of an unrecognized, severe, misunderstood, or incapacitating physical illness. It is frequently seen following: myocardial infarction, particularly in the young; the diagnosis of carcinoma; amputation; burns; and upon recognition of any chronic, socially debilitating disease, such as diabetes mellitus, epilepsy, sickle cell anemia, rheumatoid arthritis, sarcoidosis, ulcerative colitis, regional enteritis, Whipple's disease, amyloidosis, acromegaly, renal failure, paraplegia, stroke, progressive dementia, impairment or loss of sensory function secondary to cataracts, traumatic blindness, deafness, or spinal cord injury. It incapacitates at least a third of all patients who have undergone mutilative surgery (Bowers, 1969; Cairns, 1962; Colbert and Harrow, 1966; Corsellis and Brierley, 1959; Dalessio et al., 1965; Davies, 1969; Guze and Cantwell, 1964; Guze and Daenqsurisri, 1967; Korolenko et al., 1969; Lange and Poppe, 1964; Lipowski, 1967; Modlin, 1967; von Werssowetz, 1966).

Demoralization is most effectively dealt with by a physician attitude of: expectant optimism; the imparting of full and accurate information; mobilization of family support; and continued contact. Specific rehabilitation programs; referral to clubs or groups of individuals experiencing similar problems, such as the ostomy clubs; and detailed clarification of the limitations to be expected by the patient are of great assistance. It is essential that the physician encourage as much normal behavior as possible while assisting the patient to accept the chronic nature of his condition. For example, encouraging the young infarct patient to begin a carefully regulated exercise program, allaying his concerns about the potential dangers of sexual activity, discussing the specific elimination of stressors, and supporting and counseling his family, all serve to increase his control over his illness and diminish or prevent demoralization.

DEPRESSIVE STATES ASSOCIATED WITH OR SECONDARY TO CONCURRENT PHYSICAL ILLNESS

Physical disease, which alters highly valued patterns of behavior, diminishes self-esteem, induces fear, or enforces dependency, is likely to be associated with the development of a depressive reaction. In such instances, the physician's sensitivity and ability to define the patient's specific fears represents the cornerstone of successful management. Consider for a moment, the following case:

> A 75-year-old, aggressive business executive experienced a sudden and profound depression manifested by emotional lability, spontaneous tearfulness, difficulty in falling asleep, early morning awakening, constant rumination about his physical health, loss of appetite, and hopelessness, manifested by such statements as "I'd be better off dead."He was started on amitriptyline, 150 mg h.s., and within 4 days developed a psychotic organic brain syndrome that required his hospitalization. Upon discontinuation of the antidepressant, the patient's sensorium cleared and the depression re-emerged.
>
> The following history was obtained: He was the eldest of five siblings. He immigrated to America from Germany following an argument with his alcoholic father, and worked for years as a common laborer until he bought a small business that grew into a major enterprise. He prided himself on his ability to work, remain independent, and be a good father and husband. His three children are all successful and have led independent existences for the last 20 years, having little contact, except at Christmas, with their parents. The patient's wife is an invalid suffering from severe rheumatoid arthritis, which makes her unable to cook, drive, or carry out fine motor movements. The patient had a massive coronary three years previously at which time he was also found to be a dietarily controllable diabetic. Several months after his coronary, he began to experience ocular pain, noticed halos about lights, and was found to have glaucoma, which could be only marginally controlled by medication. His ophthalmologist feared surgical correction of the condition because of the patient's medical status. The decision not to operate was made 2 months

before he presented to his internist with the previously described symptoms of depression.

Discussion revealed that the patient's depression was related to his fear of impending blindness. He must be able to see if he was to effectively care for his wife! He realized that the glaucoma was being effectively controlled by medication, and that surgery was hazardous. Depression hinged on his anticipated loss of independence, his fear of being placed in a nursing home, and the subsequent loss of control over his life. Discussion and acceptance of life-style alternatives, changes of medication, and the acceptance of a somewhat reduced level of independence, produced a remission of depressive symptoms.

As the above case illustrates, incapacity caused by physical disease must be seen from the patient's perspective. The psychic significance of loss may not be apparent to the physician who sees a disease entity only in terms of its pathophysiology.

DEPRESSION ASSOCIATED WITH DEMENTIA

Dementia is a term that implies deterioration of intellectual capacity from any cause, but is distinguished from the life-long, subnormal intellectual function-

TABLE 3. DEMENTIAS PRODUCING DEPRESSIVE RESPONSES

Cerebrovascular insufficiency
Lead, arsenic, thallium intoxication
Chronic organophosphate intoxication
Idiosyncratic drug reactions
Drug intoxication
Electrolyte disorders
Generalized intracerebral mass lesions
Cerebrovascular lues
Cerebral sarcoidosis
Generalized sarcoidosis with hypercalcemia
Alzheimer's disease
Pick's disease
Jakob-Creutzfeldt disease
Huntington's chorea
Idiopathic cortical atrophy
Uremia
Hepatic failure
Chronic anoxia
Vitamin deficiencies
Normal pressure hydrocephalus

ing of retardation. It can result from any pathological process that affects cerebral hemispheric function, and is more related to the extent rather than the location or specific cause of injury. Clinically, most physicians think of dementia in its full-blown form where symptoms are easily recognizable. However, the majority of patients suffering from dementia give retrospective histories of declining mental function over several years and often present initially with symptoms of depression. Dementia may be produced by a treatable cause which, if reversed early, will prevent further deterioration (see Table 3). Depression is the most frequent specific prodrome of impaired central nervous system function; therefore the inclusion of dementia in the differential diagnosis of depressive disorders is crucial (Colbert and Harrow, 1966; Corsellis and Brierley, 1959; Davies, 1969; Guze and Cantwell, 1964; Guze and Daengsurisri, 1967; Korolenko et al., 1969; Lipowski, 1967; Hall, 1972).

The initial symptom of dementia is disturbance in the patient's capacity for problem-solving. He has trouble grasping situations, or handling new and demanding tasks, although he is frequently able to perform routine functions. Anxiety appears when the patient realizes his cognitive loss but cannot define its cause. As memory deteriorates, he becomes bewildered and perplexed. Depression now becomes fully manifest. The patient may begin to withdraw from stressful situations and his speech becomes slowed and habitual. When stressed, sudden outbursts of emotion are seen, taking the form of aggressiveness or frank tearfulness. Such *catastrophic reactions* are of short duration and provide a nidus for subsequent depressive rumination. As the dementing process continues, chronic severe depression, accompanied by anxiety states, appears. This anxiety may result from the patient's perceived loss and inability to cope, or it may be indicative of injury to the central nervous system mechanisms, which mediate emotional response and expressivity. Mental anergia and apathy may ensue, with the patient losing his animation, initiative, and energy. Performance deteriorates, while social isolation and withdrawal increase, progressing in some cases to profound psychomotor retardation or frank social unresponsiveness (Waggoner and Bagchi, 1954; Lange and Poppe, 1964).

The mental status (Bell and Hall, 1977) is helpful in differentiating true depressive reactions from dementing processes. The patient with dementia is likely to show disorientation to time, place, or person, accompanied by diminished language skills. His fund of knowledge is diminished and recent memory is impaired. He evidences restriction of attention span and is unable to perform serial subtractions. First and second order mathematical skills are also impaired. Abstract reasoning is impaired, consequently the patient experiences difficulty in defining proverbs or explaining similarities. Constructional abilities, such as drawing a clock, or copying an abstract design, are also impaired. In contrast, the depressed patient is oriented, can calculate, abstract, and construct.

A detailed medical evaulation is indicated if mental status changes suggest dementia. Such conditions as general paresis (Koch, 1964; Thomas, 1964);

hyperthyroidism (Treadway, 1969); carcinomatosis; neoplasm of the brain (Blustein and Seeman, 1972; Guvener et al., 1964; Avery, 1971; Malamud, 1967; Morse, 1920; Rubert and Remington, 1962; Selecki, 1965; Gal, 1958), or other organs; porphyria (Levere and Kappas, 1970); chronic intracerebral lesions (Thompson, 1970; Yaskin, 1931); pernicious anemia (Strachan and Henderson, 1965; Lewin, 1959; Wiener and Hope, 1959); Wilson's disease (Sternlieb and Scheinberg, 1968; Knehr and Bearn, 1956); lupus (McClary et al., 1955); or occult hydrocephalus (Adams et al., 1965), should be suspected. Poisonings and metabolic disturbances must be specifically ruled out. Physical examination may provide valuable clues, such as the Argyll-Robertson pupil of cerebral syphilis, the Kayer-Fleisher ring of Wilson's disease, localized neurological signs associated with neoplasm, the gait disorder and spastic weakness of the legs seen with hydrocephalus, the Mees lines of lead poisoning, or the glossitis and dermatitis of pellagra. If the clinical picture is in doubt, all patients should have a lumbar puncture to measure their CSF pressure and to obtain fluid for cell count, protein, electrolytes, serology, viral titers, and culture. Laboratory examination for thyroid levels, 17 hydroxy and ketosteroids, serum folate and B_12 levels, heavy metal screen, and liver and renal function tests should be performed. Electroencephalography may reveal a focal abnormality or the general slowing characteristic of delirium. C.A.T. scan or skull x-ray may define focal lesions. Pneumoencephalograms may be needed to rule out tumors of the third ventricle and occult hydrocephalus.

Careful analysis of the course and onset of the depressive state and the rapidity of progression of the dementia may be helpful in differentiating various conditions. For example, the depression and dementia associated with vascular disease is sudden in onset and progresses in an intermittent and variable fashion, while those associated with degenerative CNS disease are insidious in onset and slowly but relentlessly progressive. The dementia of general paresis is subacute and steadily progressive.

If no specific metabolic, biochemical, toxic, or neoplastic etiology can be found in a patient presenting with depression and dementia, the physician should consider those disorders that produce cerebral degeneration: Alzheimer's, Pick's, and Jakob-Creutzfeldt's diseases, or Huntington's chorea (Ehrentheil, 1957; Crapper et al., 1973; Marx, 1973; Simon, 1970; Slaby and Wyatt, 1974).

In *Alzheimer's disease* (Slaby and Wyatt, 1974; Sjogren et al., 1952; Wolsten-Holme and O'Connor, 1970), depression and progressive dementia appear in middle to late life and have few distinct characteristics. The onset is insidious and the progress slow. Depression and disturbances of recent memory are the earliest symptoms encountered. Forty percent of patients with Alzheimer's disease become delusional, while 10 to 30 percent develop auditory or visual hallucinations. Focal neurological signs are rare early in the course of the disease and do not usually become prominent until 5 to 7 years following the onset of symptoms. The most specific focal signs encountered are aphasia, apraxia, and agnosia. In advanced cases, focal and generalized seizures may occur, as well as the characteristic gait disorder produced by synchronous activation of agonist and antagonist muscles. The end stage of the disease, usually reached within 5 to 10 years, is characterized by profound dementia and a decerebrate state with flexion contractures of the limbs. Alzheimer's disease has been reported in 10 percent of psychiatric hospital patients coming to autopsy. The disease is more common in females than males and seems to have an increased incidence in boxers, patients with Down's syndrome, and postencephalitic Parkinsonism. Pneumoencephalography will usually reveal moderate dilation of the cerebral ventricles and diffuse cortical atrophy. Definitive diagnosis is made on the basis of cerebral biopsy with demonstration of characteristic neurofibrillary tangles and senile plaques. Cellular changes are most marked in the frontal and occipital lobes, which are the best sites for biopsy. Microscopic changes, however, can be demonstrated throughout the entire atrophic cortex.

Pick's disease (Lowenberg and Scharenberg, 1936; Sjogren et al., 1952) is differentiated from Alzheimer's, in that the former shows circumscribed atrophy, usually confined to the frontal and temporal lobes, while the degeneration seen with Alzheimer's is diffuse. Definitive diagnosis is based on finding the characteristic Pick cell, a degenerating neuron with a globular argyrophilic mass close to its nucleus. On biopsy, neurofibrillary tangles and senile plaques, as are seen in Alzheimer's disease, also occur. Characteristically, the depression and gait disorders seen in patients with Pick's disease are less pronounced than those that occur with Alzheimer's (Slaby and Wyatt, 1974).

Jakob-Creutzfeldt's disease is thought to be caused by a slow-growing virus, which produces dementia associated with severe depression and other psychotic manifestations (Marx, 1973). The condition is rapidly progressive, worsening day by day, until fatal termination occurs, usually within 1 year. Neurological symptoms, particularly ataxia, aphasia, paralysis, visual disturbances, and myoclonic jerking of the limbs, appear early. EEG shows loss of normal rhythm and a distinctive mixture of slow and short waves.

Huntington's chorea (Cohen, 1962; Oliphant et al., 1960) is a disorder transmitted by an autosomal dominant gene that appears during the fourth or fifth decade of life. Its onset is insidious and its course relentless, ending in death over a 12-to-15-year period. Depression, emotional lability, and agitation occur early. As the disease progresses, profound depression and apathy are common and may advance to total unresponsiveness or mutism. The absence of aphasia distinguishes the dementia of Huntington's chorea from that of Alzheimer's disease. Severe, sudden mood changes of manic proportion are common, as are discrete periods of psychotic depression accompanied by psychomotor retardation, accusatory hallucinations, and delusions of guilt. Ten percent of patients with Huntington's attempt suicide during these periods of psychotic depression. The depressive episodes are successfully treated with either electroconvulsive therapy or tricyclic antidepressants. Depression frequently alternates with periods of manic excitement. In the majority of patients, symptoms of the severe mood disorder and dementia precede the onset of choreaform movements by several months or years. Diagnosis is made on the basis of family history, or the appearance of choreiform movement.

MANAGEMENT OF DEPRESSION RELATED TO DEMENTIA

Some specific principles of management are useful when dealing with depression related to dementia (Bowers, 1969; Cairns, 1942; Colbert and Harrow, 1966; Guze and Cantwell, 1964; Guze and Daengsurisri, 1967; Lange and Poppe, 1964; Lipowski, 1967). The meticulous correction of all medical complications is of prime importance. Secondly, the patient's depression usually responds well to structured environmental support. If the environment is left unstructured, patients are likely to experience the catastrophic reactions described earlier. It is crucial that the patient be repetitively engaged, that procedures be explained, and that he be made aware of what is happening. Changes of personnel and surroundings should be minimized. Rooms should be kept well lighted and contain familiar objects, pictures, and possessions. Situations that produce stress, or require activity beyond the patient's current level of performance, should be avoided.

MEDICAL CONDITIONS DIRECTLY PRODUCTIVE OF DEPRESSION

The concept of "toxic metabolic psychosis," although extremely valuable in psychiatry, is inadequate for the description of the many disease states that present with symptoms of depression unaccompanied by clearcut signs of organic brain syndrome. Many illnesses present with purely depressive symptomatology, either prior to, or concurrent with the development of other physical signs. If the clinician is to diagnose and treat these disorders, he must be aware of their differential diagnosis (See Table 4). Although space does not permit a

TABLE 4. MEDICAL CONDITIONS PRESENTING WITH DEPRESSION

ENDOCRINE

Hyperthyroidism
Hypothyroidism
Autoimmune thyroiditis
Hyperparathyroidism
Hypothyroidism
Diabetes mellitus

TABLE 4. MEDICAL CONDITIONS PRESENTING WITH DEPRESSION (Cont.)

Hyperinsulinism of any cause
Cushing's disease (or adrenal cortical hyperplasia)
Addison's disease
Menopause

CENTRAL NERVOUS SYSTEM DISORDERS

Brain tumor
Chronic subdural hematoma
Multiple sclerosis
Wilson's disease
Alzheimer's disease
Pick's disease
Huntington's chorea
Jakob-Creutzfeldt's disease
Cerebral vascular accident

INFECTIOUS DISEASES

Tertiary syphilis
Viral encephalitis, particularly St. Louis encephalitis
Viral hepatitis-posthepatic syndrome
Mononucleosis
Influenza
Brucellosis
Malaria
Pneumonia, particularly viral
Tuberculosis
Sarcoidosis

HEPATIC DISORDERS

Inflammatory hepatitis
Early cirrhosis

PANCREATIC DISORDERS

Pancreatitis
Carcinoma of pancreas

NUTRITIONAL DEFICIENCIES

Pellagra
Thiamine deficiency
Pyridoxine deficiency
Ascorbic acid deficiency
B_{12} deficiency
Folic acid deficiency
Protein deficiency
Iron deficiency

TABLE 4. MEDICAL CONDITIONS PRESENTING WITH DEPRESSION (Cont.)

ELECTROLYTE DISORDERS

Hyponatremia
Hypokalemia
Hyperkalemia
Hypomagnesemia
Hypocalcemia
Increased plasma bicarbonate
Decreased plasma bicarbonate

SYSTEMIC DISEASE

Collagen vascular disorders
- a. Systemic lupus erythematosus
- b. Periarteritis nodosa
- c. Temporal arteritis

Amyloidosis
Gout
Psoriasis
Rheumatoid arthritis
Uremia
Ulcerative colitis
Regional enteritis
Lymphomas
Leukemias, particularly chronic myelogenous leukemia
Oat-cell carcinoma of the lung
Disseminated carcinomatosis

DRUG-INDUCED

Aliphatic phenothiazines (e.g., chloropromazine)
Reserpine
Alpha methyl dopa
Propranolol
L-dopa
Birth control pills
Benzodiazepines
Steroids
Digitalis
Disulfiram
Isonazid
Cycloserine
Ethambutol

detailed description of each of these illnesses, a brief discussion of the most common is in order. The major endocrine disorders are discussed elsewhere in the text. Suffice it to say that they frequently present with a mixed picture of anxiety and depression.

CENTRAL NERVOUS SYSTEM DISORDERS

Intracranial tumors are the third major cause for admission to neurological services in this country (Bilikiewicz and Gromska, 1963; Guvener et al., 1964; Rubert and Remington, 1962; Selecki, 1965; Waggoner and Bagchi, 1954; Avery, 1971; Blustein and Seeman, 1972; Cole, 1973; Blumer, 1970; Hobbs, 1963; Morse, 1920; Malamud, 1967; Withersty, 1974; Thompson, 1970). Of the brain tumors seen, gliomas comprise 40 to 50 percent, with their incidence being highest in the fourth and fifth decades. They are highly malignant and have a rapidly progressive course. Cerebellar medulloblastoma and astrocytoma are the most common tumors of childhood. In adults, tumors of the cerebral hemispheres are most common, particularly astrocytoma and glioblastoma multiforma. Meningiomas comprise 20 percent of intracranial neoplasms, are extremely slow-growing, and frequently present with psychiatric symptoms. When these tumors affect the frontal lobes, depression is likely and may be the only symptom seen for several years. Later in their course, impaired memory and judgment, irritability, emotional labiltiy, and perseveration occur. The convulsive disorders and speech impairment seen with tumors involving the dominant hemisphere occur late. Anosmia may be seen with tumors involving the cribriform plate and inferior frontal regions.

Parietal lobe tumors give rise to unusual sensory and motor phenomenon. As the tumor increases in size, motor and sensory focal seizures, contralateral hemiparesis, hyperreflexia, impaired sensory perception, astereognosis, Babinski's sign, and aphasia (left parietal lobe) may appear.

Occipital lobe tumors may produce visual alterations, hallucinations, or seizures. Contralateral homonomous hemianopsia occurs frequently with sparing of macular vision. Headaches and papilledema, if present, occur late.

Temporal lobe tumors may present as severe depression, or as a manic depressive or schizophreniform psychosis. Convulsive seizures of the psychomotor type are commonly present, as is aphasia, particularly when the dominant hemisphere is involved. The patient may demonstrate a contralateral homonomous visual field defect.

The most frequently observed psychiatric findings associated with brain tumor are mild to moderate recent memory defects, followed by affective disturbances, particularly depression. The depression seen in these patients is associated with increased irritability and affective lability. The patient evidences frequent episodes of crying and agitation. These initial changes are followed over months or years by a progressive loss of judgment, gradual intellectual deterioration, and disorientation. During the mid-course of his illness, the patient appears to suffer from a characteristically functional affective disorder with features of mild to moderate organic brain syndrome.

In a study of 326 patients with supratentorial neoplasms (Guvener and Bagchi, 1964), 58 percent were found to have significant early psychiatric disturbances, with depression and anxiety being the most common. The mental changes seen were not influenced by the presence or absence at some subsequent time of increased intracranial pressure, nor were they clearly related to the specific location of the tumor. There was a trend, however, for significant psychiatric symptoms to occur with tumors of the frontal and temporal lobes and with deep-seated neoplasms. Psychiatric symptoms were less common with tumors involving the parietal and occipital lobes.

The symptom analysis of these patients was particularly revealing. Disorientation occurred in only 11.9 percent, confusion in 18 percent, functional psychosis in 3.2 percent, non-specific cognitive impairment in 23.6 percent, marked emotional lability accompanied by bouts of sudden and intermittent depression in 4.6 percent, and unremitting depression in 3.6 percent. It was noteworthy that only 3.3 percent of these patients were diagnosed as having a clear-cut organic brain syndrome.

Seventy-one percent of all patients with glioblastoma experienced significant mental change. Fifty-three percent of the patients with astrocytoma or oligodendroglioma had significant mental changes, while 52 percent of those patients with meningiomas and pituitary neoplasms experienced them. The psychiatric significance of this study lies in the fact that only a small percentage of patients with brain tumor initially present with a clear-cut organic brain syndrome.

Further discussion of intracranial neoplasms is presented elsewhere in this volume.

Multiple sclerosis (Geisler and Jousse, 1963; Ivers and Goldstein, 1963; Koenig, 1968; McAlpine, 1964; Surridge, 1964) is another illness that frequently presents as depression, is often misdiagnosed, and is poorly understood psychiatrically. The majority of textbooks mention euphoria as its predominant mood change; however, this euphoria usually occurs late and may progress to a frank hypomanic state.

The most frequent psychiatric presentation of multiple sclerosis is one of moderate to severe depression with anxiety, often recurrent in nature, with each episode persisting 3 to 8 months. During the early stage of the disease, it is frequently misdiagnosed as a psychoneurotic depressive disorder or hysteria. Later, when more severe affective disturbances occur, the patient is most likely to be misdiagnosed as manic depressive. The depression is characterized by increased activity, irritability, emotional lability, and restlessness.

Multiple sclerosis is the most common of the demyelinating diseases, with the usual age of onset being between 20 and 40. The neurological symptoms seen are referrable to any part of the nervous system. The most common symptoms to occur *sometime* during its course are: unilateral blindness due to retrobulbar neuritis; nystagmus; diplopia, caused by isolated paralysis of extraocular muscles resulting from brain stem lesions; hemiparesis, secondary to pyramidal tract involvement; cerebellar ataxia of the intension type, and scanning, staccato-like speech.

The course of the illness is progressive with irregular and fluctuating periods of exacerbation and apparent remission. The etiology at present is unknown. The initial attack of the disease and subsequent relapses are frequently related to the presence of acute infections, trauma, vaccinations, serum injections, pregnancy, or somatic stress. During its course, the patient is also likely to experience episodes of incontinence, spastic paralysis, pallor of the temporal halves of the optic discs, increased deep tendon reflexes, and bilateral extensor plantar responses. Cerebral spinal fluid findings may show a first- or second-zone colloidal gold curve and elevated levels of gamma globulin. The average survival time following the onset of symptoms is approximately 30 years (Karlinner, 1956; Koch, 1964; Koenig, 1968; Malamud, 1967).

Other CNS disorders associated with primary depressive symptomatology include: chronic subdural hematoma, cerebral concussion (Modlin, 1967; Mulder and Daly, 1952), and cerebrovascular accidents (Ullman and Gruen, 1961; Timberline Conference, 1964), particularly those involving the temporal lobe.

INFECTIONS

Infectious disorders and their sequelae are a frequent and often unrecognized cause of moderate to severe depression (Azar et al., 1966; Blocker et al., 1968; Koch, 1964; Schnell et al., 1966; Schwab, 1969; Thomas, 1964; Guze and Daengsurisri, 1967; Marx, 1973). Of those infections involving the cranial cavity, *viral encephalitis* and *meningoencephalitis* (caused by the common childhood viruses), and equine encephalitis are most likely to produce psychiatric symptoms (Himmeloch et al., 1970). Emotional lability, personality disturbances, irritability, weakness, and mild confusion frequently precede the development of constitutional signs. Apathy, weakness, and depression are the major psychiatric sequelae seen following these infections. In a follow-up of patients from the St. Louis encephalitis epidemic that struck Florida in 1962, the occurrence of depression was so frequent that the study group recommended that depression be anticipated during convalescence (Azar et al., 1966).

The prevalence of *malaria* has increased significantly in this country following the Vietnam War (Blocker et al., 1968). The psychiatric manifestations of malaria (systemic and cerebral type) include personality change; frank psychotic episodes, which are most likely to occur during the recovery phase; intermittently occurring organic brain syndrome; and moderate to severe episodes of depression, which are particularly likely to occur during the postrecovery phase. The treatment of malaria with quinacrine and chloroquine also places patients at risk since both are able to induce psychotic depression (Rockwell, 1960).

The most frequent psychiatric presentation following *any severe infection* is that of a depressive syndrome, characterized by: sadness and lability of mood; easy fatigability; subjective weakness; irritability; sleep continuity disorder; and early morning awakening, accompanied by multiple somatic complaints such as headache, pain, and gastrointestinal disturbance. This constellation is most likely to occur at the end of the first or second recovery week and is particularly frequent in the young (Schwab, 1969). The syndrome occurs most often following viral pneumonia, mononucleosis, brucellosis, tuberculosis, hepatitis, and syphilis.

Mononucleosis may present as either a schizophreniform psychosis, or as a psychotic depressive disorder. In the latter instance, the depression is accompanied by somatic delusions, paranoid projective states, and hallucinations (Schnell, 1966).

Emotional disturbances occur so often in patients with *chronic brucellosis* that they are regarded as characteristic (Schwab, 1969). Anxiety is most frequent, but anxious depression also occurs in approximately one third of cases.

Apathetic depression, emotional lability, and irritability are frequently seen in association with *tuberculosis* (Schwab, 1969). Isoniazid used to treat this condition may confuse the picture by producing cognitive disturbances, emotional lability, and wide-ranging mood swings that may mimic depression or hypomania.

The constellation of severe pervasive depression, irritability, lethargy, and weakness seen in patients recovering from hepatitis occurs so frequently that the term *posthepatitis syndrome* has been coined. The depression is frequently so severe as to require psychiatric hospitalization.

Although *tertiary syphilis* is less common than it was a century ago, it is still a frequent cause of psychiatric disorder (Koch, 1964; Thomas, 1964). Classical textbooks emphasize that manic behavior, pressured speech, intellectual deterioration, and neurological changes are characteristic of general paresis. It is crucial that the physician remember that in 25 percent of cases, general paresis presents as a moderate or severe depressive disorder that may or may not be accompanied by specific neurological signs.

Neurosyphilis accounts for 20 percent of late syphilitic lesions and may present in an "asymptomatic" form. Characteristically, such patients evidence global apathetic depression and cerebral spinal fluid findings of increased cell count, positive FTA, and occasionally increased protein.

Depression is also seen in patients suffering from meningovascular syphilis. In these cases, meningeal involvement produces symptoms of headache, irritability, cranial nerve palsies subsequent to basilar meningitis, unequal reflexes, and irregular pupils that react poorly to light and accommodation (Koch, 1964; Thomas, 1964).

HEPATIC DISORDERS

Mild, moderate, and severe depressive states are frequent accompaniments of *inflammatory* and *chemical hepatitis* (Read et al., 1967) Depression occurs early in the course of cirrhosis and is seen in up to 50 percent of such patients.

Cirrhotic depression is generally of the retarded type, accompanied by symptoms of weakness, fatigue, and anxiety; these symptoms are often initially misinterpreted as signs of neurocirculatory asthenia. The depressive states seen with these conditions may persist for years prior to proper diagnosis.

PANCREATIC DISORDERS

Acute pancreatitis is frequently associated with a depressive prodrome, characterized by mood swings, emotional lability, difficulty in falling asleep with daytime hypersomnolence, confusion, cyclical thinking, and spontaneous weeping. Within a 1- to 2-week period, other signs and symptoms suggesting pancreatitis usually appear. It is not uncommon for depression to recur during recovery (Rickles, 1945; Savage et al., 1952).

Carcinoma of the pancreas is an illness specifically associated with depression. In a study of 46 patients with carcinoma of the pancreas, Fras et al. (1968) reported depression in 45; 13 patients reported associated anxiety states; and 7 experienced premonition of serious illness.

In none of these cases were non-specific personality changes present. Hopelessness, although it occurred, was never total or complete as would be expected in true psychotic depression. Feelings of worthlessness were not prominent. The depression was mild to moderate in intensity in the majority of the patients; however, several experienced depression of psychotic proportion with three reporting suicidal ideation. Twenty percent of the patients had a chief complaint of depression and were initially told they were suffering from an emotional illness. In these cases, medical workup was not initiated at the time of the first contact. Only one of the 46 cases presented with signs of organic brain syndrome.

When patients in their 50s present with symptoms of moderately severe depression, have no delusions of guilt or worthlessness, do not evidence psychomotor retardation, and have a negative history of previous depression, mania or hypomania, the diagnosis of carcinoma of the pancreas should be entertained (Fras et al., 1967; Fras et al., 1968; Karlinner, 1956; Ulett and Parsons, 1948; Yaskin, 1931).

It should be emphasized that 20 of the 21 patients presenting with depression initially evidenced no specific localizing physical findings. This, once again, underlies the need for careful medical evaluation before applying psychiatric labels.

NUTRITIONAL DEFICIENCIES

While malnutrition may be a consequence of psychiatric disorder, it may also produce psychiatric symptoms, particularly depression. The deficiencies most likely to induce depressive states include those of: niacin, thiamin, pyridoxine, ascorbic acid, B_{12}, folic acid, protein, and iron (Bram, 1969; Gordon, 1968; Jensen and Olesen, 1969; Korolenko et al., 1969; Reynolds, 1967; Strachan and Henderson, 1965; Lewin, 1959; Wiener and Hope, 1959).

The classical description of diarrhea, dermatitis, and dementia as the primary constellation of *pellagra* may be misleading. One might better think of depression, diarrhea, and dermatitis followed by dementia, as the most characteristic course. Pellagra is still a common disease in this country, and is not limited to the southern sharecropper. It is seen with increasing frequency in the urban ghetto population, the elderly, and individuals who do not eat meat, thereby not consuming enough nicotinic acid to prevent its development.

The most frequent initial psychiatric presentation of pellagra is one of agitated depression, with the subsequent development of mild confusion. Diagnosis is suggested by the presence of the above physical signs with stomatitis and glossitis, and a history of low meat, high-processed carbohydrate intake. The physician should remember that the majority of these patients have multiple vitamin deficiencies that produce changes in the ileum, reducing its ability to absorb orally administered vitamins. Consequently, treatment must be with intramuscular B complex injection.

Thiamin deficiencies will be discussed elsewhere in the text. Suffice it at this time to say that the neuropsychiatric concomitants of thiamin deficiency include peripheral neuropathy, Stokes-Adams, and Wernicke-Korsakoff syndromes. Depression is the most frequent presentation of thiamin deficiency, which should be suspected in any patient presenting with depression and paresthesias.

Ascorbic acid deficiencies are rare in the United States, but frequently occur in individuals living in other parts of the world, particularly the Indian subcontinent and Africa.

Protein deficiency states are also relatively rare in the United States; however, reports of the World Health Organization suggest that they are a frequent cause of depressive disorders in underdeveloped countries. The mechanism postulated for this depression is a lack of dietary tryptophan, which results in a deficiency of the central catecholamines.

Folic acid deficiencies are common in the United States and may produce serious psychiatric disorders simulating schizophrenia. In less severe cases, folate deficiency may present as a moderately severe retarded depression with little or no associated confusion or intellectual deterioration. Associated anemia may be absent or mild, thereby confounding diagnosis. Folate deficiencies occur most often during pregnancy, in alcoholics, patients taking anticonvulsants, and individuals on abnormal diets. Symptoms disappear rapidly with specific treatment (Bram, 1969; Gordon, 1968; Jensen and Olsen, 1969; Reynolds, 1967).

B_{12} deficiency is also specifically associated with the development of psychiatric symptoms (Reynolds, 1967; Weiner and Hope, 1959). Mental changes occur in nearly all patients with pernicious anemia, and range from

mild apathy through severe retarded depression, to states of hallucinated, agitated psychosis. The psychiatric and neurological manifestations of pernicious anemia may precede the development of hematologic change (Strachan and Henderson, 1965). Serum vitamin B_{12} assay and the Schilling's test establish the diagnosis.

Pyridoxine deficiency is specifically related to the appearance of depressive symptoms. It is most frequently seen in alcoholics and patients taking oral contraceptives or Isoniazid (Grant and Pryse-Davies, 1968).

Severe iron-deficiency anemia may produce depression. The depression of iron deficiency was initially thought to be related to anoxia; however, more recent research suggests specific iron-related biochemical changes to be a more likely cause. The etiologic mechanisms are difficult to define, since iron deficiency frequently coexists with malnutrition and vitamin deficiencies. Iron is a constituent not only of hemoglobin, but of other widely distributed enzyme systems. In addition, the majority of patients suffering from chronic iron deficiency are also zinc deplete. Zinc is necessary for the activity of carbonic anhydrase, an enzyme present in large quantities in the brain. The severity of depression associated with iron-deficiency anemia does not parallel blood hemoglobin concentration. Patients who have experienced a single depressive episode on the basis of an iron-deficiency anemia are more likely than the general population to re-experience these symptoms if they again become anemic.

ELECTROLYTE DISORDERS

The mental changes associated with disturbances of fluid and electrolyte balance are legend and will be addressed in a subsequent chapter. Specific states associated with depressive symptoms include hyponatremia, hyper and hypokalemia, hypomagnesemia, and hypercalcemia, as well as increases or decreases of plasma bicarbonate (Stenäck and Haapanen, 1967; Tyler, 1968).

Although electrolyte disorders are seen most often in hospitalized patients, secondary to surgical procedures and the administration of intravenous fluids, they also occur in ambulatory patients treated with diuretics, in alcoholics, diabetics, and patients with renal disease.

Sodium depletion occurs most commonly in patients taking diuretics and secondary to the over-zealous treatment of cardiac decompensation. Hyponatremia is the most likely cause of the so-called *"cardiac psychosis,"* which is commonly observed during the early phases of recovery from congestive heart failure. The psychiatric manifestations of hyponatremia include severe depression, apathy, or schizophreniform psychosis, all of which rapidly disappear when electrolyte balance is restored.

Hypokalemia occurs in patients treated with diuretics, as a result of prolonged steroid treatment, and in individuals suffering from diarrheal diseases. It produces severe depression and muscular weakness, both of which are rapidly reversed by replacement of potassium. The administration of intravenous solutions of dextrose and water, or sodium chloride without supplemental potassium, is a major cause of *postoperative psychosis*.

Hyperkalemia also produces depression. Although rare, it occurs in patients with uremia and those receiving aldosterone inhibitors for prolonged periods. Hyperkalemic depression is accompanied by severe muscular spasm.

Hypomagnesemia frequently presents with moderate to severe depression that may progress to a frank organic brain syndrome. A significant number of patients, however, show only depressive symptoms, which may persist unremittingly for years unless properly diagnosed. This condition occurs most commonly in chronic alcoholics and is seen in at least one half of all patients experiencing delirium tremens. Its high incidence in alcoholics is secondary to their poor dietary history and the fact that ethanol induces a profound magnesium diuresis, which persists in spite of severe total body depletion (Kalbpleisch et al., 1963).

Hypomagnesemia also occurs in individuals with prolonged vomiting, nasogastric suction, and diarrhea, as well as those with sprue syndrome. Excessive urinary loss produces it in patients with primary aldosteronism; those subjected to vigorous diuretic therapy; and those with renal tubular disease, concurrent hypercalcemia, diabetic acidosis, and alcoholism. Hypomagnesemia is frequently associated with hyperparathyroidism, hypoparathyroidism, and pancreatitis (Hall and Joffe, 1973).

Magnesium is an essential co-factor for many central nervous system enzymatic processes, particularly those concerned with energy generation such as the ATP-ADP system. It is also essential for mitochondrial phosphorylation.

Deficiency states present with mild depression and progress to moderate depression, associated with episodes of anxiety, restlessness, and agitation. Patients complain of hyperacusis and evidence a pronounced startle reflex. Disorientation occurs late, but progresses rapidly to confusion. Fifty percent of advanced cases experience auditory or visual hallucinations. Twenty-five percent experience grand mal seizures. Other symptoms that may be late in appearance include: Babinski's sign, tremor, profuse diaphoresis, profound muscular weakness, tachycardia, hypertension, arrhythmias, vasomotor changes, bilateral vertical nystagmus, and lancinating pain of the hands and feet. Replacement therapy with magnesum sulfate rapidly reverses the above symptoms and should be continued until serum magnesium levels return to the 1.6 to 2 mcg per liter range (Hall and Joffe, 1973).

Hypercalcemia is also specifically associated with depression. It represents one of the depression-inducing mechanisms for such diverse conditions as hyperparathyroidism, sarcoidosis, carcinomatosis, steroid therapy, and the milk-alkali syndrome (Petersen, 1968).

Both increased and decreased levels of *serum bicarbonate* produce a psychiatric picture of depression, anxiety, paranoid ideation, and in extreme cases, stupor. Bicarbonate shifts occur secondary to metabolic alkalosis (e.g., the ingestion of excessive amounts of sodium bicarbonate or the vomiting of gastric acid) and as a consequence of respiratory acidosis (Adams, 1957; Bowers, 1969).

COLLAGEN VASCULAR DISORDERS

The incidence of initial depressive symptoms in patients with systemic lupus erythematosus ranges from 4 to 17 percent (Dubois and Tuffanelli, 1964; O'Connor and Musher, 1966; McClary et al., 1955). Collagen vascular disease should be suspected when depression is associated with arthritis and migratory arthralgias. Such a triad occurs during the course of approximately 45 percent of lupus patients. Agitated psychotic depression or schizophreniform psychosis occur in about 12 percent of patients with lupus some time during the course of their illness. This incidence doubles for patients habitually treated with high doses of steroids. Depression also occurs in association with other collagen vascular disorders, particularly periarteritis nodosa and temporal arteritis (Ford and Siekert, 1965).

DEPRESSION ASSOCIATED WITH OTHER SYSTEMIC DISORDERS

Other systemic diseases associated with a high incidence of depressive symptomatology, either preceding or following the appearance of other physical symptoms, include: amyloidosis; gout; psoriasis; rheumatoid arthritis; systemically produced epilepsy; normal pressure hydrocephalus; pulmonary insufficiency; endocrinopathies; porphyria; Wilson's disease; ulcerative colitis; regional enteritis; uremia; lymphomas; leukemias, particularly of the chronic myelogenous type; oat-cell carcinoma of the lung; and disseminated carcinomatosis (Blumer, 1970; Cole, 1973; Guvener et al., 1964; Malamud, 1967; Thompson, 1970; Waggoner and Bagchi, 1954; Withersty, 1974; Adams et al., 1965; Adams, 1957; Petersen, 1968; Pond, 1957; Preston and Atack, 1964; Read et al., 1967; Stenbäck and Haapanen, 1967; Daly, 1968; Flor-Henry, 1969; Guze and Daengsurisri, 1967; Hossain, 1970; Korolenko et al., 1969; Levere and Kappas, 1970; Nichol, 1968; Sternlieb and Scheinberg, 1968; Tyler, 1968; Treadway, 1969; Ziegler, 1967).

DRUG-INDUCED DEPRESSION

Drug-induced depressions are being reported with increasing frequency. The psychiatric complications of drugs will be addressed in detail in subsequent chapters.

Current evidence suggests that patients with a positive family or personal history of depression are at greater risk for the development of a drug-induced depression than is the general population. A detailed history is often of value for this reason, when considering the prescription of agents likely to produce depression (See Table 4.)

REFERENCES

Adams, R. D. Neurological manifestations of chronic pulmonary insufficiency. *N. Eng. J. Med.* 257:579–590 (1957).

Adams, R. C., Fisher, C. M., Hakim, S., Ojemann, R. G., and Sweet, W. H. Symptomatic occult hyprocephalus with "normal" cerebrospinal fluid pressure: Treatable syndrome. *N. Eng. J. Med.* 273:117–126 (1965).

Avery, T. L. Seven cases of frontal tumor with psychiatric presentation. *Brit. J. Psychiat.* 119:19–23 (1971).

Azar, G. J., Bond, J. O., and Lawton, A. H. St. Louis encephalitis: Age aspects of 1962 epidemic in Pinellas County, Florida. *J. Am. Geriat. Soc.* 14:326–333 (1966).

Bell, R., and Hall, R.C.W. The mental status examination. *Am. Fam. Phys.* 16:4:145–152 (1977).

Bilikiewicz, A., and Gromska, J. Diagnostic value of mental disorders in temporal lobe tumors. *Neurol. Neurochio. Psychiat. Pol.* 13:397–404 (1963).

Blocker, W. W., Castl, A. J. and Daroff, R. B. The psychiatric manifestations of cerebral malaria. *Am. J. Psychiat.* 125:192–196 (1968).

Blumer, D. Neurological states masquerading as psychoses. *Md. St. Med. J.* 19:55–60 (1970).

Blustein, J. E. and Seeman, M. V. Brain tumors presenting as functional psychiatric disturbances. *Canad. Psychiat. Assn. J.* 17:55–59–SS–63 (1972).

Bowers, M. B., Jr. Clinical aspects of depression in a home for the aged. *J. Am. Geriat. Soc.* 17:469–476 (1969).

Bram, M. Miscellaneous advances. Neurological manifestations of folate deficiency, in *Recent Advances in Neurology and Neuropsychiatry*. L. Bram and M. Wilkinson, eds. Churchill, London, England (1969), pp. 129–146.

Cairns, H. Discussion on rehabilitation after injuries to the central nervous system. *Proc. Roy. Soc. Med.* 35:299–301 (1962).

Cohen, N. H. The treatment of Huntington's chorea with trifluoperazine (Stelazine). *J. Nerv. Ment. Dis.* 134:62–71 (1962).

Colbert, J., and Harrow, M. Depression and organicity. *Psychiat. Quart.* 40:96–103 (1966).

Cole, G. The masking of organic brain disease by a schizophrenia-like illness. *S. Afr. Med. J.* 47:731–733 (1973).

Corsellis, J.A.N. and Brierley, J. B. Observations on the pathology of insidious dementia following head injury. *J. Ment. Sci.* 105:714–720 (1959).

Crapper, D. R., Krishnsan, S. S., and Dalton, A. J. Brain aluminum distribution in Alzheimer's disease and experimental neurofibrillary degeneration. *Trans. Am. Neurol. Assn.* 98:17–20 (1973).

Dalessio, D. J., Benchimol, A., and Dimond, E. G. Chronic encephalopathy related to heart block. *Neurol.* 15:499–503 (1965).

Daly, D. Ictal affect. *Am. J. Psychiat.* 115:97–108 (1958).

Davies, G. V. Differential diagnosis of the mental disorders of late life. *Med. J. Aust.* 1:242–245 (1969).

Dubois, E. L. and Tuffanelli, D. L. Clinical manifestations of systemic lupus erythematosus. *J.A.M.A.* 190:2:104–111 (1964).

Ehrentheil, O. F. Differential diagnosis of organic dementias and affective disorders in aged patients. *Geriat.* 12:426–432 (1957).

Flor-Henry, P. Psychosis and temporal lobe epilepsy, a controlled investigation. *Epilepsia*. 10:363–395 (1969).
Ford, R. G. and Siekert, R. G. Central nervous system manifestations of periarteritis nodosa. *Neuro*. 15:114–122 (1965).
Frank, J. *Therapeutic components of psychotherapy*. C. H. Boehringer Sohn, Ingelhein am Rhein, Germany (1975) pp. 1–18.
Fras, I., Litin, E. M., and Bartholamew, L. G. Mental symptoms as an aid in the early diagnosis of carcinoma of the pancreas. *Gastroenterol*. 55:2:191–198 (1968).
Fras, I., Litin, E. M., and Pearson, J. S. Comparison of psychiatric symptoms of carcinoma of the pancreas with those in some other intra-abdominal neoplasms. *Am. J. Psychiat*. 123:1553–1562 (1967).
Gal, P. Mental symptoms in cases of tumor of temporal lobe. *Am. J. Psychiat*. 115:157–160 (1958).
Geisler, W. O. and Jousse, A. T. Rehabilitation in disseminated sclerosis. *Canad. Med. Assn. J*. 88:189–191 (1963).
Goodwin, F. K., Ebert, M. B., and Bunney, W. E., Jr. Mental effects of Reserpin in man: A review, in *Psychiatric Complications of Medical Drugs*. R. I. Shader, ed. Raven Press, New York (1972), pp. 73–101.
Gordon, N. Folic acid deficiency from anticonvulsant therapy. *Develop. Med. Child. Neurol*. 10:4972—504 (1968).
Grant, E., and Pryse-Davies, J. Effects of oral contraceptives on depressive mood changes and on endometrial monoamine oxidase and phosphatases. *Brit. Med. J*. 3:777–780 (1968).
Guvener, A., Bagchi, B. K., Kooi, K. A., and Calhoun, H. D. Mental and seizure manifestations in relation to brain tumors—a statistical study. *Epilepsia* 5:166–167 (1964).
Guze, S. B., and Cantwell, D. P. Prognosis in "organic brain" syndromes. *Am. J. Psychiat*. 120:878–881 (1964).
Guze, S. B., and Daeng Surisri, S. Organic brain syndromes. *Arch. Gen. Psychiat*. 17:365–366 (1967).
Hall, R.C.W. Psychological factors affecting routine medical care. *Md. St. Med. J*. 21:62–63 (1972).
Hall, R.C.W., and Joffe, J. R. Hypomagnesemia, *J.A.M.A*. 224:13:1749–1751 (1973).
Hall, R.C.W., and Joffe, J. R. Aberrant response to diazepam: A new syndrome. *Am. J. Psychiat*. 129:6:114–118 (1972).
Hall, R.C.W., and Popkin, M. K. Psychological symptoms of physical origin. *Fem. Patient*. 2:10:43–47 (1977).
Hall, R.C.W., and Reading, A. Steroid psychosis. *New Phys*. 20:20–23 (1971).
Hall, R.C.W., Popkin, M. K., Devaul, R., Faillaice, L. A., and Stickney, S. K. Physical illness presenting as psychiatric disease. *Arch. Gen. Psychiat*. 35:11:1315–1320, (1978).
Hall, R.C.W., Popkin, M. K., and Kirkpatrick, B. Tricyclic exacerbation of steroid psychosis. *J. Nerv. Ment. Dis*. 166:10:738–742 (1978).
Herzberg, B. and Coppen, A. Change in psychological symptoms in women taking oral contraceptives. *Brit. J. Psychiat*. 116:161–164 (1970).
Himmelhooh, J., Pincus, J., Tucker, G., and Detre, T. Subacute encephalitis: Behavioral and neurological aspects. *Brit. J. Psychiat*. 116:531–538 (1970).
Hobbs, G. E. Brain tumors simulating psychiatric disease. *Canad. Med. Assn. J*. 88:186–188 (1963).
Hossain, M. Neurological and psychiatric manifestations in idiopathic hypoparathyroidism: Response to treatment. *J. Neurol. Neurosurg. Psychiat*. 33:153–156 (1970).
Ivers, R. R. and Goldstein, N. P. Multiple sclerosis: A current appraisal of symptoms and signs. *Proc. Staff Meet. Mayo Clin*. 38:457–466 (1963).
Jensen, O. N. and Olesen, O. V. Folic acid and anticonvulsive drugs. *Arch. Neurol*. 21:208–214 (1969).
Kalbpleisch, J. M., Lindeman, R. D., Ginn, H. E., Smith, W. O. Effects of ethanol administration on urinary excretion of magnesium and other electrolytes in alcoholic and normal subjects. *J. Clin. Invest*. 42:1471–1475 (1963).

Karlinner, W. Psychiatric manifestations of cancer of the pancreas. *N. Y. J. Med.* 56:2251–2252 (1956).
Knehr, C. A. and Bearn, A. G. Psychological impairment in Wilson's disease. *J. Nerv. Ment. Dis.* 124:251–255 (1956).
Koch, R. A. Late syphilis: Modern concepts in treatment. *J. Am. Geriat. Soc.* 12:255–261 (1964).
Koenig, H. Dementia associated with the benign form of multiple sclerosis. *Trans. Am. Neurol. Assn.* 93:227–228 (1968).
Korolenko, C. P., Yevseyeva, T. A., and Volkov, P. P. Data for a comparative account of toxic psychoses of various aetiologies. *Brit. J. Psychiat.* 115:273–279 (1969).
Krupp, M. A., and Chatton, M. J. eds. *Current Diagnosis and Treatment.* Lang Medical Pub., Los Altos, California., (1973) (see applicable sections for each medical disorder.)
Lange, E., and Poppe, G. Social isolation preceding syndromes of paranoid interference in old age. *Nervenarzt.* 35:194–200 (1964).
Levere, R. D., and Kappas, A. Porphyric diseases of man. *Hosp. Pract.* 5:61–73 (1970).
Lewin, K. K. Role of depression in the production of illness in pernicious anemia. *Psychosom. Med.* 21:23–27 (1959).
Lipowski, Z. J. Delirium, clouding of consciousness, and confusion. *J. Nerv. Ment. Dis.* 145:227–255 (1967).
Lowenberg, K., and Scharenberg, K. Pick's disease. *Arch. Neurol. Psychiat.* 36:768–789 (1936).
Malamud, N. Psychiatric disorders with intracranial tumors of limbic system. *Arch. Neurol.* 17:113–123 (1967).
Marx, J. L. Slow viruses (II): The unconventional agents. *Sci.* 181:44–45 (1973).
McAlpine, D. The benign form of multiple sclerosis: Results of long-term study. *Brit. Med. J.* 2:1029–1032 (1964).
McClary, A., Meyer, E., and Weitzman, E. Observations on the role of the mechanism of depression in some patients with disseminated lupus erythematosus. *Psychosom. Med.* 17:311–321 (1955).
Modlin, H. C. Postaccident anxiety syndrome: Psychosocial aspects. *Am. J. Psychiat.* 123:1008–1012 (1967).
Morse, M. E. Brain tumors as seen in hospitals for the insane. *Arch. Neurol. Psychiat.* 3:417–428 (1920).
Mulder, D. W., and Daly, D. Psychiatric symptoms associated with lesions of temporal lobe. *J.A.M.A.* 150:173–176 (1952).
Nicol, C. F. Depression as reviewed through neurological spectacles. *Psychosom.* 9:252–254 (1968).
O'Connor, J. F., and Musher, D. M. Central nervous involvement in systemic lupus erythematosus. *Arch. Neurol.* 14:157–164 (1966).
Oliphant, J., Evans, J. I., and Forrest, A. D. Huntington's chorea: Some biochemical and therapeutic aspects. *Brit. J. Psychiat.* 106:718–725 (1960).
Petersen, P. Psychiatric disorders in primary hyperparathyroidism. *J. Clin. Endocrinol.* 28:1491–1495 (1968).
Pond, D. A. Psychiatric aspects of epilepsy. *J. Ind. Med. Prof.* 3:1441–1443 (1957).
Preston, D. N. and Atack, E. A. Temporal lobe epilepsy: A clinical study of 47 cases. *Canad Med. Assn. J.* 91:1256–1259 (1964).
Read, A. E., Sherlock, S., Laidlaw, J., and Walker, J. G. Neuropsychiatric syndromes associated with chronic liver disease and an extensive portalsystemic collateral circulation. *Quart. J. Med.* 36:135–150 (1967).
Reynolds, E. H. Schizophrenia-like psychoses of epilepsy and disturbances of folate and vitamin B_{12} metabolism induced by anticonvulsant drugs. *Brit. J. Psychiat.* 113:911–919 (1967).
Rickles, N. K. Functional symptoms as first evidence of pancreatic disease. *Ment. Dis.* 101:566–571 (1945).
Rockwell, D. A. Psychiatric complications with Chloroquine and Quinacrine. *Am. J. Psychiat.* 124:1257–1260 (1968).
Rubert, S. L., and Remington, F. B. Why patients with brain tumors come to a psychiatric hospital: A 30 year survey. *Am. J. Psychiat.* 119:256–257 (1962).

Savage, C., Butcher, W., and Noble, D. Psychiatric manifestations in pancreatic disease. *J. Clin. Exp. Psychopath.* 13:9–16 (1952).
Schnell, R. G., Dyck, P. J., Bowie, E.W.J., Klass, D. W. and Taswell, H. F. Infectious mononucleosis neurologic and EEG findings. *Med.* 45:51–63 (1966).
Schwab, J. J. Psychiatric illness produced by infections. *Hosp. Med.* 5:98–108 (1969).
Selecki, B. R. Intracranial space occupying lesions among patients admitted to mental hospital. *Med. J. Aust.* 1:383–390 (1965).
Simon, H. Physical and socio-psychologic stress in the geriatric mentally ill. *Comp. Psychiat.* 11:242–247 (1970).
Sjogren, T., Sjogren, H., and Lindgren, A.G.H. Morbuz Alzheimer and Morbus Pick: A genetic clinical and patho-anatomical study. *ACTA Psychiat. Scand.*, Suppl. 82 (1952).
Slaby, A. E., and Wyatt, R. J. *Dementia in the presenium.* T. Spring ed. Charles C. Thomas, Illinois (1974).
Stenbäck, A., and Haapanen, E. Azotemia and people. *ACTA Psychiat. Scand.* 43:9–65 (1967).
Sternlieb, I., and Scheinberg, I. H. Prevention of Wilson's disease in asymptomatic patients. *N. Eng. J. Med.* 278:352–359 (1968).
Strachan, R. W., and Henderson, J. G. Psychiatric syndromes due to avitaminosis B_{12} with normal blood and marrow. *Quart. J. Med.* 34:303–317 (1965).
Surridge, D. Investigation into some psychiatric aspects of multiple sclerosis. *Brit. J. Psychiat.* 115:749–764 (1964).
Thomas, E. W. Some aspects of neurosyphilis. *Med. Clin. N. Am.* 48:699–705 (1964).
Thompson, G. N. Cerebral lesions simulating schizophrenia: Three case reports. *Biol. Psych.* 2:59–64 (1970).
Timberline conference on psychophysiologic aspects of cardiovascular disease. *Psychosom. Med.* 26:405–541 (1964).
Treadway, C. R. Mental changes accompanying thyroid gland dysfunction. *Arch. Gen. Psychiat.* 20:48–63 (1969).
Tyler, H. R. Neurologic disorders in renal failures. *Am. J. Med.* 44:734–748 (1968).
Ulett, G., and Parsons, E. H. Psychiatric aspects of carcinoma of the pancreas. *J. Missouri Med. Assn.* 45:490–493 (1948).
Ullman, M., and Gruen, A. Behavioral changes in patients with strokes. *Am. J. Psychiat.* 117:1004–1009 (1961).
von Werssowetz, O. F. Mental and emotional readjustment of the hemiplegic patients. *Psychiat. Dig.* 27:24–37 (1966).
Waal, H. J. Propranolol-induced depression. *Brit. Med. J.* 2:50 (1967).
Waggoner, R. W., and Bagchi, B. K. Initial masking of organic brain changes by psychic symptoms. Clinical and electroencephalographic studies. *Am. J. Psychiat.* 110:904–910 (1954).
Wiener, J. S., and Hope, J. M. Cerebral manifestations of vitamin B_{12} deficiency. *J.A.M.A.* 170:1038–1041 (1959).
Withersty, D. J. Brain tumors presenting with psychiatric symptomatology: A 5 year study. *W. Ca. Med. J.* 70:51–53 (1974).
Wolsten-Holme and O'Connor, M., eds. *Alzheimer's Disease and Related Conditions.* CIBA Foundation Symposium. Churchill, London, England (1970).
Yaskin, J. C. Nervous symptoms as earliest manifestations of carcinoma of the pancreas. *J.A.M.A.* 96:1664–1668 (1931).
Ziegler, D. K. Neurological disease and hysteria: Differential diagnosis. *Int. J. Neuropsychiat.* 3:388–396 (1967).

Psychiatric Presentations of Medical Illness

CHAPTER 4

Intermittent Recurring Psychoses

GUSTAVE NEWMAN, M.D.

Many illnesses have a recurrent or intermittent course, and because of the struggle involving both psychological and physiological resistance to illness shown by most individuals, the course of almost all illnesses may, to some extent, be intermittent. The recurrent nature of the course of an illness depends upon both the direct influence of the lesion and the individual's psychological and physical response to it. Many so-called organic illnesses are known to manifest mental symptoms, but some so commonly do so that they present a diagnostic problem to most clinicians. The clinical presentation of the patient and his symptoms may suggest "psychogenic" disorder, and the patient be ineffectively treated. The following is a partial listing of some of the more common diseases whose pathogenesis is rooted in biochemical or physiological alteration of somatic processes and structures, and whose clinical course is marked by intermittent and recurrent mental changes.

Multiple sclerosis
Acute intermittent porphyria
Pheochromocytoma
Systemic lupus erythematosis
Pancreatitis
Herpes simplex encephalitis
Episodic dyscontrol syndrome

Each of these disorders will be considered separately, and an attempt will be made to provide a physiological explanation of symptoms where some evidence for providing explanations exists. Clinical clues will be provided to assist the diagnostician in raising his "index of clinical suspicion."

MULTIPLE SCLEROSIS

Multiple sclerosis (MS) is a chronic, progressive, neurological disease which is typically episodic in its gradual downhill progressive course, interspersed with temporary remissions. Although usually insidious in onset, MS may strike with awesome suddenness. *There are no typical signs and symptoms,* as almost any part or any combination of parts of the central nervous system (CNS) may be affected simultaneously. Thus, multiple, unrelated, and widespread involvement of the CNS is most characteristic (Schaumberg and Raine, 1977).

MS frequently involves the pyramidal tracts early in the illness; therefore, the patient's gait may be affected by spasticity, stiffness, or incoordination. Accompanying these symptoms of impairment of gait is hyperactivity of the deep tendon reflexes in the lower extremities. Tremor, nystagmus, and scanning speech (slowed speech with pauses between syllables or words), known as Charchot's Triad is considered a classical cluster of symptoms in MS, but it frequently does not make its appearance early in the course of the illness, nor is it universally present even in far-advanced cases. Labile emotionality or even explosive emotional dyscontrol may occur, and depression is common.

Euphoria, which may appear to the clinician to be in the service of denial of the patient's serious symptoms, occurs commonly. It is perhaps this symptom of euphoria, which appears false or inappropriate, that causes some confusion with the "belle indifference" of the hysteric and thus confounds the diagnosis. It is noteworthy that this symptom has been regarded by some authorities as evidence of thalamic damage rather than being a reactive, psychological symptom. When irregular disseminated sensory disturbances accompany the euphoria, MS is most easily mistaken for hysteria.

The misled clinician is likely to become even more convinced of the diagnosis of hysteria, when after a relatively brief span of time, the patient's symptoms begin to clear up. It is only some months or years later when the patient has a recurrence of the illness—but this time with different symptoms indicating that different areas of the CNS are affected—that the diagnosis of multiple sclerosis is entertained. It is the second episode of illness, symptomatically different from the first yet bearing some resemblence to it, which should alert the clinician to the second characteristic of this illness, namely that it is *typically episodic in nature*.

Neuropathological findings at autopsy are of widespread patches of sclerosis throughout the CNS without obvious patterning. The myelin sheathing of nerve tracts is most often affected and the neuraxis spared. Sparing of the nerve fibers makes possible the remission of neural functions subserved by those fibers. Thus, symptomatic remission is possible and occurs spontaneously, but incompletely, in most cases. Laboratory findings, including examination of the spinal fluid, EEG, and brain scan, are variable and not definitive for MS. The diagnosis is made on the basis of history and clinical findings. Treatment of MS is non-specific, although the use of corticosteroids is common because of their anti-inflammatory effect. The chronic nature of the illness mandates continued medical care, which should include supportive psychotherapy, general hygienic measures, and alertness on the part of the clinician to the development of secondary illnesses, such as genitourinary tract infections.

ACUTE INTERMITTENT PORPHYRIA

Acute intermittent porphyria (AIP) is an abnormality of pyrrole metabolism inherited as an autosomal dominant trait. Current theory is that porphyria is a group of diseases, all characterized by marked overproduction and excretion of porphyrins—the red-colored pigment in heme in the red blood cells. It is a disease of young adulthood, more frequent in women than in men; and appears to occur more often in persons of North European ancestry, such as Anglc-Saxon, German, and Scandivanian.

AIP is an uncommon illness, estimated to occur in only one per 100,000 population. Symptoms are often vague and always recurrent. Collicky, severe abdominal pain is the most common symptom, but may exist without muscular guarding ("soft abdomen"), so that to the clinician, the complaints appear disproportionate and exaggerated in relation to the physical findings on examination of the abdomen. Vomiting is common and may be prolonged and severe, suggesting a psychogenic cause. The patient may have either diahrrea or constipation. The psychic symptoms vary considerably from anxiety and emotional lability to acute, frank, delusional psychosis.

Disorientation and confusion is *not* common, except in the most severe cases. When it occurs, it is indicative of severe CNS involvement and is thought to predict even more serious symptoms such as seizures or coma (Becker and Kramer, 1977). Clinical evidence indicates that an episode may be precipitated by the ingestion of one of a number of common drugs. Among the medications implicated are barbiturates, estrogens, sulfanomides, and greiseofulvin. Diagnosis is made by the laboratory finding of porphobilinogen in the urine, which is said to be uniformly present during acute attacks.

There is no specific treatment for porphyria, although acute attacks can sometimes be aborted by administration of carbohydrates, either orally or intravenously. Becker and Kramer (1977) suggest that intravenous hematin is more reliable than carbohydrate-loading in suppressing an attack of AIP. Psychiatric symptoms may be managed with phenothiazines, which often give more relief for the abdomenal pain than do opiates. When the diagnosis is established, obviously barbiturates, glutetheamide, estrogens, sulfanomides, and greiseofulvin are to be avoided in the interest of prevention of subsequent attacks.

Demyelination of the cerebral cortex has been described (Gibson and Goldberg, 1956), in addition to demyelination of peripheral nerves, in those afflicted with the disease. Axones may be affected, as well as myelin sheathing; and both types of lesions have been found in the same patient. Postmortem examination usually shows minimal brain involvement, which is not well correlated with psychiatric symptoms, suggesting that a cerebral "biochemical lesion" resulting from the abnormality of pyrrole metabolism may be causal to the mental changes (Becker and Kramer, 1977).

PHEOCHROMOCYTOMA

A pheochromocytoma is a catecholamine-producing tumor arising from cells of the sympathetic nervous system. It tends to occur in young persons, with most diagnoses occuring in patients of age 5 to 25.

Hypertension, the most common physical finding, is typically paroxysmal and is produced by an outpouring of epinephrine or norepinephrine into the systemic circulation. The paroxysmal attack is usually abrupt and produces symptoms of anxiety with tachycardia, sweating, feelings of apprehension, and frequently pounding headache. The intense symptoms of anxiety produce mental disorganization in some patients, and a transient, acute psychosis may supervene. Between attacks, the blood pressure is found to be lower than at the time of the paroxysm, and may even approach normal levels.

The diagnosis is established by biochemical assay of the catecholamines, uniformly found to be elevated in the 24-hour urine collection. Provocative or blocking tests of the catecholamine response have been used, employing challenging doses of histamine or regitine with measurement of elevation or depression of blood pressure, respectively. The use of these tests has been discouraged because of the risk attendant to the production of hypertensive crisis and asthmatic or hypotensive attacks (Engelman, 1975). Definitive treatment is achieved by surgical removal of the hormone-secreting tumor.

SYSTEMIC LUPUS ERYTHEMATOSIS

Systemic lupus erythematosis (SLE) is a chronic illness, involving multiple organ systems and characterized by exacerbations and remissions. The disease is of unknown cause, but immunological mechanisms are involved and SLE serum contains antinucleoprotein antibodies and may contain anti-DNA antibodies. Females are affected in a 9:1 proportion to males. Onset is most common in the second to fifth decades of life.

SLE commonly presents as a slowly progressive, intermittent disease with joint and muscle pain, but it may be explosive in onset with fever, skin rash, cough, and chest pain with pulmonary and myocardial involvement. The CNS is commonly involved, and the kidneys almost invariably so. Necrotizing vasculitis of the medium-sized arterioles of the brain is a common pathological finding at autopsy. This inflammatory reaction of the vascular structures of the brain is thought to give rise to the psychic symptoms that are common. Among such symptoms, emotional dyscontrol is most prominent while depression or dysphoric mood is common.

One study (Guze, 1970) showed SLE patients to have more psychiatric symptoms than general medical patients in the same hospital. The observed symptoms ranged from anxiety to schizophreniform psychosis with hallucinations and delusions, but with clear sensorium, thus making the differential from true schizophrenia difficult.

In a pair of reports (Baker, 1973); Baker et al., 1973) from the National Institute of Health, 17 SLE patients were studied intensively from both a physiological and psychiatric viewpoint. Seven patients (41 percent) had a total of 11 episodes of psychiatric complication. Most commonly observed (45 percent) was a mixed syndrome, characterized by a combination of organic symptoms plus affective or schizophreniform symptoms. "Pure" affective syndromes were second most common (36 percent), but pure organic and pure schizophreniform syndromes were also observed. According to these authors, psychiatric episodes in SLE patients *do not* represent an intensification of pre-existing psychopathology. There was no correlation found between psychotic episodes and the severity of the disease as judged by laboratory tests, nor was there any correlation between psychiatric symptoms and the duration or dosage of corticosteroid therapy. Thus, the authors suggest that dosage of corticosteroids *not* be reduced because of the development of psychopathology in patients with SLE.

In another study (Feinglas et al., 1976), 51 percent of 140 patients with SLE had significant neuropsychiatric problems during the course of their illness. Organic features were present in 22 of the 24 patients who demonstrated psychiatric symptomatology. Seventy-one percent of the patients with neuropsychiatric symptoms had an abnormal EEG, while only 8 percent had abnormal brain scans. Among the clinical findings, only vasculitis and thromocytompenia correlated with neuropsychiatric symptoms. Only 2 of 140 patients were judged to have had corticosteroid-induced psychosis, a low risk considering the benefits of steroids to many SLE patients.

Because the onset is insidious and often first manifested by neuropsychiatric symptoms, the diagnosis of SLE is frequently missed in its earlier stages. Emotional disturbance, particularly mood disturbance accompanied by anemia, fever, and a skin rash on any part of the body, should alert the clinician to suspect SLE. Usual laboratory procedures are often helpful. Microscopic examination of the urine commonly reveals hematuria or renal red-cell casts (Samter, 1971) in SLE patients. Special laboratory examination of the peripheral blood may confirm the diagnosis by revealing characteristic "lupus cells." Autoimmune antibodies are also detectable in serum and are preferred by many internists for confirmation of the diagnosis. Current treatment is usually by immunosuppression with corticosteroids. However, since lupus encephalopathy is not consistently responsive to such treatment (Johnson and Richardson, 1968), concurrent psychotherapeutic and psychopharmacologic treatment with antipsychotic medication is often indicated.

PANCREATITIS

Pancreatitis is known to be associated with alcohol abuse, and when a patient with an alcoholic history presents acutely ill with fever and abdominal pain radiating to the back, it presents little problem in diagnosis. However, neither fever nor abdominal pain need be present, or prominent, and the patient may present with only an acute hallucinatory psychosis. In one study (Shuster and Iber, 1965), hallucinatory phenomena were found to be more common with pancreatitis than was diabetes, gastroentestinal malabsorption, or pancreatic calcification, which are all commonly associated with it. The patients with pancreatitis were compared with a control group of patients who also had alcoholic histories but who had pneumonia in contrast to pancreatitis. Fifty-three percent of the pancreatitis patients had acute hallucinosis as compared to only 13 percent of the pneumonia patients. It thus appeared that hallucinosis could not be explained on the basis of alcoholism alone, nor on alcoholism accompanied by febrile illness, and must then in some way be related to disturbed pancreatic function and its effects on the total organism.

Recurrent vague abdominal pain with dysphoric mood may be all the clinician has to go on, and since these symptoms suggest a mildly depressed patient asking for analgesic drugs, the diagnosis may be easily missed. A careful history pointing to excessive use of alcohol over a sustained period of time in a patient with these symptoms can alert the physician to the possibility of pancreatitis (Snodgrass, 1974). Although x-rays may reveal calcification of the gland, elevations of pancreatic enzymes in serum and urine are more useful in making the diagnosis. Serum lipase, and both serum and urinary amylase are freqeuntly elevated in pancreatitis. Laboratory examination of the stool for excess fat when the patient has eaten a diet of *known* fat content is also hlepful (Kowlessar, 1975) in revealing the reduced enzyme output of the pancreas.

HERPES SIMPLEX ENCEPHALITIS

According to one authority in neurology, herpes simplex encephalitis (HSE) is the single most important cause of viral encephalitis in the United States (Merritt, 1973). HSE may attack persons of any age and is not particularly a disease of children as are other types of encephalitis. Approximately half of the reported cases of HSE occur in persons over 20 years of age.

Although the onset is frequently abrupt and manifested by fever and seizures, HSE may first present with a variety of mental symptoms, including *recurrent organic psychosis* (Shearer, 1964) and *catatonic stupor* (Raskin and Frank, 1974). In those cases in which the course of the illness is slower and less acute, the patient is very likely to manifest mental and emotional symptoms *before* clear-cut neurological symptoms appear (Himmelhock et al., 1970). Close observation has frequently revealed a *fluctuating mental status,* with patients moving from lucidity to disorientation from day to day. Aggressive, assaultive, and bizarre behavior has been reported early with neurological manifestations, such as disturbed speech including aphasia, and sensory paresthesias developing later (Breeden et al., 1966). When unrecognized and untreated, however, HSE patients are quite likely to develop seizures, with one study (Meyer et al., 1970) reporting seven of eight cases manifesting generalized seizures.

Recovery was reported in four of six patients treated with iododeoxyuridine (IDU). The Breeden group (Breeden et al., 1966) had earlier reported on the possible effectiveness of this substance in the treatment of HSE, which had previously been recognized as a highly lethal disease with a mortality rate approaching 70 percent.

Nahmias and Starr (1977) refer to HSE as the most common form of nonepidemic encephalitis and more often lethal than any other kind of encephalitis in the United States. They warn against the toxicity of IDU in the treatment of HSE and suggest that adenine arabinoside (Ara-A) may be equally effective but less toxic.

In suspected cases, careful neurological examination with attention to organic signs is helpful in making the diagnosis as is a lumbar puncture, which typically reveals increased spinal fluid protein and increased numbers of lymphocytes. The EEG commonly shows slowing with spikes, and one investigator (Elian, 1975) has suggested that the progress of the illness may be followed by serial EEG's. Because of the treatability of this illness, the diagnosis of HSE should be kept in mind with any patient suspected of having encephalitis with fluctuating mental status.

EPISODIC DYSCONTROL SYNDROME

The episodic dyscontrol syndrome is the descriptive title applied to the behavior of a group of patients manifesting intermittent, violent behavior and abnormal electroencephalographic changes (Bach-y-Rita, 1971). The onset of the violent behavior usually begins in the teens or early 20s and is manifested primarily in physical attacks on others, which may or may not be provoked. The onset of the attacks suggests a convulsive disorder: Auditory or visual illusions, nausea, and numbness of limbs are reported by approximately one half of such patients. About half of the patients also reported headache and drowsiness following the violent episodes. Many have reported severe headache *without* associated violence, as well as an altered state of consciousness usually manifested in the form of brief staring spells. Only a small proportion of such patients report amnesia following an episode of dyscontrol. More commonly, the episode is remembered and the patient expresses extreme remorse for his behavior, in contrast to violent patients with character disorders who rationalize their behavior or claim amnesia for the event.

Mark and Ervin (1970) note four characteristics defining the patient with episodic dyscontrol: (1) a history of physical assault, (2) extreme sensitivity to alcohol, i.e., susceptibility to pathological intoxication, (3) a history of impulsive sexual behavior including sexual assault, and (4) a history of traffic violations and serious automobile accidents.

Maletzky (1973) found 14 of 22 patients with episodic dyscontrol to have abnormal EEG's with slowing (theta activity) and spiking in the temporal region. He confirmed Mark and Ervin's data regarding the sensitivity of these persons to alcohol, finding that all of his 22 patients had increased frequency and severity of dyscontrol episodes while drinking alcohol. He also noted a high frequency of suicidal ideation and ineffective treatment by usual methods available to psychiatrists. Maletzky treated all his cases with diphenylhydantoin (Dilantin) 100 mg three times daily, and reported that 19 of the 22 patients achieved a therapeutic response with cessation or marked reduction in the frequency and severity of the episodes of dyscontrol. The emotional dyscontrol is thought to be related to epilipetogenic foci in the limbic system or in the temporal regions. Although Maletzky did not believe the patients in his series had obvious brain disease, he thought a case could be made for "some form of temporal epileptic equivalent."

Marinacci (1963) has found that alcohol did more than intoxicate the individual with episodic emotional dyscontrol. It appeared to trigger or facilitate temporal lobe epileptoid states, and he found he was able to activate a temporal lobe dysrhythmia with alcohol in a group of patients who had previously had normal EEG's.

Evidence seems to be accumulating which may factor out a definite syndrome of neurogenic behavioral dyscontrol from the undifferentiated group of character disorders and "borderline states" who also manifest behavioral disorders. (Gross, 1971). (As with temporal lobe epilepsy, reliance upon a single procedure, such as the EEG, can lead to diagnostic confusion.) Although violence and aggression do occur in those with temporal lobe epilepsy, Goldstein (1974) states it is perhaps no more frequent than in the general population. Multidimensional research is urged by Plutchik et al. (1976) who favor the use of behavioral indices that can be generated by instruments such as Monroe's dyscontrol scale (Monroe, 1970).

REFERENCES

Bach-Y-Rita, G., Lion, J. R., and Ervin, F. R. Episodic dyscontrol: A study of 130 violent patients. *Am. J. Psychiat.* 127:1473–1478 (1971).

Baker, M. Psychopathology in systemic lupus erythematosis. I. *Semin. Arthrit. Rheum.* 3/2:95–110 (1973).

Baker, M. Hadler, N. M., Whitaker, J. N., Dunner, D. L., Gerwin, R. D., and Decker, J. K. Psychopathology in systemic lupus erythematosis. II. *Semin. Arthrit. Rheum.* 3/2:111–126 (1973).

Becker, D. M., and Kramer, S. The neurological manifestations of porphyria: A review. *Med.* 56:411–423 (1977).

Bennett, R., Hughes, G.R. V., Bywaters, E.G.L., and Holt, P.J.L. Neuropsychiatric problems in systemic lupus erythematosis. *Brit. Med. J.* 4:342–345 (1972).

Breeden, C. J., Hall, T. C., and Tyler, H. R. Herpes simplex encephalitis treated with 5-10do-2'-deoxyuridine. *Ann. Int. Med.* 65:1050 (1966).

DuBois, E. L., ed. *Lupus Erythematosis*. McGraw-Hill Book Co., New York (1966), and 2nd ed. So. Cal. Press, Los Angeles, California (1974).

Elian, M. Herpes simplex encephalitis. *Arch. Neurol.* 32:39–43 (1975).

Engelman, K. The adrenal medulla and sympathetic nervous system, in *Textbook of Medicine,* 14th ed. P. B. Beeson and W. McDermott, eds. W. B. Saunders, Philadelphia, Pennsylvania (1975), pp. 1787–1795.

Feinglas, E. J., Arnett, F. C., Dorsch, C. A., Zizic, T. M., and Stevens, M. B. Neuropsychiatric manifestation of systemic lupus erythematosis: Diagnosis, clinical spectrum, and relationship to other features of the disease. *Med.* 55:323--339 (1976).

Gibson, J. B. and Goldberg, A. The neuropathology of acute porphyria. *J. Pathol. Bact.* 71:495 (1956).
Goldstein, M. Brain research and violent behavior. *Arch. Neurol.* 30:1–35 (1974).
Gross, M. D. Violence associated with organic brain disease, in *Dynamics of Violence*. J. Fawcett, ed. Am. Med. Assn., Chicago, Illinois (1971), pp. 85–91.
Guze, S. B. The occurrence of psychiatric illness in systemic lupus erythematosus. *Am. J. Psychiat.* 123:1562–1570 (1967).
Harvey, A. M. Shalman, L., Tumulty, P., Conley, C. L., and Schoenrich, E. H. Systemic lupus erythematosis: Review of the literature and clinical analysis of 138 cases. *Med.* 33:291 (1954).
Himmelhoch, J., Pincus, N., Tucker, G., and Detre, T. Sub-acute encephalitis: Behavioral and neurological aspects. *Brit. J. Psychiat.* 116:531–538 (1970).
Holman, H. R. Systemic lupus erythematosis, in *Immunological Diseases,* 2nd ed. M. Samter, ed. Little, Brown and Co., Boston, Massachusetts (1971) pp. 995–1013.
Johnson, R. T., and Richardson, E. P. The neurological manifestations of SLE. *Med.* 47:337 (1968).
Kowlessar, O. D. Diseases of the pancreas, in *Textbook of Medicine, 14th ed. P. B. Beeson, and W. McDermott, eds. W. B. Saunders, Philadelphia, Pennsylvania (1975), pp. 1250–*1252.
Maletzky, B. M. The episodic dyscontrol syndrome. *Dis. Nerv. Syst.* 34:178–185 (1973).
Mannik, M., and Gilliland, B. C. Systemic lupus erythematosis, in *Principles of Internal Medicine,* 7th ed. T. R. Harrison, ed. McGraw-Hill Book Co., New York (1974), pp. 385–390.
Marinacci, A. A. A special type of temporal lobe (psychomotor) seizure following ingestion of alcohol. *Bull. L. A. Neurol. Soc.* 28:241–250 (1963).
Mark, V. H., and Ervin, F. R. *Violence and the Brain.* Harper and Row, New York (1970).
Merritt, H. H. *A Textbook of Neurology,* 5th ed. Lea and Febiger, Philadelphia, Pennsylvania (1973), pp. 84–86.
Meyer, J. S., Bauer, R. B., Rivera-Olmo, V., Nolan, D. C., and Lerner, A. M. Encephalitis: Neurological manifestations and use of idoxuridine. *Arch. Neurol.* 23:438–450 (1970).
Monroe, R. R. *Episodic Behavior Disorders.* Harvard Univ. Press, Cambridge, Massachusetts (1970).
Nahmias, A. J., and Starr, S. E., in *Infectious Diseases,* 2nd ed. P. D. Hoeprich, ed. Harper and Row, Hagerstown, Maryland (1977).
Plutchik, R., Climent, C., and Ervin, F. R. Research strategies for the study of human violence, in *Issues in Brain/Behavior Control.* W. L. Smith and A. Kling, eds. Spectrum Publications, New York (1976), pp. 69–94.
Raskin, D. E., and Frank, S. W. Herpes encephalitis with catatonic stupor. *Arch. Gen. Psychiat.* 31:544–546 (1974).
Schaumburg, H. H., and Raine, C. S. Multiple sclerosis in the neurology of myelin disease, in *Myeline.* P. Morell ed. Plenum Press, New York (1977), pp. 326–330.
Schuster, M. M., and Iber, F. L. Psychosis with pancreatitis. *Arch. Int. Med.* 116:228–233 (1965).
Shearer, M. L., and Finch, S. M. Periodic organic psychosis associated with recurrent herpes simplex. *N. Eng. J. Med.* 271:494–497 (1964).
Snodgrass, P. J. Pancreatitis, in *Principles of Internal Medicine,* 7th ed. T. R. Harrison, ed., McGraw-Hill Book Co., New York (1974), pp. 1567–1579.

Psychiatric Presentations of Medical Illness

CHAPTER 5

Delusions, Depersonalization, and Unusual Psychopathological Symptoms

ARTHUR M. FREEMAN, III, M.D.

In this chapter, delusions, depersonalization, and several other subjective states will be described as they present in a number of nonpsychiatric illnesses. In addition, a possible mechanism for the formation of persecutory delusions and the relationship between delusions and depersonalization will be discussed.

DELUSIONS

A delusion is defined by Jaspers (1968) as an unshared, outlandish belief that is maintained in spite of logical argument or subsequent experience. A delusion is then a false belief that is difficult to falsify. In this section, we will consider persecutory, depressive, grandiose, somatic, and unusual delusions, which are associated with a variety of illnesses. These illnesses, including epilepsy, infections, neoplasms, toxic and metabolic disturbances, to name a few, may present with delusions to the physician. Usually, these delusions do not represent an exacerbation of underlying psychopathology brought on by the stress of illness. More typically, the individual has no striking premorbid psychiatric history, but becomes delusional as a direct consequence of the medical illness. Delusions may or may not accompany other psychiatric or general medical symptoms, thus complicating the diagnostic process.

Persecutory Delusions

Illnesses in Which Persecutory Delusions are Associated with CNS Pathology

Temporal Lobe Epilepsy. Temporal lobe epilepsy has long been known to be associated with paranoid psychoses. Slater and Beard (1963) found that epileptics develop paranoid schizophrenia-like psychoses with a frequency much greater than chance expectation would allow. They postulated a causal relationship between epilepsy and psychosis. Flor-Henry (1972) specified that in epileptics, involvement of the dominant temporal lobe is far more likely to be associated with paranoid schizophrenic symptoms than involvement of the nondominant temporal lobe, which is more often associated with affective symptoms. Sigal (1976) has also postulated that some paranoid psychoses are produced by dominant temporal lobe seizure activity.

Some support for the causal relationship between epilepsy and paranoid states is suggested by the action of anticonvulsant and antipsychotic drugs. Wengert and Hartford (1971) and Sherwin (1976) have both demonstrated that drugs which control seizures can exacerbate psychotic episodes in epileptics, whereas drugs which control psychoses may lower the seizure threshold.

Slater and Beard (1963) related persecutory delusions to an early onset of temporal lobe epilepsy. Standage (1973) found that his male patients who become psychotic developed seizures between age 14 and 17.

Pond (1957) describes the main difference in the paranoid psychosis of epileptics and nonepileptics as a warm affect that is generally preserved, in contrast to the affective blunting seen in nonepileptic schizophrenics. Another differential point is that in temporal lobe epileptics, the premorbid personality is usually not schizoid.

Some temporal lobe epileptics who do not develop chronic persecutory delusions may have transient delusions during a psychomotor seizure (Wengert and Hartford, 1976). Other patients may fall short of delusional formation and experience only suspiciousness, misperceptions, and auras of fear (Andy, 1976).

Systemic Lupus Erythematosis. The incidence of mental disturbance in lupus may be as high as 50 percent and may take several forms: organic brain syndrome, affective psychosis, or schizophreniform psychosis (Sandok, 1972). Feinglass et al. (1976) found that 25 percent of his patients with psychiatric manifestations of lupus had paranoid ideation. In 63 percent of the patients he studied, psychiatric symptoms either preceded the diagnosis or occurred in the first year of diagnosed disease. Feinglass deemphasizes the influence of steroid therapy on symptom formation, as 82 percent of his patients developed psychiatric symptoms while they were on no steroids or low-dose therapy. Bennett (1972) describes an interesting case of lupus in which the psychiatric symptoms antedated other symptoms of the disease by two years. MacNeill et al. (1976), Baker (1973), and Denko (1977) have all reported cases of lupus with associated persecutory delusions.

Normal Pressure Hydrocephalus. Rice and Gendelman (1973) reported that of their five patients with normal pressure hydrocephalus, three had persecutory ideation. In one of these patients, the persecutory delusions and behavioral difficulties were the compelling reasons for seeking treatment. Price and Tucker (1977) reported a patient who presented with persecutory delusions and depression and was not diagnosed as having normal pressure hydrocephalus until 22 months later.

The usual presentation of this syndrome is in an elderly patient who develops apathy, psychomotor retardation, forgetfulness, and unsteadiness of gait, followed by incontinence.

Marchiafava-Bignami Disease. This disease is associated with chronic alcoholism and has the pathology of symmetrical degeneration of myelin in the central portion of the corpus callosum. Usually, there are focal neurologic symptoms, as well as dementia, depression, and persecutory delusions (Dale, 1975).

Encephalitis. Many forms of encephalitis, including herpes encephalitis, may present with psychiatric symptoms before neurologic signs appear. Misra and Hay (1971) reported three cases misdiagnosed as schizophrenia. One woman presented only with irritability, depression, and persecutory ideation. Wilson (1976) reported another patient, eventually diagnosed as having encephalitis, who presented with incontinence and persecutory delusions.

Neurosyphilis. Gowardman (1970) reported a patient hospitalized for three years with persecutory delusions before neurosyphilis was diagnosed. The Kahn test was positive, but the Wasserman test was negative and CSF was normal. Slurred speech and ataxia may be helpful signs in leading to a consideration of this illness.

Cerebral Malaria. Blocker et al. (1968) reported that three patients during the recovery period of Falciparum malaria developed auditory hallucinations and persecutory delusions. The patients were afebrile, but were believed to have their symptoms secondary to malarial cerebral involvement.

Subacute Bacterial Endocarditis. Jones et al. (1969) studied 110 cases of subacute bacterial endocarditis and found that 21 developed a toxic encephalopathy. The symptoms included paranoid ideation, which was severe enough in a few cases to lead to psychiatric hospitalization.

Endocrinopathies and Metabolic Disorders Associated with Persecutory Delusions

Myxedema. Clower et al. (1969) examined the population of a large state hospital, and found a number of patients with psychotic states secondary to previously undiagnosed hypothyroidism. He estimated the incidence of psychotic symptoms in myxedema to be in the range of 15 to 25 percent. Common symptoms included disorientation, hallucinations, and persecutory delusions. One of his patients was diagnosed as having paranoid schizophrenia, and another as having psychotic depression with paranoid delusions. When treated for the thyroid disorder, the patients' delusions disappeared. Olivarius and Roder (1970) report that paranoid suspiciousness and auditory hallucinations are quite common in myxedema, and cite numerous reports linking myxedema with paranoid states.

Hyperthyroidism. No psychotic picture is typical of hyperthyroidism, as patients may present as having organic brain syndrome, involutional melancholia, mania, paranoid states, or schizophrenia with persecutory delusions (Koran and Hamburg, 1975).

Bewsher (1971) proposed that a rapid alternation in thyroid status, rather than the absolute level of thyroid hormone, may be the causative factor in thyroid psychoses. He cited the case of a patient who developed a psychosis, characterized by paranoid delusions, 6 days after completing a 3-week course of treatment for hyperthyroidism. She was considered euthyroid at the onset of psychosis.

Cushing's Syndrome. Regenstein et al. (1972) described seven patients with psychopathology secondary to Cushing's syndrome, of whom three had paranoid symptoms. Psychoses may be seen in as many as 25 percent of patients with Cushing's syndrome, with paranoid ideation found quite commonly in this group.

Addison's Disease. The usual presentation of Addison's disease is with lethargy and depression, but occasionally the patient may present with a paranoid state (Koran and Hamburg, 1975).

Hyperparathyroidism and Hypoparathyroidism. Excessive secretion of parathyroid hormone from parathyroid adenoma or hyperplasia causes hypercalcemia. The usual presentation of hypercalcemia is with lassitude, irritability, and anxiety, but some patients display paranoid ideation (Dale, 1975; Karpati and Frame, 1964). This may also be seen with hypoparathyroidism (Denko and Kaelbing, 1962; Snowden et al., 1976).

Vitamin B-12 Deficiency. Hart and McCurdy (1971) described a patient with pernicious anemia who presented with incontinence, hallucinations, and paranoid ideation. The psychosis cleared within 8 days of treatment with cyanocobalamin.

Typically, these patients present as depressed, but sometimes persecutory ideation is prominent. This is thought to be related to cerebral involvement with patchy areas of demyelination and degeneration (Dale, 1975).

Sodium Depletion. Sodium depletion may occur in the course of several medical illnesses. It is sometimes overlooked, and may lead to an acute psychotic reaction, such as in a case reported by Burnell and Foster (1972). Their patient presented with disorientation, hallucinations, and paranoid suspiciousness. Other electrolyte disturbances, especially of potassium, may also present with paranoid ideation.

Drugs that May be Associated with Persecutory Delusions

Angrist (1978) describes a sequence of symptoms of *amphetamine intoxication* leading to the development of persecutory delusions. Sometimes persecutory delusions are seen in patients using amphetamine inhalants (Kane and Florenzano, 1971). *Levodopa* therapy, as reported by Celesia and Barr (1970), may be associated with paranoid ideation. Klawans (1978) found that 3 percent of patients treated for 2 years or more developed a paranoid delusion with no other qualities of thought disorder present. *Tricyclic antidepressants* may also precipitate an attack of psychosis with predominantly paranoid ideation. *LSD* and *cannabis* are well known for producing paranoid ideation.

Depressive Delusions

Several endocrinopathies have been reported to present with depressive delusions. Tonks (1977) has noted that the most common picture of mental disorder in *Cushing's syndrome* is a depressive illness with delusions. Koran and Hamburg (1975) have also described a clinical picture that includes depressive delusions in *Addison's disease, hyperthyroidism,* and *hypopituitarism.* Price and Tucker (1977) reported a case of *normal pressure hydrocephalus,* initially misdiagnosed as psychotic depression.

Grandiose Delusions

Baker (1973) reported that in two of seven patients with psychiatric syndromes secondary to *lupus,* delusions of grandeur were prominent. Maletzky (1976) described one case of *pathological intoxication* in which the patient developed grandiose delusions.

Gowardman (1970) reported a case of grandiose delusions in a patient with *neurosyphilis.* Koran and Hamburg (1975) described a manic picture with grandiose delusions in *Addison's disease, Cushing's syndrome,* and *hyperthyroidism.*

Somatic Delusions

Baker (1973) reported a case of *lupus* in which somatic delusions occurred. Parasitophobia is a delusional state in which there is the belief that one's skin is infested by insects. Pope (1970) described a patient with a *B-12 deficiency,* whose parasitophobic somatic delusions responded immediately to treatment for the deficiency. Levin (1946) reported a number of cases of somatic delusions secondary to *bromide intoxication.* Several women believed that they were pregnant with dogs or insects. One patient thought her abdomen contained a copperhead snake. Somatic delusions have also been associated with *pentazocine intoxication* (Blazer and Haller, (1975).

Unspecified Delusions

Sack (1979) reports that a number of illnesses can manifest ''schizophrenia-like'' symptoms, presumably including delusions. These are: *acute intermittent porphyria, Wilson's disease, Niemann-Pick disease, homocystinuria, diabetes (hypoglycemia), alcoholism (pathological intoxication), uremia, hepatic encephalopathy, pellagra, toxoplasmosis, brain abscess, granulomatous meningitis, congestive heart failure, hypertensive encephalopathy, presenile and senile dementias, Wernicke-Korsakoff encephalopathy,* and primary metastatic *cerebral neoplasms.*

Capgras Phenomenon

The Capgras phenomenon is the delusional belief that someone close to the individual is actually an impostor. Although most cases in the literature have been described in association with paranoid schizophrenia, 7 of the 46 cases reported in the English literature since 1933 have been found to have an organic etiology. According to Merrin and Silberfarb (1976), it is likely that at least five of those diagnosed as schizophrenic had organic factors contributing to their condition. Five patients reported by MacCallum (1973) had Capgras delusions with the following underlying conditions: *bronchopneumonia* (with the use of an inhalant solution), *basilar migraine, alcoholic paranoid state, abscess* (in a patient with diabetes and low serum folate), and *malnutrition.* Hay et al. (1974) has reported a case in which a patient had abnormal cerebral development due to *pseudohypoparathyroidism,* whose Capgras followed ECT. Another case is reported by Nikolovsky and Fernandez (1978) of a boy with recurring Capgras following *Varicella encephalitis.*

Postpartum Delusions

Melges (1968) found that postpartum psychoses usually occur within the first week postpartum, but may occur earlier. The clinical picture includes confusion, disorientation, and delusions that may involve the idea that the baby is dead or defective in some way. The birth may be denied, and ideas of persecution may also be expressed. Fifty-one percent of Melges' sample was diagnosed as schizophrenic. He stated that the delusions and other psychotic symptoms occurred as a result of identify diffusion rather than a delirium.

Lycanthropy

Lycanthropy, the delusion of being changed into a wolf, has been known since antiquity. Patients having such a delusion, according to Surawicz and Banta (1975), have been described consistently through the ages as pale, having poor vision, being dehydrated, and falling frequently. Of their two cases, one was secondary to LSD and strychnine, and the other was found to have an organic brain syndrome. Severe depersonalization, hysteria, and paranoid schizophrenia were diagnoses given these patients by earlier clinicians, but the current authors believe that modern lycanthropes have an organic basis for their condition.

DEPERSONALIZATION AND DEREALIZATION

Depersonalization, or the experience of the self as changed or unreal, is often a terrifying experience. It can be either transient or protracted. It usually occurs with derealization, the sense of the environment having changed. These symptoms are associated not only with a variety of psychiatric illnesses (they may precede delusions in some patients), but may be seen in a variety of physical illnesses.

Illnesses in which Depersonalization and Derealization may be a Presenting Symptom

Temporal Lobe Epilepsy

Wengert and Hartford (1971) noted that episodic phenomena of depersonalization and derealization; and automatisms of searching, swallowing, and fumbling in various pockets are highly suggestive of temporal lobe epilepsy. Slater and Beard (1963) reported that feelings of depersonalization and derealization often lead to delusions in patients with temporal lobe epilepsy. This is particularly true for somatic delusions. One of their patients could feel light playing through his eyes into his skull, which he believed to be empty.

Walton (1977) observed that in some patients with lesions of the temporal lobe, intense depersonalization experiences can lend to autoscopic phenomena or visual hallucinations in which the individual believes that he is observing himself from outside.

Encephalitis

Wilson (1976) described a patient who presented with the feeling that she was "living in a dream." She had felt "unreal" for 2 weeks prior to admission. She was also despondent, agitated, and confused. Eventually, she was diagnosed as having herpes simplex type I encephalitis.

Basilar Migraine

MacCallum (1973) noted that depersonalization can be seen in association with basilar migraine. His case showed the overlap of the symptom of depersonalization with the Capgras phenomenon in a patient with basilar migraine.

Systemic Lupus Erythematosus

Baker (1973) reported that 2 of his 17 patients with systemic lupus erythematosus had episodes of depersonalization. One of the patients described "unreal feelings . . . very strange, acting not at all like himself . . . like something about me was very different from my normal self."

Pentazocine Psychosis

Blazer and Haller (1975) found that depersonalization and derealization may be among the presenting symptoms of pentazocine psychosis.

Marijuana-Related Depersonalization and Derealization

Mild to intense depersonalization and derealization experiences are integral to the "marijuana high." Depersonalization was documented in a group of normal volunteers intoxicated with tetrahydrocannabinol (Melges, 1970).

OTHER UNUSUAL SUBJECTIVE EXPERIENCES

Symptoms Found in Temporal Lobe Epilepsy

One highly characteristic ictal memory disturbance in temporal lobe epilepsy is that of *déjà vu* (the peculiar experience of false familiarity of people and places), and, less commonly, *jamais vu* (the failure to see as familiar, well-known people and places (Glaser, 1975). Other symptoms are mentioned by Sherwin (1976), and include: *deja pensée* (false familiarity with thoughts), *deja entendu* (false familiarity with voices), *dreamy states* (in which familiar objects and people may seem peculiar and unreal to the patient), and *forced thinking* (in which the patient's consciousness is suddenly interrupted by the feeling of a forced channeling of thoughts).

Body-Image Disturbances

General Medical Patients

Taggart (1977) describes two symptoms of body-image disturbance in medically ill patients. The first, *body estrangement,* is a form of depersonalization in which the entire body, or any part of it, is experienced as unreal or unfamiliar. The second, *personification,* is an extension of body estrangement in which a person treats a body part as a separate person, unattached to himself. These symptoms may become present weeks after discharge from the hospital.

Temporal Lobe Epilepsy

In temporal lobe epilepsy, distortions of the body image involve the experience of feeling disconnected, fragmented, malformed, or incomplete. Often, a feeling of fear is associated with the distortion of the body image (Glaser, 1975).

Parietal Lobe Lesions

Lesions of the parietal lobe may cause *anosognosia* (denial of illness) and impairment of spatial integration with associated *autotopagnosia* (the inability to relate individual parts of the body to one another, or the inability to recognize body parts). Distortion of the body image and other spatial distortions may initially suggest the diagnosis of hysteria (Solomon, 1975; Allison, 1970).

Phantom Experiences

Gangale (1968), in a review of phantom phenomena, notes that consciousness of an amputated member may occur following the loss of a nose, breast, or penis, and in conditions other than amputations, such as hemiplegia, or a lesion of the brachial plexus. Often it involves unpleasant sensations, such as itching, tingling, or pain. The nonpainful phantom, which is more common, involves a tingling that may even be pleasant. Usually the phantom involves only the distal portion of the amputated member, which is thus experienced as shorter than the unaffected unit in cases of extremity amputation.

Pain from a phantom can be experienced as cramping, squeezing, burning, shooting, or lancinating. The mechanism of phantom experiences is not well understood. From 85 to 95 percent of amputees experience phantom phenomena, but painful phantoms occur in less than 2 percent.

Conomy (1973) noted that in patients with spinal cord trauma, all experienced a disordered sensation of the placement of their limbs in space early in the course of their illness, often at the instant of spinal cord injury. The sensation of their legs being stationed in a position other than that visually perceived, often persisted.

Bromage (1974) reported that brachial plexus anesthesia of the upper limb and subarachnoid, or epidural anesthesia, of the lower limb resulted in a phantom-limb experience in 86 percent of the brachial plexus-blocked patients and 10 percent of the epidural-blocked patients. The phantoms assumed neutral joint positions between 40 and 70 percent of available joint motion, and were not influenced by the actual position of the limb. In some cases, when the patient was allowed to look at the limb, the phantom moved to assume the actual position of the limb.

Taggart (1977) described the resolution of phantom limb experiences occurring by a mechanism known as "telescoping," or a gradual disappearance of the sensation proceeding from proximal to distal. Distal parts may thus "telescope" into the stump, as sensation is lost in proximal parts. This may result in a phantom hand being attached to an upper-arm stump. The patient may experience the phantom as being inside the stump. Such phantoms have lasted from a few months to 30 years.

Subjective Experiences in Postpartum Patients

Melges (1968) studied 100 patients with postpartum psychiatric disturbances. Usually the onset was between the third and seventh day postpartum. It included *delirioid phenomena,* or confusion often marked by uncertainty and indecision; *temporal disorientation* and associated *depersonalization; déjà vu; dreamy states;* and *misidentifications.*

PERSECUTORY DELUSIONS AND DEPERSONALIZATION: PROPOSED MECHANISMS

The onset of persecutory delusions has been linked to the threat of a loss of control over the self (Melges and Freeman, 1975). This is clearly a possible mechanism in organic brain syndromes, during which the patient becomes terrifyingly aware of the loss of control over his thought processes. The first stage is usually a *premonition* that something is amiss, followed by a sense of being *pursued* or watched. This, in turn, leads to the defense mechanism of *projection* (in time as well as space), which the person attempts to predict what his pursuers will do to him. The final stage is one of *presumption,* or what Cameron (1963) has called "*sudden paranoid crystallization.*" At this point, persecutory delusions become fixed and a "*paranoid pseudocommunity*" is blamed as the group behind the conspiracy.

Distortions of time may play a major part in the formation of delusions in patients with various illnesses and intoxications. In normal subjects who develop paranoid ideation under the influence of hashish, *temporal disorganization* is initially induced (Melges et al., 1970). This term refers to alterations in the rate, sequential ordering, and goal directedness of thought processes, but does not necessarily entail disorientation to calendar time. Aberrant temporal processes, such as racing of thoughts, difficulties with keeping track of goal-relevant sequences, or indistinction between past, present, and future, may occur in intoxications, temporal lobe epilepsy, postpartum states, and other conditions. These distortions present a significant threat to the individual's sense of control over himself, and thereby may prompt suspicions of control by others. A "sudden paranoid crystallization" may result from temporal blurring of past, present, and future in which memories, perceptions, and expectations seem to be linked together and point to a global conspiracy directed against the self.

Clinicians have believed for some time that temporal distortions are related to the phenomenon of depersonalization. Schilder (1950) wrote that "every negation of one's self is connected with troubles in the perception of time." *Temporal disintegration* (impaired goal-directedness and temporal indistinction) has been shown to be substantially correlated with depersonalization in acutely ill psychiatric patients and in normal subjects intoxicated with tetrahydrocannabinol (Freeman and Melges, 1977; Melges et al., 1970). *Body image distortions* have also been demonstrated to be correlated with temporal disintegration in these two groups, and it is probable that the same mechanism pertains to depersonalized patients with medical illnesses and intoxications. For example, in patients intoxicated with phencyclidine, depersonalization is common, and the ability to estimate the passage of time is impaired (Yesavage and Freeman, 1978).

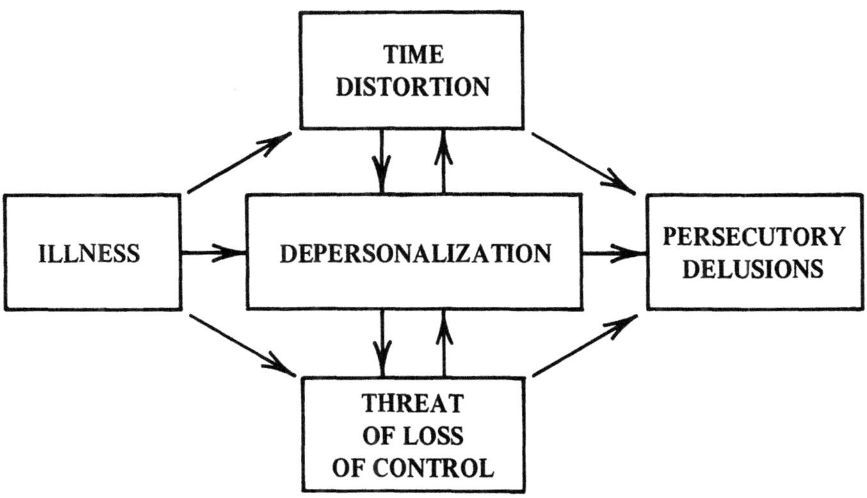

Figure 1. Formation of Persecutory Delusions

Illnesses such as temporal lobe epilepsy, organic brain syndromes, and schizophrenia may induce time distortions, depersonalization, and the threat of loss of control. These are mutually interacting processes, all of which may precede persecutory delusions.

It has been proposed that temporal disorganization, depersonalization, and persecutory ideation are processes that are sequenced in time during acute psychiatric illness (Freeman and Melges, 1978). Interviews with patients who have persecutory delusions as part of a psychiatric or general medical illness suggest that the time distortion is primary, and is followed by depersonalization. As shown in Figure 1, this may lead to persecutory ideation in which some elements of the depersonalization experience are incorporated into the delusions.

SUMMARY

While not exhaustive, this chapter represents an attempt to bring together some medical illnesses that may present with, or be associated with, delusions, depersonalization, and other symptoms. A few illnesses, such as temporal lobe epilepsy and lupus, are generally entertained in differential diagnoses of certain psychopathological states. Other illnesses and other psychological symptoms are not so frequently encountered. As psychiatrists enter into even more fruitful dialogue with other physicians, they will define more clearly the psychological manifestations of general medical illnesses. Psychiatric diagnoses will also become defined more clearly. Thus, in the future, we may reasonably expect that the presence of a delusion will not lead automatically to a diagnosis of schizophrenia.

REFERENCES

Allison, R. S. Parietal lobes: Clinical and pathological aspects of their dysfunction. *Ulster Med. J.* 39:1–20 (1970).

Andy, O. J. Psychomotor-psychic seizures treated with bilateral amygdalotomy and orbitotomy. *S. Med. J.* 69:88–93 (1976).

Angrist, B. M. Toxic manifestations of amphetamine. *Psychiat. Ann.* 8:13–18 (1978).

Baker, M. Psychopathology in systemic lupus erythematosus. I. Psychiatric observations. *Sem. Arthrit. and Rheum.* 3:95–110 (1973).

Bennett, R., Hughes, G.R.V., Bywaters, E.G.L., and Holt, P.J.L. Neuropsychiatric problems in systemic lupus erythematosus. *Brit. Med. J.* 4:342–345 (1972).

Bewsher, P. D., Gardiner, A. Q., Hedley, A. J., and Maclean, H.C.S. Psychosis after acute alteration of thyroid status. *Psychol. Med.* 1:260–262 (1971).

Blazer, D. G., and Haller, L. Pentazocine psychosis, a case of persistent delusions. *Dis. Nerv. Syst.* 36:404–405 (1975)-

Blocker, W. W., Kastl, A. J., and Daroff, R. B. Psychiatric manifestations of cerebral malaria. *Am. J. Psychiat.* 125:192–196 (1968).

Bowers, M. B., and Freedman, D. X. Psychoses associated with drug use, in *American Handbook of Psychiatry,* 2nd ed. M. F. Reiser, ed. Basic Books, Inc., New York (1975), pp. 356–370.

Bromage, P. R., and Melzack, R. Phantom limbs and the body schema. *Canad. Anesthes. Soc. J.* 21:267–271 (1974).

Burnell, G. M., and Foster, T. A. Psychosis with low sodium syndrome. *Am. J. Psychiat.* 128:10:133–134 (1972).

Cameron, N. *Paranoid Reactions in Personality, Development, and Psychopathology.* Houghton Mifflin Co., Boston, Massachusetts, (1963), pp. 470–515

Celesia, G. G., and Barr, A. N. Psychosis and other psychiatric manifestations of levodopa therapy. *Arch. Neurol.* 23:193–200 (1970).
Clower, C. G., Young, A. J., and Kepas, D. Psychiatric states resulting from disorders of thyroid function. *Johns Hopkins Med. J.* 124:305–310 (1969).
Connell, P. *Amphetamine Psychosis*. Maudsley Monograph, No. 5. Oxford University Press, London, England (1958), p. 5.
Conomy, J. P. Disorders of body image after spinal cord injury. *Neurol.* 23:842–850 (1973).
Dale, A.J.D. Organic brain syndromes associated with disturbances in metabolism, growth, and nutrition, in *Comprehensive Textbook of Psychiatry II*, 2nd ed. A.M. Freedman, H.I. Kaplan and B.J. Saddock, eds. Williams & Wilkins, Baltimore, Maryland (1975), pp. 1078–1085.
Denko, J. D. Problems of diagnosis and treatment of patients with lupus psychosis. *Am. J. Psychother.* 31:125–137 (1977).
Denko, J.D. and Kaelbing, R. The psychiatric aspects of hypoparathyroidism. *Acta. Psychiat. Scand.* 38:1 (1962).
Feinglass, E. J., Arnett, F. C., Dorsch, C. A., Zizic, T. M., and Stevens, M. B. Neuropsychiatric manifestations of systemic lupus erythematosus: Diagnosis, clinical spectrum, and relationship of other features to disease. *Med.* 55:323–339 (1976).
Fisher, R. M. Psychiatric symptoms of patients having neurosurgical lesions. *J. Med. Soc. N.J.* 73:963–967 (1976).
Flor-Henry, P. Ictal and interictal psychiatric manifestations in epilepsy specific or non-specific? *Epilepsia* 13:773–783 (1972).
Freeman, A. M. and Melges, F. T. Temporal disorganization, depersonalization, and persecutory ideation in acute mental illness. *Am. J. Psychiat.* 135:123–124 (1978).
Freeman, A. M. and Melges, F. T. Depersonalization and temporal disintegration in acute mental illness. *Am. J. Psychiat.* 134:679–681 (1977).
Gangale, J. P. A review of the phantom sensation phenomenon. *Virg. Med. Monthly* 95:425–429 (1968).
Glaser, G. H. Epilepsy, neuropsychological aspects, in *American Handbook of Psychiatry, 2nd ed.* M.F. Reiser, ed. Basic Books, Inc., New York (1975), pp. 314–355.
Gowardman, M. G. Problems of diagnosis and management of neurosyphilis in psychiatric hospital: Report of 10 cases. *N. Zeal. Med. J.* 72:178–182 (1970).
Hart, R. J., and McCurdy, P. R. Psychosis in vitamin B-12 deficiency. *Arch. Int. Med.* 128:596–597 (1971).
Hay, G. C., Jolley, D. J., and Jones, R. G. A case of the Capgras syndrome in association with pseudo-hypoparathyroidism. *ACTA Psychiat. Scand.* 50:73–77 (1974).
Jaspers, K. Delusion and awareness of reality. *Int. J. Psychiat.* 6:23–38 (1968).
Johnson, R. T., and Richardson, E. P. The neurological manifestations of systemic lupus erythematosus. *Med.* 47:337–369 (1968).
Jones, H. R., Siekert, R. G., and Gevaci, J. E. Neurologic manifestations of bacterial endocarditis. *Ann. Int. Med.* 71:21–28 (1969).
Kane, F., and Florenzano, R. Psychosis accompanying the use of bronchodialator compounds. *J.A.M.A.* 215:2116 (1971).
Karpati, G. and Frame, B. Neuropsychiatic disorders in primary hyperparathyroidism. *Arch. Neurol.* 10:397 (1964).
Klawans, H. L. Levo-dopa induced psychosis. *Psychiat. Ann.* 8:19–29 (1978).
Koran, L. M., and Hamburg, D. A. Psychophysiological endocrine disorders in *Comprehensive Textbook of Psychiatry II*, 2nd ed. A.M. Freedman, H.I. Kaplan and B.J. Saddock eds. Williams & Wilkins, Baltimore, Maryland (1975), pp. 1673–1684.
Levin, M. Transitory schizophrenias produced by bromide intoxication. *Am. J. Psychiat.* 103:229–237 (1946).
Lewis, D. O. Delinquency, psychomotor epileptic symptoms, and paranoid ideation: A triad. *Am. J. Psychiat.* 113:12:1395–1398 (1976).
MacCallum, W.A.G. Capgras syndrome with an organic basis. *Brit. J. Psychiat.* 123:639–642 (1973).

MacNeill, A., Grennan, D. M., Ward, D., and Dick, W. C. Psychiatric problems in systemic lupus erythematosus. *Brit. J. Psychiat.* 128:442–445 (1976).

Maletzky, B. M. Diagnosis of pathological intoxication. *J. Stud. Alc.* 37:1215–1228 (1976).

Melges, F. T. Postpartum psychiatric syndromes, in *Psychosomatic Medicine*, M.F. Reiser, ed. Vol. 30, No. 1, Hoeber Medical Division, Harper and Row, New York (1968), pp. 95–108.

Melges, F. T. et. al. Temporal disintegration and depersonalization during marijuana intoxication. *Arch. Gen. Psychiat.* 23:204–210 (1970).

Melges, F.T., Tinklenberg, J.R., Hollister, L.E. et al. Marihuana and temporal disintegration. *Science* 168:1118 –1120 (1970).

Melges, F. T., and Freeman, A. M. Persecutory delusions: A cybernetic model. *Am. J. Psychiat.* 132:1036–1044 (1975).

Melges, F. T. et al. Temporal disintegration and depersonalization during marijuana intoxication. *Arch. Gen. Psychiat.* 23:204–210 (1970).

Merrin, E. L., and Silberfarb, P. M. The Capgras phenomen. *Arch. Gen. Psychiat.* 33:965–968 (1976).

Misra, P. C., and Hay, G. G. Encephalitis presenting as acute schizophrenia. *Brit. Med. J.* 1:532–533 (1971).

Nikolovski, O. T., and Fernandez, J. V. Capgras syndrome as an aftermath of chicken pox encephalitis. *Psychiat. Opin.* 15:39–43 (1978).

Olivarius, B de F., and Roder, E. Reversible psychosis and dementia in myxedema. *ACTA Psychiat. Scand.* 46:1–13 (1970).

Pond, D. A. Psychiatric aspects of epilepsy. *J. Ind. Med. Prof.* 3:1441–1451 (1957).

Pope, F. M. Paraistophobia as the presenting symptom of vitamin B-12 deficiency. *Practitioner.* 204:421–422 (1970).

Price, T.R.P., and Tucker, G. J. Psychiatric and behavioral symptoms of normal pressure hydrocephalus. *J. Nerv. Ment. Dis.* 164:51–55 (1977).

Regenstein, Q. R., Rose, L. I., and Williams, G. H. Psychopathology in Cushing's syndrome. *Arch. Int. Med.* 130: 114–117 (1972).

Rice, E., and Gendelman, S. Psychiatric aspects of normal pressure hydrocephalus. *J.A.M.A.* 223:409–412 (1973).

Sack, R. L. Schizophrenia and manic-depressive disease, in *Psychiatry for the Primary Care Physician*. A.M. Freeman, R.L. Sack, and P.A. Berger, eds. Williams & Wilkins, Baltimore, Maryland (1979).

Sandok, B.A. Temporal arteritis. *J.A.M.A.* 222:1405 (1972).

Schilder, P.F. *The Image and Appearance of the Human Body*. International Universities Press, New York, (1950).

Sherwin, I. Temporal lobe epilepsy: Neurological and behavioral aspects. *Ann. Rev. Med.* 27:37–47 (1976).

Sigal, M. Psychiatric aspects of temporal lobe epilepsy. *J. Nerv. Ment. Dis.* 163:5:348–351 (1976).

Slater, E., and Beard, A. W. The schizophrenic-like psychoses of epilepsy. *Brit. J. Psychiat.* 109:95–150 (1963).

Snowden, J.A., Macfie, A.C., and Pearce, J.B. Hypocalcemic myopathy with paranoid psychosis. *J. Neurol. Neurosurg. Psychiat.* 39:48 (1976).

Solomon, S. Anatomy and physiology of the central nervous system, in *Comprehensive Textbook of Psychiatry II*, 2nd ed., A.M. Freedman, H.I. Kaplan, and B.I. Saddock, eds. Williams & Wilkins, Baltimore, Maryland (1975) pp. 212–220.

Standage, K. F. Schizophreniform psychosis among epileptics in a mental hospital. *Brit. J. Psychiat.* 123:231–232 (1973).

Surawicz, F. G., and Banta, R. Lycanthropy revisited. *Canad. Psychiat. Assn. J.* 20:537–542 (1975).

Taggart, M. Body image, looking beyond the mirror. *J. Pract. Nurs.* 27:25–35 (1977).

Tonks, C. M. Psychiatric aspects of endocrine disorders. *Practitioner.* 218:526–531 (1977).

Walton, J. N. *Brain's Diseases of the Nervous System,* 8th ed. Oxford University Press, New York (1977), pp. 1171–1172.

Wengart, J. W., and Hartford, J. T. Psychiatric aspects of temporal lobe epilepsy. *Neb. Med. J.* 56: 301–304 (1971).
Wilson, L. G. Viral encephalopathy mimicking functional psychosis. *Am. J. Psychiat.* 133:165–170 (1976).
Yesavage, J. A., and Freeman, A. M. Acute phencyclidine intoxication: Psychopathology and prognosis. *J. Clin. Psychiat.* 39:664–666 (1978).

Psychiatric Presentations of Medical Illness

CHAPTER 6

Hallucinations

RICHARD A. DeVAUL, M.D.
RICHARD C. W. HALL, M.D.

INTRODUCTION

Hallucinations are considered a cardinal symptom of psychiatric illness and are often thought to be synonymous with psychosis; yet these phenomena occur more frequently as a symptom of serious medical illness (postsurgical delirium, epilepsy, drug intoxication), or as an inconsequential or normal event (hypnagogic hallucination). A brief look at the history of scientific interest in hallucinations and at developments in the theory of hallucination etiology will serve as background for discussion of their clinical significance.

History

While references to "visions" date back to antiquity, modern investigations of hallucinations are considered to have begun with the work of Jean Esquirol in the 1830s. Esquirol differentiated hallucinations from illusions by defining the former as a perception without an object, and the latter as a misinterpretation or distortion of a perceived object (Esquirol, 1845). He also was the first to note the similarities between reveries, dreams, and hallucinations.

In the latter decades of the nineteenth century, widespread use of hashish and other hallucinogens stimulated research into the hallucinatory experience. Clinical investigation of drug-induced hallucinations spread throughout Europe and to the United States with major results reported from experimentation with hashish (Ludlow, 1857) and mescaline (Kluver, 1926).

In the early twentieth century, Freud's psychosocial theory of dreams and hallucinations supplemented the pharmacological reports (Freud, 1900, 1911, 1924, and 1932). Freud viewed hallucinatory activity as evidence of regression to a primitive level of psychic development. He postulated that hallucinations in the infant provide temporary but immediate gratification of intense desire or need. He considered their presence in adults as evidence of an extreme disruption of ego function and a return to an infantile state where fantasy and reality are undifferentiated. He believed that the content of hallucinations, like that of dreams, offered insight into the functions of the unconscious and subconscious.

These historic trends in research continue today—clinical investigation centers primarily around artificially induced hallucinations, analytic interest in the content of hallucinations as a reflection of intrapsychic processes, while descriptive interest persists in defining the relationship of altered perception to various clinical conditions. Unfortunately, such emphases in the literature have fostered the notion that hallucinations are most often associated with "nonmedical" conditions, i.e., hallucinogen abuse and mental disorders; while, in terms of total occurrence, hallucinations are most often the sequelae of medical disease.

Definition

For our purposes, a hallucination will be defined as *a perception without an external stimulus*. Two subtypes, the functional hallucination and the pseudohallucination, deserve mention. In an attempt to differentiate hallucinations from dream states, Jaspers (1963:p. 66) defined a true or functional hallucination as a "false perception which occurs simultaneously with an accurate perception of reality." This refinement, as we will later see, is useful in distinguishing between organic and functional disorders known to have hallucinations as symptoms. Jaspers defined pseudohallucinations as images that: lack concrete realtiy, appear in inner subjective space, are incomplete sensory elements compared with real perceptions, and dissipate and must be recreated. Others have summarized these attributes by saying that pseudohallucinations are perceptual experiences known to be unreal when experienced. Much disagreement remains concerning pseudohallucinations (Fish, 1971; Fischer, 1975; Hartmann, 1975; Horowitz, 1975; Savage, 1975; Sedman, 1966; Siegel and Jarvik, 1975); but clinically they have little differential diagnostic or prognostic significance.

ETIOLOGY

Theories concerning the etiology of hallucinations rely heavily upon contributions from both neurophysiology and psychoanalysis. Neurophysiologic theories stem from formulations by British neurologist Hughlings Jackson (1958). He considered the phenomena of hallucinations and illusions as a "release or disinhibition" of lower nervous center activity secondary to impairment of higher nervous center control.

L. Jolyon West's (1975) more refined and comprehensive "perceptual release theory" acknowledges Jackson's theory and offers a neurophysiological explanation for the content of hallucinations. Conceptualizing the brain as an information processing machine, West believes that all experience leaves a trace on the brain; and that these neural traces then join and intermix with new information at an unconscious level to form the basis for thought, memory, dreams, and hallucinations.

The work of Penfield and Perot (1963) supports this aspect of West's theory. They found that hallucinations produced by electrostimulation of the brain frequently contained images and feelings identified by the patient as traces of his past. According to the perceptual release theory, certain areas of the cortex (called the "interpretive cortex" by Penfield and Perot) scan and screen incoming stimuli. At the same time, this cortical activity and the inflow of incoming data provide a check on the release into awareness of neural trace images. In sleep, when both cortical interpretive activity and sensory stimulation are diminished, neural trace images are released; that is, dreams occur. If cortical awareness is maintained but the check supplied by normal sensory input is relaxed or absent, hallucinations may result. Hallucinations associated with sensory deprivation and isolation are thus explained, as are phantom limb phenomena and the hallucinations of "Black Patch" disease. Conversely, hallucinations can result from sensory overload, when subcortical arousal or the intensity of external stimuli overwhelms the ability of the interpretive cortex to keep up with the presentation of data.

Roland Fischer (1975) agrees that a low ratio of cortical interpretive activity to subcortical activity creates a prehallucinatory condition. In addition, he suggests that interaction between the left and right hemispheres of the brain influences this process. Nonverbal, visual-spatial, and intuitive-cognitive functions are controlled by the nondominant (usually the right) hemisphere, and verbal-ideational cognitive and reality-testing functions are controlled by the dominant (usually the left) hemisphere. Communication between the two integrates their functions; the ratio of activity between the two varying, Fischer thinks, with the different cognitive processes—meditation, concentration, reverie, creative thinking, and so on. Any condition that results in an increased rate of nondominant hemisphere activity predisposes to hallucination. The work of Penfield and Perot lends support to this hypothesis inasmuch as their subjects demonstrated a high rate of nondominant hemisphere activity during hallucinations produced by electrical brain stimulation. Fischer believes, then, that both the ratio of right to left hemisphere activity and the ratio of cortical to subcortical activity play a part in determining the tendency to hallucinate.

Psychodynamic theory explains the release into awareness of hallucinated material as a disruption of ego function. Hallucination may offer immediate resolution of a psychodynamic conflict, resulting from an overwhelming but unacceptable need or wish. In addition to supplying immediate satisfaction, the hallucination furnishes a defense against taking real action to fulfill such a need. For example, a hallucination of destruction may indulge the aggressive impulse while inhibiting a real aggressive act with its attendant consequences.

In sum, hallucination theory holds that alterations in function of the interpretive cortex and changes in sensory input or subcortical arousal may lead to hallucinosis, and that the tendency to hallucinate is increased by the presence of psychodynamic conflict. Predictably then, causes for hallucinations are varied and include sensory and sleep deprivation, intense emotion, suggestion, and disorders of the central nervous system.

Sensory and Sleep Deprivation

That normal subjects experience hallucinations and impaired cognitive function when subjected to sensory deprivation has been well documented (Schulman et al., 1967). Visual hallucinations usually predominate in such cases, with the subjects being able to describe the experienced imagery (Hebb, 1961; Heron, 1961). Extensive investigation of acute sensory deprivation in ophthalmologic patients who required patching of both eyes for several days (Weisman and Hackett, 1958; Ziskind, 1964, 1965), led to the following observations regarding Black Patch delirium:

1. Sensory deprivation causes predictable mental irregularities.
2. Symptoms occurred during changes in the patients' states of wakefulness.
3. Changes in arousal could be documented by EEG changes.
4. Mental symptoms could be modified by changes in sensory input.

Like Black Patch disease, phantom limb phenomena, the most common of kinesthetic hallucinations, result from sensory deprivation. They follow most limb amputations and occur less frequently in cases where a limb has been denervated peripherally or by spinal cord transection. The size and shape of the hallucinated body part may vary considerably, the sensation often attended by pain and discomfort refractory to treatment. Studies of sensory deprivation have provided insights into the mechanism of hallucination, as well as offering important clinical aids to the management of patients whose treatment may necessitate sensory deprivation (i.e., patients in intensive care and those with special syndromes).

Extended periods of sleeplessness may induce hallucinations, presumably because of decreased cortical awareness with a decreased ability to interpret sensory data (West, 1962). Fleeting, hallucinated images may appear after 2 to 3 days of sleep deprivation, with prolonged periods of hallucinosis and dissociation occurring after 100 to 200 hours (West, 1975).

Hallucinations often take place in the interval between wakefulness and sleep. They are called hypnogogic, if they occur as the subject falls asleep; and hypnopompic, if they occur as the subject awakes. EEG recordings demonstrate a loss of alpha rhythm during the episodes. Unlike dreams, in which the subject ordinarily participates, these perceptions seem to be forced upon the subject who often feels paralyzed and unable to respond. They vary in form from elementary to complex and may be auditory, visual, or multisensory. Although hypnogogic and hypnopompic hallucinations may be part of normal experience, they are frequently reported by patients with a range of psychiatric diagnoses and/or organic disorders (McDonald, 1971) and are common symptoms of narcolepsy.

Hypnosis, Suggestion and Emotion

Hallucinations can be induced by hypnosis, suggestion, or intense emotion. Normal subjects can be persuaded to hallucinate either by hypnosis or encouragement (Barber, 1964). Suggestion is probably the mechanism for hallucination in hysterical disturbances. Hypnotic and suggestion-induced hallucinations are most often visual or auditory, and generally consist of frightening experiences that relate to typical childhood fears. In auditory hallucinations so induced, the subject may hear his parents calling him by name. The hallmark of these hallucinations is the close relationship of their content to childhood fantasies and psychodynamic issues. Intense emotions like those associated with depression may also be accompanied by auditory hallucinations. The hallucinated voices in these instances are usually interpreted as voices of the conscience and tend to repeat self-derogatory phrases like "bad person" (Fish, 1967).

Central Nervous System Disorders

Whether or not a focal lesion of the central nervous system will produce hallucinations depends upon the overall condition of the brain, the emotional state of the patient, psychodynamic factors, and the specific nature of the lesion. Our present ability to predict the location of central nervous system lesions by symptoms owes much to the work of Penfield and Perot (1963), who investigated both spontaneous hallucinations and those produced by electrostimulation. By probing temporal, parietal, and occipital lobes in conscious subjects and recording the responses, Penfield and Perot were able to map areas of response in the different sensory modes. Their cartography of experiential responses is summarized in the following paragraphs.

Stimulation of different points on the temporal lobe produced single mode or multisensory hallucinations of all types except those of somatic distortion. Visual hallucinations were experienced following stimulation of the lateral surface of the nondominant temporal lobe. So-called panoramic or scenic hallucinations with both visual and auditory perceptions were elicited by stimulation of the first temporal convolution of either hemisphere. Hallucinations of noise were produced by stimulation of Brodmann's areas (41, 42) located in the first temporal convolution. Organized voices occurred with stimulation of the lateral surface of the first temporal convolution of either hemisphere. Part of the central field for smell and taste also falls in the temporal lobe. Gustatory hallucinations resulted from deep stimulation of the Sylvan fissure at the transverse gyri.

Stimulation of the parietal cortex and adjacent cortical areas produced parasthesias and unpleasant sensations, including distortions of body image. The phantom limb phenomenon, discussed earlier, is the most common of these somatic hallucinations.

Visual hallucinations occurred with stimulation of the visual projection area of the calcarine fissure, and optic radiations of the occipital lobe. Stimulation of Brodmann's areas (17, 18, 19) gave rise to visions of lights, geometric figures, and zigzag lines, in contrast to the complex visual hallucinations evoked by stimulation of the posterior temporal lobe.

It is important to remember that although these responses can be elicited by stimulation of the cortex, they are not *caused* by the cortical stimulation. Rather, the electrical stimulation of specific cortical areas allows specific sensory data to be released into awareness. Identifying the locations which, upon stimulation lead to hallucinations of a given type, has aided in the diagnosis of focal pathology. *Organically produced hallucinations usually occur in association with other mental state changes suggestive of cognitive impairment. Such changes may be clinically inapparent unless specifically tested for* (Bell and Hall).

TYPES OF HALLUCINATIONS

Below, in chart form, are the main types of clinically significant hallucinations by sensory mode, their descriptions, and the pathologies of which they have been known to be symptomatic. Note that all types may be found in organic, toxic, or functional disorders.

Visual Hallucinations

Nature of perception:

Simple patterns (dots, flashes of light, zigzag lines), organized patterns, or complex objects, people, scenes, and panoramas.

Occur in:

Organic and emotional disorders. More commonly indicators of organic and toxic states than of functional psychoses.

Nature of Perception	Description	Common Etiologies
Simple	Lines, dots, flashes of light	Psychedelic drug use, epilepsy, migraine, advanced syphilis retinal disease, temporal arteritis
Small insects, spiders, rats	Usually unpleasant and attended by fear or suspicion	Characteristic of delirium tremens
Miniature human beings (Lilliputian hallucinations)	Entertaining scenes (i.e., miniature circus on bedside stand)	Organic and toxic states
Scenes and panoramas	Often accompanied by auditory perceptions, frequently religious content	Temporal lobe epilepsy
Autoscopy, mirror-image phenomenon	Patient reports seeing himself and is certain of identification	May occur in depression or emotional illness, but more frequently in epilepsy, focal lesions and brain stem infections

Auditory Hallucinations

Nature of perception:

Simple sounds (buzzing, bells), music, voices, and complicated communications.

Occur in:

Organic or emotional disorders. Hallucinated voices, particularly those speaking complicated sentences, are more characteristic of schizophrenia than of organic or toxic states.

Nature of Perception	Description	Common Etiologies
Noise	Buzzing, bells	Salicylism, middle-ear disease, auditory nerve injury and deafness, acoustic neuroma, organic psychosis, schizophrenia

Nature of Perception	Description	Common Etiologies
Voices	In clouded sensorium	Toxic and organic states
	In clear sensorium often speaking in sentences with abusive or sexual content	Functional psychosis
Echo de pensée	Hearing one's thoughts spoken aloud	In absence of clouded sensorium, considered pathognomonic of schizophrenia
Multisensory		Structural problems of the brain, such as temporal lobe epilepsy

Gustatory/Olfactory Hallucinations

Nature of perception:

Hallucinations of taste and smell, far more often of unpleasant tastes and smells than of agreeable ones.

Occur in:

Organic, toxic, or emotional disorders, more often organic.

Nature of Perception	Description	Common Etiologies
unpleasant odor	Isolated	Migraine, temporal lobe epilepsy
	Accompanied by salivation, chewing and sniffing movements	Temporal lobe epilepsy
	Accompanied by hallucinations in other senses	Organic lesions, or, if associated with bizzare thought content and auditory hallucinations, schizophrenia (Rupert 1961)
Gustatory and olfactory	Ill-defined, difficult to distinguish from delusional ideation	May occur in depression

Pain, Touch and Deep Sensation

Nature of perception:

Tactile and somatic sensations varying from pain to hallucinations of insects on or in the body (zoopathy).

Occur in:

Organic, toxic, and emotional disorders, more often organic and toxic.

Nature of Perception	Description	Common Etiologies
Pain	Bizarre twisting and tearing	Schizophrenia, epilepsy, migraine
Tactile zoopathy	Insects crawling over skin, e.g., "cocaine bug"	Toxic states
Somatic zoopathy	Infestation of body by insects	Organic states, schizophrenia
Phantom limb	Hallucinated presence of missing body part	Follows amputation (sometimes denervation) of body part or limb
Epigastric discomfort	Feeling of fullness rising upward from stomach, epigastric pain	Migraine, temporal lobe epilepsy

CLINICAL CONSIDERATIONS

Reversible organic brain syndrome (delirium) is the most common source of hallucinations in the medical population. While as many as 20 to 30 percent of all hospital patients may experience delirium at some time in their hospital stay, this condition frequently goes unrecognized, or is mistakenly treated as an emotional disorder. Caused by a diffuse metabolic impairment of the cerebrum, delirium is a nonspecific indicator of inadequate cerebral function (Engel and Romano, 1959; DeVaul, 1976).

Clinically, it is identified by evidence of global cognitive impairment—short-term memory deficit, disorientation for time and place, compromised judgment and intellectual function, and diminished awareness. The degree of dysfunction tends to fluctuate, so that in mild cases completely lucid intervals may alternate with periods of frank confusion. With progressive dysfunction, secondary symptoms including hallucinations, delusions, incoherence, sleeplessness, and hyperactivity are seen.

The diagnosis of delirium is suggested by the presence of the primary cerebral dysfunction symptoms, which are frequently overlooked, due to the more dramatic and troublesome secondary symptoms. In hallucinations caused by organic brain syndromes, the primary symptoms of delirium are usually present, and, if they are, the hallucination cannot be correctly attributed to an emotional disorder.

Like hepatic or renal insufficiency, delirium can result from almost any systemic illness or trauma, central nervous system disease, toxic drug effect, or drug withdrawal state (Table 1). Often, several general physiologic problems combine to produce delirium. In a patient who is anemic, hypoxic and over-medicated, for instance, the three conditions together may lead to the onset of clinical delirium. Once it has developed, delirium may progress, resulting in permanent brain damage or even death, or may clear completely with return of normal brain function. Early identification with prompt determination of the underlying cause is requisite to recovery.

Differential Diagnosis of Hallucination Etiology

Although the mode and content of the hallucinations themselves are not specific for emotional or organic etiology, some generalizations can be made. Elementary hallucinations (noises rather than voices, zigzag lines, or flashing lights) are more often observed in organic conditions such as migraine and epilepsy. Complex auditory hallucinations occurring in isolation are the only type of hallucination suggestive of an emotional disorder, but even these may also be seen in organic disease.

In the medical patient, hallucinations generally indicate a serious condition: delirium, focal brain disease, toxic psychosis, or infrequently, a functional psychosis such as schizophrenia. Focal brain disease (epilepsy, tumor) can usually be suspected from history and confirmed by neurological tests (CAT scan, EEG). Toxic psychoses generally present with delirium, but those that present with a clear sensorium (e.g., cocaine and amphetamine psychoses) can usually be detected by a history of drug use and by urine screens. This leaves the critical differential diagnosis of delirium, or functional psychosis. As Jaspers (1963) specified, a functional or emotional hallucination is one that takes place simultaneously with a true perception of reality. In other words, the patient accurately perceives his immediate environment and, superimposed on this, the hallucination.

Hallucinations secondary to delirium, on the other hand, usually occur along with frank primary symptoms of delirium. Patients with delirium are confused and unable to perceive accurately or remember where they are. The delirious patient who is in a lucid interval is an exception to this rule as are those certain patients with toxic psychosis just mentioned. In the case of the delirious patient, observation over time, or a review of the nursing notes, will bring to light the characteristic alternation of confusion with lucid intervals.

Information about the onset of the illness can be an aid to the differential diagnosis. In psychiatric disorders, bizarre and inappropriate behavior, which careful history-taking can uncover, precedes the actual psychotic break. Most deliria, in contrast, occur quite suddenly with a prior history of completely normal behavior. Sudden onset, then should be considered a sign of an organic problem unless proven otherwise (DeVaul and Zisook, 1977).

The course of the illness may also supply a clue. The emotionally disturbed patient will demonstrate sustained evidence of psychosis, unlike the fluctuating delirium and clear-headedness of the organic patient. Finally, the EEG is of particular aid. A typical EEG in delirium shows a diffuse slow pattern in the dominant activity ranges, occasionally with superimposed, intermittent, fast waveforms. This sign of metabolic encephalopathy generally persists during the delirium and returns to normal with its resolution. This differential is exceedingly important because, as stated earlier, prompt recognition of organic brain syndrome and early, proper management are critical to its reversal. Large doses of antipsychotic drugs, appropriately used for the treatment of hallucinations of functional psychoses, may prolong or aggravate an organic brain syndrome.

Like any nonspecific symptom, hallucinations are indicators of a more widespread dysfunction, disease, or disorder. In the medical patient, the origin is most likely to be an organic dysfunction or toxic reaction. Information assembled from patient history, clinical presentation, close observation, and the appropriate tests and screens will usually suggest the correct clinical diagnosis.

TABLE 1. DELIRIUM: COMMON MEDICAL CAUSES*

SYSTEMIC	
Metabolic:	Cardiac insufficiency, pulmonary insufficiency, hepatic failure, renal failure, electrolyte imbalance, malnutrition, vitamin deficiencies, metabolic effects secondary to carcinoma, trauma, infection, and allergic reactions
Endocrine:	Adrenal insufficiency, Cushing's disease, pituitary insufficiency, diabetes and other causes of hyper- and hypo-glycemia, hyper- and hypothyroidism, hyper- and hypo-parathyroidism
Drug-Related:	Withdrawal syndromes (especially alcohol, barbiturates, sedatives, narcotics), acute and chronic intoxication (especially from steroids, L-DOPA, bromides, alcohol, sedatives, barbiturates, minor tranquilizers, narcotics, and anticholinergics)

TABLE 1. DELIRIUM: COMMON MEDICAL CAUSES* (cont.)

CENTRAL NERVOUS SYSTEM

Vascular:	Embolism, ischemia, hemorrhage, collagen vascular disease
Trauma:	Concussion, subdural hematoma, hemorrhage
Tumor:	Primary and metastatic carcinoma
Infections:	Meningitis and encephalitis (viral, bacterial, fungal spirochetal), abscess

*These conditions do not necessarily result in delirium, and other causes of delirium exist.

REFERENCES

Barber, T. X. Towards a theory of 'hypnotic' behavior: Positive visual and auditory hallucinations. *Psychol. Rec.* 14:197–210 (1974).

Bell, R., and Hall, R.C.W. The mental status examination. Am. Fam. Phys. 16:145–152 (1977).

De Vaul, R. A., and Zisook, S. Reversible organic brain syndrome: Clues to quick recognition. *Med. Times.* 105:9d–15d (1977).

De Vaul, R. A. Acute organic brain syndromes: Clinical considerations. *Tex. Med.* 72:51–54 (1976).

Engel, G. L., and Romano, J. Delirium: A syndrome of cerebral insufficiency. *J. Chron. Dis.* 9:260–277 (1959).

Esquirol, J.E.D. *Mental Maladies: A Treatise on Insanity.* E. K. Hunt, trans., 1845, rpt. Hafner Pub., New York (1965).

Fischer, R. Cartography of inner space, in *Hallucinations: Behavior, Experience, and Theory.* R. K. Siegel and L. J. West, eds. John Wiley and Sons, New York (1975), pp. 197–239.

Fish, F. *Clinical Psychopathology, Signs and Symptoms in Psychiatry.* John Wright and Sons, Ltd., Briston, England (1971).

Freud, S. The Interpretation of Dreams (1900), in *The Standard Edition of the Complete Psychological Works of Sigmund Freud,* Vols. 4, 5. The Hogarth Press, London, England (1974).

Freud, S. Psycho-analytic notes upon an autobiographical account of a case of paranoic (dementia paranoides) (1911), in *The Standard Edition of the Complete Psychological Works of Sigmund Freud,* Vol. 12. The Hogarth Press, London, England (1974), pp. 1–80.

Freud, S. The loss of reality in neurosis and psychosis (1924), in *The Standard Edition of the Complete Psychological Works of Sigmund Freud,* Vol. 19. The Hogarth Press, London, England (1974), pp. 183–191.

Freud, S. New Introductory Lectures on Psychoanalysis (1932), in *The Standard Edition of the Complete Psychological Works of Sigmund Freud,* Vol. 22. The Hogarth Press, London, England (1974).

Hartmann, E. Dreams and other hallucinations: An approach to the underlying mechanism, in *Hallucinations: Behavior, Experience, and Theory.* R. K. Siegel and L. J. West, eds. John Wiley and Sons, New York (1975) pp. 71–79.

Hebb, E. O. (Discussion of) S. J. Freedman's Sensory deprivation: Facts in search of a theory. *J. Nerv. Ment. Dis.* 132:40–43 (1961).

Heron, W. Cognitive and physiological effects of perceptual isolation, in *Sensory Deprivation.* P. Solomon, P. E. Kubzansky, P. H. Leiderman, J. H. Mendelson, R. Trumbull, and D. Wexler, eds. Harvard Univ. Press, Cambridge, Massachusetts (1961).

Horowitz, M. J. Hallucinations: An information-processing approach, in *Hallucinations: Behavior,*

Experience, and Theory. R. K. Siegel and L. J. West, eds. John Wiley and Sons, New York (1975), pp. 163–195.

Jackson, J. H. *Selected Writings*, Vol. 2. J. Taylor, ed. Basic Books, Inc., New York (1958).

Jaspers, K. *General Psychopathology*. J. Hoenig, and M. W. Hamilton, trans. Univ. of Chicago Press, Chicago, Illinois, (1963).

Kluver, H. Mescal visions and eidetic vision. *Am. J. Psychol.* 37:502–515 (1926).

Ludlow, F. *The Hasheesh Eater*. Harper and Brothers, New York (1857).

McDonald, C. A clinical study of hypnagogic hallucinations. *Brit. J. Psychiat.* 118:543–547 (1971).

Penfield, W. and Perot, P. The brain's record of auditory and visual experiences. *Brain.* 86:595–696 (1963).

Rubert, S. L., Hollender, M. H., and Mehrhof, E. G. Olfactory hallucinations. *Arch. Gen. Psychiat.* 5:313–320 (1961).

Savage, C. W. The continuity of perceptual and cognitive experience, in *Hallucinations: Behavior, Experience, and Theory*. R. K. Siegel and L. J. West, eds. John Wiley and Sons, New York (1975), pp. 257–286.

Schulman, C. A., Richlin, M., and Weinstein, S. Hallucinations and disturbances of affect, cognition, and physical state as a function of sensory deprivation. *Percept. Mot. Skills.* 25:1001–1024 (1967).

Sedman, G. A comparative study of pseudohallucinations, imagery, and true hallucinations. *Brit. J. Psychiat.* 112:9–17 (1966).

Siegel, R. K., and Jarvik, M. E. Drug-induced hallucinations in animals and man, in *Hallucinations: Behavior, Experience, and Theory*. R. K. Siegel and L. J. West, eds. John Wiley and Sons, New York (1975), pp. 81–161.

Weisman, A. D., and Hackett, T. P. Psychosis after eye surgery. *N. Eng. J. Med.* 258:1284–1289 (1958).

West, L.J. A clinical and theoretical overview of hallucinatory phenomena, in *Hallucinations: Behavior, Experience, and Theory*. R.K. Siegel and L.J. West, eds. John Wiley and Sons, New York (1975), pp. 287–311.

West, L. J. Janszen, H.H., Lester, B.K., and Cornelison, F.S. The psychosis of sleep deprivation. *Ann. N. Y. Acad. Sci.* 96: 66–70 (1962).

Ziskind, E. A second look at sensory deprivation. *J. Nerv. Ment. Dis.* 138, 223–240 (1964).

Ziskind, E. An explanation of mental symptoms found in acute sensory deprivation: Researches 1958–1963. *Am. J. Psychiat.* 121: 939–946 (1965).

Psychiatric Presentations of Medical Illness

CHAPTER 7

Hysterical Symptoms

RICHARD A. DeVAUL, M.D.

INTRODUCTION AND HISTORY

The definition of hysteria and its history as a subject of medical interest are inextricably bound. Questions of nosology, etiology, and the clinical validity of hysterical symptoms persist; questions that bear witness to a history of diverse thinking about the mechanisms and range of the clinical disorder. The Greek term "hysteria" was an attempt to designate etiology (wandering womb) rather than to define the nature of the symptom (paralysis or anesthesia, for example). The later designations of conversion and dissociative reactions, naming the mechanisms thought to produce the symptom, followed the precedent.

Clinical observations and hypotheses about hysteria began to accumulate from English and French practitioners in the eighteenth century. Prior to that, in the mid-1600s, Sydenham had marked the range of hysterical symptoms which, he said, could mimic all known diseases. Mesmer (1733–1815) established the relationship between hysteria and altered states of consciousness demonstrating the clinical use of hypnosis in its treatment. Contributions to the understanding of the symptoms were made by Sir Benjamin Brodie, Robert Brudenell Carter, and J. R. Reynolds, all Englishmen. But much of the early, sustained work and communication among researchers on hysteria took place in France under Jean-Martin Charcot (1825–1893) and his student Pierre Janet (1859–1947). The Charcot school, while acknowledging a psychological component to hysterical symptomology and, therefore, its amenability to treatment by hypnosis, believed that degenerative nervous system disease was the cause. In fact, they considered suggestibility and the ability to be hypnotized as pathologic results of the organic disease and as pathognomonic of hysteria.

Janet's explanation for the production of hysterical symptoms derived from his conceptualization of consciousness. He postulated that consciousness is a product of many mental processes, which, under normal circumstances, are integrated. Hysterical symptoms occur when, as a result of degeneration of the nervous system, the mental functions become dissociated from one another and produce effects that are not mediated by conscious awareness. He referred to this dysfunction as *dissociation*.

H. Bernheim, working apart from the Charcot school, believed that suggestibility and dissociative phenomena did not require nervous system degeneration but were psychological events. When Freud went to France, he was greatly influenced by Bernheim's success in treating hysteria with hypnosis. Like Bernheim, Freud accepted Janet's theory of dissociation and rejected the idea that organic disease was the cause. Instead, on the basis of histories obtained under hypnosis, Freud began to think that memory of a traumatic event (or, as he later recognized, an unbearable idea) had been cut off from the patient's awareness because of its moral or ethical repugnance. The hysterical symptom, manifest later, appeared to be an unconscious or unwilled somatic expression of the psychological conflict surrounding the trauma. Freud introduced the concept of conversion, explaining that emotional energy unreleased at the time of trauma was converted into somatic expression and discharged by way of the voluntary nervous system. Hence the designation *hysterical conversion*.

Breuer, who collaborated with Freud in early work on hysteria (Breuer and Freud, 1895) hypothesized, like Freud, that feelings engendered by trauma and dissociated from consciousness were responsible for the symptoms. But Breuer contended that the affect was unavailable to conscious awareness because the trauma had precipitated a *hypnoid* state. The affect was *state-bound* and could be released by ushering the patient back into the hypnotic state.

At this stage in its development, the study of hysteria did not differentiate between those manifestations which today are called conversion reactions and those which are called dissociative reactions. All abnormal symptoms of the nervous system that occurred without demonstrable cause were called hysteria. Likewise, the not-incompatible theories of dissociation and conversion were used interchangeably as possible explanation for the phenomena. Some current thinking considers the split between conversion and dissociation to have been arbitrary, and favors return to a single theoretical model, which would probably be that of dissociation*.

This rather lengthy introduction has been necessary because the history of the specific topic of our present concern, *hysterical neurosis, conversion type,* merges

*Merskey (1978) claims that "on theoretical grounds there is no real need to distinguish conversion and dissociative symptoms" (p. 306), and that the "mental mechanism that permits this method of symptom production he is speaking of conversion is called dissociation because feelings and symptoms are split off or separated fro each other" (p. 305). Nemiah (1975), Cleghorn (1969), and West (1967) agree that dissociation is the mechanism of conversion symptom formation.

prior to the middle of the twentieth century with the larger diagnostic category *hysteria,* or *conversion hysteria,* under which were lumped the dysmnesic states (amnesia, fugue, somnambulism, multiple personality), motor disturbances, sensory disturbances, disease simulation and, to a lesser degree, abnormally dramatic behavioral characteristics. As a result of observations of war neuroses and trauma during the two world wars, the American Psychiatric Association replaced the designation *hysterical conversion* with the two psychopathologies *conversion reaction* and *dissociative reaction* in its first Diägnostic and Statistical Manual of Mental Disorders (DSM, 1952). The former term referred to localized functional sensory/motor disorders, and the latter, to the fugue states and amnesias. In the DSM II (1968) the term *hysteria* returned; the current nomenclature being *hysterical neurosis, conversion type* and *hysterical neurosis, dissociative type.* Dysmnesic states are seldom confused with medical illnesses and will not be of major concern here.

In the period between the wars, work was being done that distilled out a further concept of hysteria. In 1930, Fritz Wittels published the first psychoanalytic description of the hysterical character (Wittels, 1930). As Lazare (1971) points out, psychiatric literature prior to that time had focused on symptoms rather than on character. The line of investigation initiated by Wittels eventually led to two areas of continuing theoretical debate: (1) whether there is a connection between the personality type described as hysterical by Wittels and others (Reich, 1933; Marmor, 1953; Chodoff and Lyons, 1958; Ziegler and Imboden, 1962; Ziegler et al., 1963; Halleck, 1967; Lazare, 1971; Nemiah, 1975) and the development of conversion symptoms, and (2) whether a history of conversion symptom development constitutes, in itself, a disease entity or syndrome (Purtell et al., 1951; Perley and Guze, 1962; Guze and Perley, 1963; Slater, 1965; Cleghorn, 1969; Woodruff, 1971; Guze, 1974; Reed, 1975; *Lancet,* 1977). We will consider these conditions insofar as they are demonstrated in the clinical situation, after looking more closely at the nature and range of hysterical neurosis, conversion type.

HYSTERICAL NEUROSIS, CONVERSION TYPE

Definition and Conceptual Model

The DSM II (1968) definition of hysterical neurosis, conversion type is not itself uncontroversial. In stating that the disorder affects the special senses or the voluntary nervous system only, it implicitly accepts the dichotomy between psychophysiological symptoms and conversion symptoms established by Franz Alexander (1943). Alexander's distinction between vegetative or organ neuroses (psychophysiological responses of the autonomic nervous system to stress) and conversion hysteria (voluntary nervous system responses to emotional conflict) has been contested, initially by Rangell (1959), Engel and Schmale (1967), and Engel (1968). Engel agreed with Alexander that only those body parts and functions are available for the conversion process which are "capable of being perceived consciously or unconsciously, and thereby giving rise to perceptual memory traces which can be used by the ego to symbolize and express hidden wishes" (Engel, 1968: p. 319). He disagreed, however, that only functions of the major sense organs and voluntary motor system are so perceived. Engel argued that visceral processes could be perceived, or gain symbolic representation, and thereafter become available for the conversion process. The nausea that results in vomiting provides an obvious example. Engel is quick to add that the vomiting itself is not a conversion reaction, but that the sensation of nausea that precedes and produces it, is. Laboratory and biofeedback studies (Miller and Banuazzi, 1968; Miller, 1969; Barr and Abernethy, 1977) have demonstrated that visceral responses can indeed be altered under reward motivation. Engel sees wish fulfillment or psychological need satisfaction as the reward in his model of conversion, so that fantasy of injury to a body part or function coupled with some previous sensation associated with that bodily part or function could enable it to become involved in conversion symptomology.

In a series of three articles on contemporary conversion reactions, Ziegler and Imboden (1960, 1962) and Ziegler et al., (1963) define conversion reactions as "specific, relatively persistent physical symptoms or syndromes which exist in the absence of sufficiently causative physiological pathology; they constitute an unconscious simulation of illness by the patient, who is convinced of their somatic origin; and they enable the patient to remain relativley unaware of conflicts, stresses, or inadequacies that would otherwise be emotionally disturbing" (Ziegler et al., 1963: p. 308).

Neurophysiological Model

Freud's theory, that psychic potential transmuted into somatic energy produces hysterical symptoms, has been of greater metaphorical than neurophysiological service. The point is taken up by Ziegler and Imboden (1962), who cite scientific evidence from several disciplines in disputing the existence of a unique psychic energy. They claim that the "libidinal" or "instinctual" energy hypothesis can be retired without sacrificing the psychodynamic model, in which dissociation of affect from conscious awareness is followed by symbolic somatic expression of the affect. In a neat statement of the case, which bears direct quotation, Nemiah explains that conversion of affect to sensorimotor symptoms may be no different from the translation of any idea into a volitional motor act. He says, "The problem of how the mental act of volition is related to its corresponding physical bodily movement has been a puzzle to philosophers since Descartes. Conversion is simply the same process taking place in a state dissociated from awareness" (Nemiah, 1975: p. 1214).

West's model of dissociation (West, 1967), drawing on neurophysiological thought from Janet to Hughlings Jackson to Magoun, can be used to foster understanding of hallucinations and classical conversion reactions as well as dissociative type hysterical reactions. In West's model, the brain is viewed as an information-processing machine that integrates incoming information on the one hand with the internal store of data and awareness on the other. Needless to say, much scanning and screening of stimuli is carried out by the brain so that we are only "conscious" of a very small part of the unprocessed real world at any given time. The structure that carries out the scanning and screening is the ascending reticular activating system, and the data it handles include emotions and memories as well as sensory information. When psychological demands so dictate, West says that this system is able to narrow the focus of awareness on a particular aspect of reality, causing an "emergency misapplication of the information-processing mechanisms" (West, 1967: p. 890).

Comparative studies of EEG readings during stimulation of limbs affected and nonaffected by hysterical anesthesias (Lader, 1973) have detected a lowering of peripheral receptor activity and some central inhibition along afferent nerve pathways, substantiating West's theory that the information-processing system is malfunctioning. It should be noted that incomplete understanding of the ascending reticular activating system, and other neural structures and pathways that figure in West's discussion, require his theory to be recognized as just that—a theory. Nemiah (1975), for one, feels that, based on the available information, the psychodynamic model is the most useful for describing and dealing with hysterical reactions.

Psychodynamic Model

The current psychodynamic coneptualization of conversion hysteria expands Freud's final formulation that energy from repressed oedipal conflicts is converted and discharged through a somatic symptom, which at one and the same time expresses the drive symbolically and protects the patient from a conscious awareness of it. It is now recognized that pregenital, particularly oral, dependency conflicts may trigger hysterical responses; and that symptom production may be perpetuated to gratify dependency needs, to communicate distress, or to facilitate the individual's adaption to his or her environment (Ziegler and Imboden, 1960, 1962; Ziegler et al., 1963; Nemiah, 1975).

In their conceptual model of conversion reactions, Ziegler and Imboden (1960, 1962) and Ziegler et al., (1963) emphasize the role played by the symptom in helping patients to deal with "dysphoric affect," a term they prefer to the more restrictive "anxiety." By assuming the role of persons with organic illness, patients communicate emotional distress in a way that does not compromise their self image. At the same time, they distract themselves from the perception of dysphoric affects. Symptom display is determined further, the authors explain, by the patients' understanding of the physical illness* and the suitability of specific symptoms for symbolic expression of their fantasies.

---

*Babinski and Froment (1918) demonstrated how the physician's suggestion during history-taking can cause elaboration of hysterical symptoms.

DIAGNOSIS AND CLINICAL CONSIDERATIONS

Warnings against the temptation to diagnose hysteria by the mere absence of physical, laboratory, and x-ray examination are the common denominator of diagnostic instruction in the literature—old and recent. Slater (1965) quotes Charlton Bastian's late nineteenth century reference to diagnosis of hysterical paralysis as, "a negative verdict" that often has more to do with the practitioner's lack of knowledge than with the patient's condition.

In 1922 Henry Head's address on "The Diagnosis of Hysteria" (Head, 1922) reiterated the need for positive evidence in hysterical diagnoses. Head then described, one by one, the clinically replicable, positive signs by which hysterical aphonias, tremors, spasms, paralyses, abasias, pain, analgesias, dysopias, visceral symptoms, amnesias, and fugues could be detected. Head's positive signs were observed reactions of the affected body part to physical manipulation. As such, they were relatively free of the clinician's subjectivity, possible frustration, and perhaps even anger (Leeman, 1975) in the face of diagnostic uncertainty.

Today, however, pain and simulation of bodily disease are replacing the dramatic and more easily recognized conversion displays described by Head (Ziegler and Imboden, 1960; Engel and Schmale, 1968; Cleghorn, 1969; Nemiah, 1975; Merskey, 1978). In fact, Merskey claims that the "classic anesthesias, paralyses, amnesias, blindnesses and so forth, are now extremely rare except in certain clinical settings. . . ." (1975: p. 306). This situation has made management of patients with pain complaints of no obvious physiologic origin a perplexing, often frustrating, matter. Although never simple or sure, some methods of dealing with possible conversion symptoms are more satisfying for the patient and physician, than others.

A careful medical evaluation, including a thorough medical history, examination, and relevant laboratory tests, will usually document the lack of obvious physiologic cause. At this point in the diagnostic process, consideration should be given to two characteristics of conversion display.

First, the patient with conversion symptoms typically insists, with conviction and urgency, that the discomfort is caused by some disease or organic dysfunction as yet undetermined. The insistence persists despite reassurances that would normally satisfy the average or even anxious patient (Ziegler et al., 1963; De Vaul and Faillace, 1978). Often, the patient's continued assertions lead the physician either to question the thoroughness of the evaluation, or to attempt to prove the diagnosis to the patient with the aid of unnecessary tests and procedures. This attempt is not only costly in time and money and uncomfortable, but is also as doomed to failure as any attempt to prove a negative.

The second and more signal characteristic of conversion reactions is that the symptom usually performs a function, that is, it is goal-oriented. The patients' pains or disabilities prevent them from performing undesirable activities, or from accepting unwanted responsibilities. So indicative is goal-orientation of hysterical conversion reactions that, in its absence, a physical cause should be sought further. Such was the case in the following history.

Case 1

A 15-year-old male with "drop attacks" of recent and sudden onset presented to an evaluating neurologist. The boy would fall suddenly to the ground during various athletic activities. Medical history and neurological evaluation (including CAT scan and EEG) were normal. Psychiatric evaluation brought to light expected adolescent conflict, but uncovered, remarkably, no situation or activity with which the boy's symptom interfered. The fact of his continued competition in track and participation in all school activities despite the embarrassing attacks gave cause for further neurological assessment, which subsequently revealed evidence of a seizure disorder.

Additional aids for determining whether a symptom is of psychological origin include psychiatric evaluation, hypnosis, and the Amytal interview. Placebo medications are often misused in the differential diagnosis of conversion symptoms. The placebo effect derives from suggestion and from the expectations inherent in the doctor-patient relationship, and has been proven effective in relieving pain and discomfort from organic as well as emotional sources. For this reason, placebos are of little differential diagnostic usefulness and may even jeopardize the success of constructive medical interventions by undermining the patient's trust in the physician.

Like placebo trail, psychological testing is, unfortunately, not a reliable tool for establishing the hysterical origin of a symptom. The MMPI is most widely used for this purpose, with elevation in the scale 3 and a "conversion V" pattern considered to be evidence of hysterical problems. However, the same pattern is frequently seen in chronic medical problems of organic origin and should not be considered to be specific for hysterical conversions. Even when, based upon physical findings and careful consideration of how the symptom fits into the patient's daily life, the physician judges that a symptom is probably hysterical, this does not preclude the coexistence of medical illness. There may be hysterical elaboration of an organically caused pain or an organic illness, and conversion reaction may exist side by side. Slater reported being most surprised by the "gravity of after-history and the frequency of misdiagnoses" in a follow-up survey of patients who had received diagnoses of "hysteria" at The National Hospital in London (1965: p. 1398). Evidence that symptom formation is the result of an hysterical process indicates only that the symptom will not respond to medical treatment even if an accompanying underlying disease process is treated. This is exemplified in the following case.

Case 2

A 22-year-old, recently married woman presented to the OB/Gyn clinic with a history of pelvin pain and overt marital problems. Psychiatric evaluation confirmed the conversion nature of the pain symptom. Because of objective pelvic findings, a laparoscopy was performed and endometriosis diagnosed. Satisfactory treatment of the endometriosis resulted in no change in the symptomatic pain complaint.

Two final points deserve mention before we leave the subject of conversion symptoms per se. The first concerns the confusion of early central nervous system disease with conversion symptoms. The symptoms of organic brain syndrome and the transitory sensorimotor disturbances of early multiple sclerosis may easily be mistaken for hysterical reactions (Ziegler et al., 1963; Nemiah, 1975; Merskey and Buhrick, 1975). Merskey and Buhrich found the incidence of organic brain syndrome to be so high among index patients with conversion symptoms, that they inferred a causal, if indirect, relationship between the organic lesions and the hysterical reactions.

Secondly, research frequently uncovers organic etiologies for symptoms traditionally thought to be conversion or hysterical reactions. In a recent symposium, Merskey (1978) draws attention to the fact that organic and chemical causes have been found for such classically accepted conversion symptoms as globus hystericus, tics, torticullis, and other abnormal movements. Not only must practitioners be aware of these newly treatable illnesses, but their reclassification forces us to recognize that lack of sufficient knowledge may be responsible for the labeling of other organic abnormalities as "hysterical."

In sum, "conversion-like" symptoms are always secondary to another process. They are commonly seen in a wide range of medical illnesses (particularly organic brain syndrome and chronic illness), in a variety of psychiatric disorders (particularly depression), and in relation to many stressful life situations. The physician, after thorough physical examination and appropriate tests, followed by thoughtful consideration of the patient's manner of presentation and use of the symptom in daily life, must recognize the pseudo nature of conversion symptoms when they exist and not treat them somatically. Medical treatment of conversion symptoms can postpone identification of the underlying cause (physiologic or psychologic), which may require treatment in itself. Conversely, a diagnosis of conversion hysteria should not be made in the absence of careful examination and the presence of the positive inclusion criteria listed above.

THE HYSTERICAL PERSONALITY AND ILLNESS BEHAVIOR

It has been impossible to avoid reference to the hysterical personality in discussing conversion-type hysterical neurosis. As already mentioned, personality was not the focus of hysteria research before Wittels. At the same time that the sensational aspects of hysteria were being studied (and exhibited as public spectacle), however, Freud and his followers were describing personality traits with dominant points of fixation, which they said resulted from inhibition of libidinal development at different stages. Of the behavioral responses so described, those deriving from dependency and dread of loss of love object seemed to fit with many of the character delineations accompanying case studies of hysterics. And so, Chodoff and Lyons (1958) surmise, the dependent and manipulating behavior style became associated with personality descriptions of those being treated for hysterical reactions (most of them women) to produce the present sketch of "the hysteric," a caricature of feminine dependency and coquetry.

Much academic interest has been directed toward explaining the psychodynamics of hysterical or histrionic behavior and has resulted in such designations as "true hysterics," "so-called good hysterics," "healthy" or "sick hysterics" and "hysteroid personalities."* In 1958, Chodoff and Lyons surveyed the literature and put together a composite of the "hysteroid personality, which has become well accepted. "Hysterical personality," they say, "is a term applicable to persons who are vain and egocentric, who display labile and excitable but shallow affectivity, whose dramatic, attention-seeking and histrionic behavior may go to the extremes of lying and even pseudologic phantastica, who are very conscious of sex, sexually provocative yet frigid, and who are dependently demanding in interpersonal situations" (p. 736). This method of relating to the world and of dealing with conflict is found almost exclusively in women, for reasons that Chodoff and Lyons attribute in part to the aforementioned historical coincidence, and in part to the fact that the behavior is more acceptable (and even reinforced) in women.

Whether or not hysterical personality types can be expected to develop more conversion symptoms than does the general population has been investigated, discussed widely, and answered variously (Chodoff and Lyons, 1958; Ziegler and Imboden, 1962; Slater, 1965; Halleck, 1967; Cleghorn, 1969). When they do seek medical care, whether for complaints of organic, psychophysiological or conversion origin, these patients can present management problems for the physician. Their demanding and dependent behavior, partially legitimized by the presence of medical complaints, can best be viewed as an attempt to obtain reassurance that the physician will take care of them. Strategies for medical management of this patient group are outlined elsewhere (Kahana and Bibring, 1964; De Vaul et al., 1977). In general, the physician should demonstrate willingness to continue as primary physician to the patient, even though further evaluation and treatment may be required from a second physician, psychiatrist, or counselor. The physician should also make it clear that disappearance of the symptom will not bring an end to the patient-doctor relationship.

A final category embraces those patients who have histories of frequent medical contacts with an unusually high number of treatments—medical, surgical, and pharmacological. These people have been loosely referred to as hysterics, even though very often their symptoms are not conversion-type reactions, strictly speaking, and they are not necessarily of the personality type designated as hysterical. Although a single diagnostic label may not suffice for the classification of this diversified group, certain medical and psychological profiles can be helpful in identifying them. Purtell et al., (1951) and their followers (Robins et al., 1952; Perley and Guze, 1962; Guze and Perley, 1963; Woodruff et al., 1971; Guze, 1974) consider the recurrent multiple medical complaints to be a diagnostic entity in itself, which they call Briquet's syndrome, after theFrench physician who first

*Developments in the theories concerning the hysterical personality are well summarized by Lazare (1971).

suggested the syndromatic approach to the diagnosis of hysteria in 1859. The syndrome, as they describe it, is characterized by early development (usually before age 20) of many medical complaints in different body systems and locations. It occurs almost exclusively in women and generally includes sexual maladjustment. Engel (1959) describes a group, similar in many respects to those just discussed, as pain-prone personalities. His psychodynamic viewpoint emphasizes the underlying need to suffer, which manifests itself in the polysymptomatic syndrome. A group somewhat more inclusive than the Briquet's group is medically described by De Vaul and Faillace (1978) as patients with persistent pain and illness insistence. Common to members of this patient group is the unconscious use of simulated illness behavior and pseudomedical symptoms as mechanisms for avoiding personal or interpersonal stress.

Clinical recognition of these patients is important because, although they may have no higher incidence of illness than the general population, they put themselves at risk for medical and surgical treatments and iatrogenic drug dependence (Engel, 1959; Perley and Guze, 1962; Guze and Perley, 1963; Woodruff et al., 1971; De Vaul and Faillace, 1978). Once identified, they should be viewed as similar to patients with conversion symptoms. The symptom here is also secondary and should not be allowed to obscure the medical or psychological condition, which demands management.

CONCLUSION

In dealing with symptoms of no obvious organic etiology, physicians must guard against two possibilities—one at the opposite end of the treatment continuum from the other. On the one hand, they should not become part of the cycle of symptom treatment/failure/ more symptom treatment established by those with conversion symptoms, simulated illness, and pain syndromes. On the other hand, they must make every effort to discover an organic etiology for every complaint with which they are presented. While theories of hysteria in all its manifestations are valid for understanding symptom formation and the mechanisms used by certain people in dealing with stress, anxiety or dysphoria, allowing this understanding to interfere with medical evaluation is dangerous. Neither being an hysteric, nor having a history of medical symptoms, conversion, or otherwise, exempts a person from becoming ill.

ACKNOWLEDGMENTS

I would like to thank Faith L. Jervey for her help in the preparation of this chapter.

REFERENCES

Alexander, F. Fundamental concepts of psychosomatic research: Psychogenesis, conversion, specificity. *Psychosom. Med.* 5:205–210 (1943).

Babinski, J., and Froment, J. *Hysteria or Pithiatism.* J. D. Rolleston, trans. University of London Press, Ltd., London, England (1918).

Barr, R., and Abernethy, V. Conversion reaction :Differential diagnosis in the light of biofeedback research. *J. Nerv. Ment. Dis.* 164:287–292 (1977).

Breuer, J., and Freud, S. Studies in hysteria (1895), in *The Standard Edition of the Complete Works of Sigmund Freud,* Vol. 2 The Hogarth Press, London, England (1955).

Briquet's syndrome or hysteria; (edit). *Lancet.* 1:1138–1139 (1977).

Chodoff, P., and Lyons, H. Hysteria, the hysterical personality, and "hysterical" conversion. *Am. J. Psychiat.* 114:734–743 (1958).

Cleghorn, R. A., Hysteria—multiple manifestations of semantic confusion. *Canad. Psychiat. Assn. J.* 14:539–550 (1969).

De Vaul, R. A., and Faillace, L. A. Persistant pain and illness insistence. *Am. J. Surg.* 135:828–833, 1978.

De Vaul, R. A., Zisook, S., and Stuart, H. J. Patients with psychogenic pain. *J. Fam. Pract.* 4:53–55 (1977).

Diagnostic and Statistical Manual of Mental Disorders (DSM). Am. Psychiat. Assoc. Washington, D. C. (1968).

Diagnostic and Statistical Manual of Mental Disorders (DSM). Am. Psychiat. Assn. Washington, D. C. (1952).

Engel, G. L. A reconsideration of the role of conversion in somatic disease. *Comp. Psychiat.* 9:316–326 (1968).

Engel, G. L. Psychogenic pain and the pain-prone patient. *Am. J. Med.* 26:889–918 (1959).

Engel, G. L., and Schmale, A. H. Psychoanalytic theory of somatic disorder. *J. Am. Psychoanal. Assn.* 15:344–365 (1967).

Guze, S. B. Hysteria (Briquet's syndrome), in *Psychiatric Diagnosis.* R. A. Woodruff, D. W. Goodwin, and S. B. Guze, eds. Oxford University Press, New York (1974), pp. 58–74.

Guze, S. B., and Perley, M. J. Observations on the natural history of hysteria. *Am. J. Psychiat.* 119:960–965 (1963).

Halleck, S. L. Hysterical personality traits. *Arch. Gen. Psychiat.* 16:750–757 (1967).

Head, H. An address on "The Diagnosis of Hysteria." *Brit. Med. J.* 1:827–829 (1922).

Kahana, R. J., and Bibring, G. L. Personality types in medical management, in *Psychiatry and Medical Practice in a General Hospital.* N. E. Zinberg ed. International University Press, New York (1964), pp. 108–122.

Lader, M. The psychophysiology of hysterics. *J. Psychosom. Res.* 17:265–269 (1973).

Lazare, A. Hysterical character in psychoanalytic theory. *Arch. Gen Psychiat.* 25:131–137 (1971).

Leeman, C. P. Diagnostic errors in emergency room medicine: Physical illness in patients labeled "psychiatric" and vice versa. *Int. J. Psychiat. Med.* 6:533–540 (1975).

Marmor, J. Orality in the hysterical personality. *J. Am. Psychoanal. Assn.* 1:656–675 (1953).

Merskey, H. Disorders of conscious awareness: Hysterical phenomena. *Brit. J. Hosp. Med.* 19:305–309 (1978).

Merskey, H., and Buhrich, N. A. Hysteria and organic brain disease. *Brit. J. Med. Psychol.* 48:359–366 (1975).

Miller, N. E. Learning of visceral and glandular responses. *Sci.* 163:434–445 (1969).

Miller, N. E., and Banuazzi, A. Instrumental learning by curarized rats of a specific visceral response, intestinal or cardiac, *J. Comp. Physiol. Psychol.* 65:1–7 (1968).

Nemiah, J. C. Hysterical neurosis, conversion type, in *Comprehensive Textbook of Psychiatry II,* 2nd ed. Vol. I. A. M. Freedman, H. I. Kaplan, and B. J. Sadock, eds. Williams & Wilkins, Baltimore, Maryland (1975), pp. 1208–1220.

Nemiah, J. C. Hysterical neurosis, dissociative type, in *Comprehensive Textbook of Psychiatry II*, 2nd ed., Vol. 1. A. M. Freedman, H. I. Kaplan, and B. J. Sadock, eds. Williams & Wilkins, Baltimore, Maryland (1975), pp. 1220–1231.

Perley, M. J., and Guze, S. B. Hysteria—the stability and usefulness of clinical criteria. *N. Eng. J. Med.* 266:421–426 (1962).

Purtell, J. J., Robins, E., and Cohen, M. E. Observations on clinical aspects of hysteria. *J.A.M.A.* 146:902–909 (1951).

Rangell, L. The nature of conversion. *J. Am. Psychoanal. Assn.* 7:632–662 (1959).

Reed, J. L. The Diagnosis of "hysteria." *Psychol. Med.* 5:13–17 (1975).

Reich, W. *Character Analysis*. V. R. Carfagno, trans. Farrar, Straus, and Giroux, New York (1972), pp. 204–209.

Robins, E., Purtell, J. J., and Cohen, M. E. Hysteria in men. *N. Eng. J. Med.* 246:667–685 (1952).

Slater, E. Diagnosis of "hysteria." *Brit. Med. J.* 1:1395–1399 (1965).

West, L. J. Dissociative reaction, in *Comprehensive Textbook of Psychiatry*. A. M. Freedman, and J. I. Kaplan, eds. Williams & Wilkins, Baltimore, Maryland (1967), pp. 885–899.

Wittels, F. The hysterical character. *Med. Rev. Rev.* 36:186–190 (1930).

Woodruff, R. A., Clayton, P. I., and Guze, S. B. Hysteria: Studies of diagnosis, outcome, and prevalence. *J.A.M.A.* 215:425–428 (1971).

Ziegler, J. J., and Imboden, J. B. Contemporary conversion reactions II: A conceptual model. *Arch. Gen. Psychiat.* 6:279–287 (1962).

Ziegler, J. J., and Imboden J. B. Contemporary conversion reactions: A clinical study. *Am. J. Psychiat.* 116:901–910 (1960).

Ziegler, J. J., and Imboden, J. B., and Rodgers, D. A. Contemporary conversion reactions III: Diagnostic considerations. *J.A.M.A.* 186:308–311 (1963).

Section III
PSYCHIATRIC PRESENTATION OF SPECIFIC DISORDERS

CHAPTER 8

Psychiatric Manifestations of Infectious Diseases

JOHN J. SCHWAB, M.D.

BACKGROUND

Although the "conquest of the epidemic diseases" (Winslow, 1943) has been one of the magnificent triumphs of twentieth century medicine, the morbidity produced by these once dreaded diseases continues to be great. From 1900 to 1970, mortality from the infectious diseases in the United States dropped more than 90 percent, but the National Health Interview Survey conducted in 1974 reported about 70,000,000 cases of acute infective and parasitic diseases—the rate was 19.8 per 100 population (Hoeprich, 1977). Despite advances in antibiotic therapy, immunization, sanitation, and other therapeutic and preventive measures, these illnesses are responsible for a tremendous number of days of disability. Some of that disability and a great deal of human anguish is produced by the psychiatric aspects of the infectious diseases, a seriously neglected topic.

Emotional distress and more discrete psychiatric disorders are predecessors, concomitants, and sequelae of infectious diseases. For centuries, the threat of an epidemic of infectious disease has produced anxiety, and at times, panic in the general population. Such fears persist; for example, during the recent localized outbreak of Legionnaires' Disease in New York City, the emergency telephone service that was established responded to 60,000 inquiries within 3 days, although less than 70 possible cases of the disease had been found. Such widespread anxiety is reminiscent of the fear that gripped the cities of Europe and the United States just 100 or 200 years ago when they were threatened by epidemics, or at least outbreaks, of the plague, smallpox, or yellow fever.

Major Associated Psychiatric Disorders

The major psychiatric disorders associated with the infectious diseases are anxiety, delirium, or depression—anxiety prior to, or coincident with the onset of the disease; delirium during its course; and often depression as a complication. In addition, an infectious disease contracted during pregnancy, infancy, or early childhood, is a significant cause of mental retardation, epileptiform disorders, and even unusual psychiatric illnesses. Furthermore, the possibility that the "slow" viruses are responsible, in part, for Creutzfeld- Jakob disease and Alzheimer's presenile dementia indicates that the relationship between infectious diseases and disorders of the central nervous system may be much more complicated and extensive than we had previously thought (Dale, 1975; *Clinical Psychiatry News*, 1978). Thus, the psychiatric disorders associated with the infectious diseases encompass a broad range of symptoms and emotional illness.

In his classic *General Psychopathology*, Karl Jaspers (1972) states that "almost all physical illnesses have at some time provoked psychic disturbance; from the *symptomatic* point of view, an enormous variety of clinical states, and indeed almost all clinical symptoms, can at some time be provoked by exogenous causes (exceptions up to now are, for instance, paranoid syndromes in the narrower sense)" (p. 476). Also, the emotional illnesses produced by the infectious diseases may be complicated by the effects of newer medications, steroids, alcohol, or drugs. As a consequence, the psychiatric disorders may appear in vaguer and less specific forms than previously, and the clinical picture may be atypical or even bizarre. These complexities can make diagnosis difficult.

In this chapter, I shall present a description of the psychiatric disorders associated with the more common infectious diseases, mention some of the rarer psychiatric disturbances caused by infective agents, and look briefly at some of the newer findings in this area. Conventionally, the psychiatric disorders are classified into two major categories: (1) those associated with intracranial infections, and (2) those associated with systemic infections.

PSYCHIATRIC DISORDERS ASSOCIATED WITH INTRACRANIAL INFECTIONS

Bacterial, viral, and other infectious agents that invade the central nervous system can produce meningitis, encephalitis, or brain abscess. But central nervous system infections are seldom circumscribed. Meningitis usually involves some degree of encephalitis; an encephalitis generally causes some degree of meningeal irritation; and a brain abscess becomes encapsulated only after the surrounding brain tissue has been inflamed.

Arthropod-Borne Viruses

Since the advent of the antibiotic era, the feared bacterial infections of the central nervous system, particularly meningococcal meningitis, have been supplanted in frequency by the viral encephalitides. The most common of these are the arthropod-borne encephalitides, such as Western Equine encephalitis, Eastern Equine encephalitis, St. Louis encephalitis, Japanese B encephalitis, and the Australian and Russian forms. These agents produce a relatively similar clinical picture characterized by anxiety, irritability, headache, fever, somnolence, and some degree of confusion. In addition to nuchal rigidity, in severe cases, tremor, dysarthria, muscle weakness, and paralysis may ensue. And generally, these encephalitides are followed by periods of lassitude and depression. Thus, the psychiatric aspects are not limited to the acute stage of the infectious illness, but persist as emotional sequelae.

The epidemic of St. Louis encephalitis that occurred in Florida in the late 1960s illustrates the most common psychiatric features of this group of diseases. The epidemic afflicted many elderly people; mortality increased with advancing age. Emotional complaints typical of neurasthenia were reported as being the most common sequelae regardless of the age of the patient or the severity of the illness. Many patients remained disabled for months after the illness had subsided. Weakness and depression were such common residuals that they should be anticipated in order to provide effective management during convalescence and to allay the concerns of patients and their families. Unless the patients and their families are warned that such psychiatric sequelae are common, the depressive episode may become even more severe—compounded by frustration about failure to recover quickly, fears of prolonged disability, and intrafamilial or other interpersonal problems.

Childhood Diseases

Common viral infections, such as measles and mumps, are reported to produce meningoencephalitis in from 1 to 10 percent of cases. But many authorities believe that the incidence of subclinical involvement of the central nervous system is more frequent than previously realized. At the time of the acute illness, the child usually complains of headache and irritability, and shows some degree of nuchal rigidity, somnolence, and sometimes, focal neurological signs.

Chicken-pox encephalitis has recently been reported as the cause of a rare psychiatric disorder, the Capgras syndrome. Nikolovski and Fernandez (1978) describe the case of a 15-year old white boy who had been healthy until he developed varicella at the age of 9; he was comatose for 1 month. For the next 6 years, he believed that his parents had been "switched" on him. The delusion waxed and waned in severity. Other symptoms were a difficulty with concentration, poor performance at school, and facial tics that were considered to have a postencephalitic origin. Although a single case report of such a rare syndrome may appear to have more immediate than general interest, it reminds us that the infections of the brain are capable of producing a wide variety of unusual as well as common psychiatric symptomatology.

The association between rubella (German measles) during the mother's pregnancy and the high incidence of congenital defects has prompted a number of prospective studies of children born with congenital rubella. Chess (1974) reports that a study of 223 patients with congenital rubella, who were examined at the age of 4 and again at the age of 8, showed that the incidence of emotional disturbances of childhood, particularly autism, was much greater than in children in the population at large. About 10 years ago, Van Krevelen (Makita, 1975) proposed the concept of "autism infantum," a syndrome characterized by oligophrenia and an affective defect, presumably caused by rubella during the pregnancy of the mother.

Recently, Ziring (1978) published a comprehensive review of the "Psychiatric Sequelae of the 1964–65 Rubella Epidemic." He mentions that transplacental infection of the fetus is exceedingly comn n and occurs even when the mother's symptoms are subclinical or minimal. Furthermore, the virus persists in the child's tissues; 10 percent of children born to mothers who had rubella were found to be shedding the virus from the throat when they were 1 year old.

The children who were born during the 1964–65 rubella epidemic are now adolescents. The New York City-based rubella project has been following about 600 of them. Many have had neurological disorders and about 74 are mentally retarded, but Ziring cautions against giving a "hopeless prognosis." When these children received treatment, and as they passed through the developmental stages of childhood and early adolescence, many of them improved significantly. Even in early childhood, between the ages of 3 and 5, some of these children demonstrated marked improvement in their learning skills.

Medications of choice for the treatment of these children's behavior disorders are the phenothizines, such as Thorazine or Mellaril, that diminish the severe hyperactivity that is a major feature of the clinical syndrome. However, the physician should be careful about giving medications that lower the seizure threshold since many of these children are subject to epileptiform disorders. In addition to learning, behavioral, and seizure disorders, other clinical manifestations found in these children were hearing loss; eye disorders, such as congenital cataracts and glaucoma; cardiovascular disease; urogenital disorders; and an unusually high incidence of endocrine disturbances, such as diabetes mellitus and disease of the thyroid.

Ziring (1978) concludes his interesting article with the statement: "[T]he nature of the disorder contracted by the infants born following the 1964–65 rubella epidemic is now being manifested in new physical and psychological signs as they reach adolesence. . . . [These young people] are continuing to teach us about the pathogenesis and clinical manifestations of congenital infections" (p. 69).

Other Viral Infections

The dermotropic viruses that cause herpes simplex and herpes zoster can also produce encephalitis or meningitis. The mortality rate from herpes simplex encephalitis is very high, and persisting neurological disabilities occur. The antiviral agent, idoxuridine, is reported to be a potential specific treatment (Dale, 1975).

A recent Israeli study of psychiatric patients showed that those with psychotic depressions had high serum antibody levels to the virus of herpes simplex, but not to measles or rubella. Among the schizophrenics, the level of neutralizing herpes simplex antibodies was also high, but lower than that of the psychotically depressed. The investigators emphasize that false positive immune responses produced by psychotropic and other medications may complicate this type of research (Rimon and Halonen, 1977).

Herpes zoster may be manifest in its prodromal stages by complaints of nervousness and irritability that the family labels "neurotic." Also, many patients with herpes zoster exhibit general nervousness, lack of stamina, insomnia, and a whining crabbiness for 1 to 2 months after the skin conditions have cleared.

Epidemic neuromyasthenia is reported by Shelokov (1977) as one of the aspects of the coxsackie and echo viral infections. The symptoms are headache, fatigue, lowered mood, myalgia, some muscular weakness, and paresthesias. This neuromyasthenic syndrome has been noted in many parts of the world. Apparently it affects more women than men, particularly in the acute stages; chronic psychiatric sequelae have been reported in chronic cases. Shelokov suggests that chronic psychoneurosis may be a residual of sporadic or epidemic cases of these infections.

The Chronic "Slow" Viral Infections

Increasing attention is being given to the longer-term effects of viral infections of the central nervous system—the psychiatric as well as the neurologic syndromes that may become apparent years or even decades after the person suffered from the acute infection. During the last 10 years, investigators have found the chronic "slow" viral infections are possibly the responsible etiologic agents for Creutzfeld-Jakob disease and also Alzheimer's presenile dementia. Creutzfeld-Jakob disease has been successfully transmitted from the human to the chimpanzee (*Clinical Psychiatry News,* 1978). Formerly, this rare affliction was thought to be a degenerative disease of the central nervous system, but recent laboratory findings and Heston's description of an association among Alzheimer's disease, Down's syndrome, and myeloproliferative diseases indicate that they may be produced by the effect of viral agents superimposed on a hereditary susceptibility (*Clinical Psychiatry News,* 1978).

Jarvik's report (*Clinical Psychiatry News,* 1978) to the 1978 session of the California Medical Association mentioned that Yugoslavian investigators have associated dementia with an alteration in the immune system; 69 percent of a group of patients with cerebral atrophy were found to have delayed skin hypersensitivity reactions to human brain protein. The possibility that a viral agent is one of the essential etiological agents for such baffling diseases raises hope that the presenile dementias can be prevented, or at least treated successfully, sometime in the not-too-distant future.

Another serious, but fortunately rare, "slow" viral disease is subacute sclerosing panencephalitis (SSPE; inclusion body encephalitis of Dawson) that develops about 4 to 17 years after a clinical attack of measles. It is a progressive, almost invariably fatal encephalopathy that is manifested by personality changes, mental deterioration, involuntary movements, and death within a year or two.

Although there is some presumptive evidence that "slow" viruses are etiologic factors that contribute to the development of serious mental illnesses, the evidence is scanty, and the "slow" virus hypothesis is still a tenuous one. At the Yale University Child Study Center, investigators (Young et al., 1975) found no cerebrospinal fluid abnormalities in 15 children with autism; they conclude that the immunoglobulin levels offered no support for the "slow" virus hypothesis. Thus, opposing points of view about the significance of the "slow" viruses are supported by contrasting findings. Nevertheless, this is an important area of investigation that is just beginning to be evaluated by the advanced scientific methods that can now be employed.

The Virus Hypothesis and Schizophrenia

At the 1975 Totts Gap (Pennsylvania) Colloquium on the Biology of Schizophrenia, Wolf and Berle (1975) suggested that "slow" viruses might explain the penetrance of a schizophrenic genetic trait. In their discussion of a possible viral etiology of schizophrenia, Torrey and Peterson (1976) maintain that viruses are probably responsible for only one subgroup of schizophrenia. An English study of 106 patients referred to the psychiatric inpatient and outpatient units of a general hospital showed that only eight (7 percent) had serum antibody titers to a number of viruses studied (Chacon et al., 1975). These investigators conclude that viral infections are not major factors causing or precipitating the major mental illnesses. At our current level of understanding, it is possible that viruses could account for the genetic patterns observed in chronic forms of schizophrenia, but this line of inquiry requires vigorous and rigorous research (Bigelow et al., 1975).

Mental Retardation

Congenital toxoplasmosis and bacterial meningitis, as well as the various viral agents that have been discussed, are associated with both mental retardation and epileptiform disorders. Although the successful treatment of the bacterial meningitides has reduced many of the complications of these formerly dreaded diseases, it is not known whether the number of cases of mental retardation among the survivors has decreased significantly. Increasing interest in the longer-term effects of the infectious agents on the central nervous system suggests that illnesses such as uncomplicated measles may have mental sequelae (Fog et al., 1968; Stein and Susser, 1974).

In one study, children with a history of measles demonstrated less reading readiness when they entered school than did a control group. In Stein and Susser (1974), Panum (1940) points out that the effects of even the common childhood diseases may depend on the "interaction of the infectious agent and host characteristics" (p. 470). Children who came from middle and upper socioeconomic strata seemed to suffer much less from the sequelae of infectious diseases such as mental retardation, than did those reared in poverty and deprivation.

Citing Dauer et al. (1968), Stein and Susser state: "Social changes have improved host resistance and immunity, effected environmental control, and provided the techniques to prevent or to treat such infectious diseases as syphilis, bacterial meningitis, pertussis, meales, mumps, and rubella" (p. 471).

Furthermore, a better understanding of the encephalitides, toxoplasmosis, common childhood diseases, and cytomegalovirus should lower the incidence of mental retardation and other sequelae. But, the long recognized association between lower social class status and mild mental retardation shows clearly that a reduction of the psychiatric and neurologic sequelae of the infectious diseases of the childhood period depends on an improved quality of life—a lessening of material and cultural deprivation—as well as a greater understanding of virology.

Syphilis of the Central Nervous System

Prior to World War II, general paresis was responsible for almost 10 percent of all admissions to state hospitals in the United States. With the advent of penicillin therapy, the psychiatric and neurologic disorders produced by syphilis have diminished dramatically. In fact, many recent graduates of our medical schools have never seen a case of "dementia paralytica," which was once so common. The number of cases of venereal disease in the United States, however, continues to be very great—the median number of reported cases from 1973 to 1977 was about 700,000, of which about 15,000 were syphilis (U.S.DHEW, 1978). When a disorder such as general paresis has diminished in frequency so dramatically, there is always danger that the occasional case will be overlooked. Recently, Raskind and Eisdorfer (1976) reported that of 216 elderly psychiatric patients, 13 had a positive VDRL test. Eleven of these had a history of syphilis. Such results indicate that there is still a relatively high incidence of past or present syphilitic infection in geriatric psychiatric patients.

The typical symptoms of paresis are: euphoria, delusions of grandeur; some paranoid suspiciousness; and as the disease progresses, confusion, apathy, and neurological symptomatology. Classical neurological signs are the pupillary irregularity, the responses of the pupil to accommodation but not to light (Agryll Robertson), tremors, weakness, and paralyses. Diagnosis depends, of course, on blood and spinal fluid studies.

Malaria

Malaria, which everyone thought had virtually disappeared in the United States, began to be diagnosed more frequently in the early 1970s, coincident with the shuttling of Americans back and forth to the Far East during the Vietnam conflict. The number of civilians in the United States diagnosed as having malaria in 1977 was 466, triple the number diagnosed in 1972 (U.S.DHEW, 1978: p. 332). The recent increase is attributed to the large number of tourists and businessmen going to Asia, Africa, Central America, and the Caribbean. Blocker (1968) and his colleagues, have pointed out that the cerebral anoxia accompanying malaria produces personality disturbances, as well as many neurologic signs and symptoms of brief duration that may be difficult to differentiate from functional psychoses. The correct diagnosis of mental symptomatology caused by malaria depends upon the psychiatric and psychometric evaluations, which reveal transient memory loss, difficulty with recall and concentration, and disorientation, as well as a negative past history for psychiatric illness. Prognostically, patients with functional psychoses tend to remain psychiatrically ill for considerably longer periods of time than do those suffering from a personality disturbance caused by malaria. Furthermore, the clinician should be aware that the use of quinacrine and chloroquine for the treatment of malaria and other illnesses can produce a toxic psychosis.

Brain Abscess

Although brain abscess is now a much rarer condition than it once was, an occasional case is still observed in public hospitals. It is found more commonly in chronic alcoholics, individuals who have been living in poverty, and those not receiving adequate medical care than in other groups of our population. Usually the patient with a brain abscess presents with many of the features of a chronic brain syndrome such as disorientation, memory loss, and confusion. Focal neurological signs may be present. The physician should be aware that the abscess may be encapsulated, and that the patient may not reveal characteristic signs of systemic infection such as fever or leucocytosis. Only a high degree of awareness will enable the physician to undertake the necessary X-ray and laboratory studies that point to the possibility of a brain abscess.

SYSTEMIC DISEASES

Depending upon ego strength, general physical condition, and both the severity and disruptive effects of the illness, any person can become psychiatrically ill when afflicted with an infectious disease or afterward. Whether the disease is bacterial, viral, or fungal is not nearly so important in terms of the psychiatric manifestations as is the quality of the patient's premorbid physical and mental health, quality of life, and his or her capacities for adaptation. Certain general principles increase our understanding of the emotional aspects of the systemic diseases. These are:

1. It is unwise to maintain hard and fast convictions about susceptibility. Generally, the elderly and the chronically ill are more likely to develop psychiatric disorders when they are stricken with an infectious illness than are young adults. But the widespread use and abuse of medications (particularly tranquilizers and stimulants), alcoholism, and drug abuse are factors that contribute substantially to the development of psychiatric disorders when an individual is suffering from an infectious disease.
2. The psychiatric manifestations of the infectious diseases are frequently vague and at times bizarre, not coinciding with textbook descriptions. The clinical patterns are produced by premorbid personality conflicts, stressors at home or at work, and both direct and side effects of chemotherapeutic agents used to combat the infection as well as other medications.
3. Multiple etiologic factors combine to produce the psychiatric disorders associated with infections. Treatment must be directed toward a host of forces, rather than solely toward the infectious agent.
4. Psychiatric disorders following infectious diseases are much more common than generally recognized. In particular, many patients show transient personality disorders, or especially, semichronic depressive episodes for months following a serious infectious disease.
5. Delirium occurring during the course of an infectious illness is the most common psychiatric manifestation of a systemic infection and is a complication of the infectious diseases that too often is neither diagnosed correctly nor treated adequately.

Some Specific Systemic Diseases

Psychiatric disorder is associated with the following systemic illnesses.

Pneumonia

Because it is so often a disease of the elderly who may be chronically ill, the hospitalized patient with pneumonia is particularly susceptible to delirium. Delirious reactions are seen more frequently in patients with bacterial pneumonia, whereas depressive conditions are more commonly observed in patients with viral pneumonia.

Infectious Mononucleosis

The psychiatric manifestations of infectious mononucleosis usually appear during convalesence when the patient is inactive and complains of weakness and easy fatigability. Many of these patients suffer for months from a depressive-like syndrome as a sequel to mononucleosis. The relationship between it and depression, however, is complicated. Investigators at the Mayo Clinic (Harvey et al., 1976) warn that the classic signs of acute psychosis may overshadow the typical symptoms of mononucleosis. Hendler and Leahy's (1978) recent report of two cases of infectious mononucleosis describes the psychiatric sequelae. Both patients suffered depression following the illness; their performance at school deteriorated; and they had EEG abnormalities. Hendler and Leahy suggest that the central nervous system (CNS) involvement following infectious mononucleosis is "similar to minimal brain dysfunction, since both conditions respond to amphetamine-like substances, are associated with difficulty in school, and may be secondary to viral diseases that affect the CNS" (p. 844).

Brucellosis

Emotional disturbances, particularly irritability, depression, lassitude, chronic anxiety, and a neurasthenic state, have been reported so often as sequelae to brucellosis that they are usually dismissed as "merely part of the illness." Although brucellosis is now uncommon in the United States, the emotional symptoms that appear as a chronic mixed anxious-depressed state require vigorous treatment. Patients who have had brucellosis almost always should be placed on vigorous mental and physical rehabilitation programs.

Tuberculosis

This dire, previously common disease has been known historically for its emotional and behavioral manifestations. Fortunately, only slightly more than 20,000 cases per year have been reported in the United States during the 1970s (U.S.DHEW, 1978: p. 334); although during the late 1960s, it was feared that the frequency was increasing, especially among inhabitants of the inner cities. Early in the course of the disease, the patient may appear to be irritably and apathetically depressed, but later may exhibit flushed bouts of excitement that border on hypomanic episodes. Or, sometimes the patient may display a lighthearted optimism that has an unreal quality. Toxicity from isoniazid may be manifested by euphoria, memory disturbance, and an emotional lability, as well as by neurologic signs. The psychiatric aspects of tuberculosis are not limited solely to the patient. Because of the sinister history of the disease, relatives and peers can become excessively anxious, not only about the patient, but also about possible contagiousness. Despite the triumphs of microbiology, a frightening "mystique" continues to surround tuberculosis—consumption is still a feared disease and the word itself is often mentioned only in a hushed whisper.

Hepatitis

About 35,000 cases of hepatitis are reported annually in the United States (U.S. DHEW, 1978: p. 334). The sequelae are so definitely a feature of the course of the overall illness that they have been labeled the posthepatitic syndrome. Major manifestations of this syndrome are lethargy, weakness, irritability, and lowered mood. Often these depressive features are so prominent that the main task of convalescence is to remobilize the patient's energies toward optimism and activity, away from the self-preoccupation and sadness of depression.

A Polish study (Stankiewicz et al., 1975) of 70 female hepatitis patients, age 20 to 40, showed that none were psychotically ill, but that 48 exhibited asthenic reactions. Of these, 29 continued to have manifestations of anxiety and emotional insecurity after the acute hepatitis had subsided. No correlation could be found between the presence of psychiatric symptomatology and the severity of the hepatitis (except for those treated with steroids). The investigators believe that infectious hepatitis disposes to asthenic and anxious syndromes.

MAJOR PSYCHIATRIC DISORDERS MANIFESTED BY INFECTIOUS DISEASES

Anxiety

As we have seen, anxiety is associated with fears of infectious diseases, particularly new or strange ones for which there are no definitive therapies. Also, manifest anxiety is one of the earliest symptoms of delirium that develops during the course of an infectious illness. And, chronic anxiety syndromes, characterized by neurasthenia, can be the sequelae not only of diseases such as brucellosis, but also of many chronic or complicated infective processes.

The anxiety usually appears as apprehension, difficulty with concentration, and particularly, as asthenia. Awareness of its ubiquity and a sensitivity to the patient's emotional distress enable the physician to detect the anxious patient speedily and precisely. Successful treatment calls for listening to the patient's fears and worries—rational and irrational—and explaining what is happening and why. The ensuing clarification and realistic reassurance help the patient to employ his or her intellectual defenses. The rapport between the doctor and the patient increases the patient's level of self-esteem and ability to cope. Use of intellectual defenses, increased self-esteem, awareness that anxiety is a part of the human condition (neither an abnormality nor a "weakness"), and improved coping lower the patient's anxiety level and promote healthy attitudes toward the self as a patient and toward doctors, other hospital personnel, and family and friends.

Generally, adequate nighttime sedation and/or diazepam (Valium) 5 mg t.i.d. or q.i.d. are symptomatically beneficial. They are most effective when the physician has worked with the patient to achieve a greater understanding of the source of the anxiety and to develop a relationship characterized by mutual respect and confidence.

Delirium

Typically, delirium begins gradually on about the third or fourth day after the patient has become acutely ill. But the time of its appearance varies according to the patient's age, general physical condition, previous use of alcohol and/or drugs, and the presence of psychiatric illness prior to the onset of the infectious disease. The presence of delirium is always indicative of biochemical, metabolic, or structural impairment of brain function. During an infectious disease, delirious behavior may parallel the temperature elevation; however, dehydration, lack of sleep, sensory deprivation, electrolyte imbalance, impaired cardiovascular dynamics, the strangeness of the hospital setting, sedatives, tranquilizers, antibiotics, steroids, or other drugs, influence both the onset and the course of delirium. Early diagnosis is critical; it is directly associated with a better prognosis.

Diagnosis and Clinical Picture

Prompt diagnosis is dependent upon finding a disturbance of consciousness produced by the impairment of brain function. The early stage of delirium is characterized by apprehension, restlessness, some disturbance of the sleep pattern, difficulty in concentration, and generally, anxiety about diagnosis and prognosis. Difficulty with evaluating the passage of time is an early clue; the patient may complain that it has been hours since the nurse entered the room while, in reality, it has been only a few minutes. The physician who is alert to the subtler symptoms of early delirium can ask the patient to gauge the passage of 1 minute, or how long the patient thinks the doctor has been in the room. Other signs of early delirium are the patient's inability to follow the hospital routine, mild agitation, and the appearance of slight confusion in the evening.

Obvious confusion, disorientation, and other evidence of perceptual and cognitive insufficiency, such as hallucinations and delusions, are clear indicators that the patient is in the deepening stage of frank delirium. Stupor or convulsions are usually signs of advanced, possibly irreversible, delirium. When the patient with an infectious disease suddenly becomes delirious, the physician should always suspect drug effects, alcoholism, or both. The EEG provides an excellent diagnostic clue to the presence of delirium and also can be used as an indicator of the patient's progress. In delirium, the EEG is characterized by diffuse slowing with a predominance of six to eight per second frequency; as the delirium deepens greater slowing can be observed.

Differential Diagnosis

In a great number of cases, delirium is still misdiagnosed as acute schizophrenia. Differential diagnosis is crucial for patient management. Symptoms such as agitation, confusion, some degree of disorientation, hallucinations, and delusions may be seen in both conditions. However, in delirium these symptoms usually develop over a 12- to 48-hour period and progress in severity more quickly and consistently than in acute schizophrenia. On the other hand, acute schizophrenia is characterized by a slower onset of the symptomatology, inconsistent or erratic development of the symptoms, and a longer prodromal period in which overt anxiety and some bizarre behavior are evident. The patient's age is also a differential factor; almost all patients suffering from their first acute schizophrenic episode are younger than age 35, whereas most patients who develop delirium are older. If the patient has no previous history of a psychiatric disorder, the symptomatology is almost always caused by delirium, not schizophrenia. But when there is a history of previous psychiatric illness, extreme nervousness, or the frequent use of tranquilizers, a clear-cut diagnosis of either delirium or schizophrenia cannot be made without psychiatric consultation. When the physician is in doubt about the diagnosis, the patient should be placed on the treatment program for delirium until the final diagnostic decision is made.

Management

When the physician suspects that the patient is delirious, the following procedures should be carried out as quickly as possible:

1. Reevaluate the patient's general condition by physical examination, laboratory tests, and a mental status examination. These are absolutely necessary in order to detect contributory causes of the delirium. The results of the various examinations should be noted to provide a baseline for gauging changes.

2. Review all orders; discontinue all sedatives; limit medications to only those that are absolutely essential.
3. Protect the patient from harm or from suicide by removing dangerous objects and by locating the patient near the nursing station where he or she is under close observation.
4. Evaluate the patient's perceptual acuity; provide spectacles, hearing aid, etc.
5. Explain all procedures in simple terms.
6. When possible, keep one person (nurse, attendant, or relative) with the patient as much as possible.
7. Simplify environment; keep a dim light on at all times, but be careful that the light does not cast unusual shadows on the walls.
8. Attempt to maintain the patient's orientation by having someone read the daily newspaper, mention the time of day, identify self, etc.
9. For medication, use phenothiazines, such as chlorpromazine (Thorazine); or butyrophenones, such as haloperidol (Haldol). Generally, if the patient has had no adverse reaction, such as hypotension following the initial dose of a chloropromazine, the dosage can be quickly raised to 300 to 400 mg per day. If a test dose of a chloropromazine produces an adverse effect, or if it is contraindicated, administer 5 to 10 mg of haloperidol intramuscularly every 1 to 2 hours until the patient's symptoms have subsided; usual dosage is about 20 to 40 mg per 24 hours (Moore, 1977). Another alternative is 50 to 100 mg of chlordiazepoxide (Librium) every 6 hours.
10. Anticonvulsants may be indicated; if an analgesic is needed, small doses of meperidine (Demarol) are preferred. Vitamins can be helpful, particularly for the elderly or the chronically ill patient.

Depression

The depressive syndrome—characterized by complaints of lowered mood, sadness, and weakness; difficulty eating and sleeping; irritability and pessimism; and, multiple somatic symptoms such as chronic headaches or gastrointestinal dysfunction—is the most frequent psychiatric illness following infectious diseases. Although the timing is variable, the symptoms of depression generally appear during the first week or two of the recovery phase. In the beginning, the depression may resemble a slight relapse, or it may be shrugged off as only a slight delay in convalescence. At such times, however, the patient's general physical condition should be reevaluated to determine whether another physical illness or a physical complication is contributing to the continued lack of well-being. When the patient's physical condition is consistent with recovery from the illness, the patient should be encouraged to become more active because restrictions on activity tend to focus the patient's attention on the weakness and incapacity following the infectious disease, and contribute to the depression.

Diagnosis

The diagnosis of depression depends upon accurately appraising the symptoms, being sensitive to the patients' depressed feelings, and maintaining constant awareness of the relationship between depression and the infectious diseases. The diagnosis of depression following an infectious illness cannot be made solely on the basis of the expressed symptomatology, because symptoms such as irritability, fatigability, headaches, and gastrointestinal dysfunctions cover a wide range of human reactivity and may be residuals of the infectious illness and/or reactions to hospitalization and medical care. Therefore, sensitivity to the patient's feelings of sadness and lowered mood that is evoked in the physician when he or she meets the patient may be one of the most significant clues to the patient's depression. This sensitivity can be enhanced by constant awareness that depression has manifold relationships with the infectious illnesses, preceding, accompanying, or more usually, following them. Furthermore, in order to diagnose the depression of convalescence following infectious illnesses, the physician should be alert to familial or other interpersonal difficulties, problems at work or financial strain, and the patient's often unrealistic goals for full recovery of activity. Also, to achieve precision in diagnosis, the physician should question the patient about recent object loss, make a careful evaluation of the patient's reaction to illness, and maintain a holistic approach, which recognizes the reality of psychological as well as physical distress.

Management

The following guidelines enable the physician to speed the patient's recovery from a depressive episode following an infectious illness:

1. Design a graduated program of physical and mental activity that mobilizes the patient in accordance with his or her physical condition.
2. Hold a conference with the spouse or other family members (with the patient in attendance) in order to clarify the patient's and others' expectations of the degree of activity and obtain consensual agreement about it. At such time, also discuss the implicit, if not expressed, worries about relapse and further invalidism.
3. Use occupational and recreational therapies while the patient is in the hospital to increase the patient's interest in activities and provide tangible evidence that he or she is productive. Gear these tasks to the patient's capabilities, for when the patient is unable to carry them out successfully, a sense of failure develops and the depression tends to deepen. Continue such therapeutic activities during convalescence at home.
4. Prescribe an antidepressant medication such as amitriptyline (Elavil) or imipramine (Tofranil) in dosage of 75 to 150 mg per day.

5. Provide for adequate nighttime sedation. Improved sleep patterns are excellent indicators of the lifting of the patient's depression. Administering amitriptyline in a single bedtime dosage often provides sufficient sedation.
6. Manipulate the environment; often a vacation or change of routine is especially beneficial.
7. Be aware that there is always danger of suicide, particularly late in convalescence when the patient fears that he or she has not really recovered from the infectious illness. Frequently, the suicidal, depressed patient indicates that the situation appears to be hopeless and that "there is no way out." Such threats should not be taken lightly; something constructive should be done at once. Generally, when the patient's depression is impeding convalescence, producing difficulties at home, and is sufficiently severe to produce concern about suicide, it is best to hospitalize the patient for definitive antidepressant therapy.

CONCLUSION

The relationships between infectious diseases and mental illnesses have impressed psychiatrists for at least a century. Particularly in Europe, astute clinicians have thought that patients with asthenic states were unusually susceptible to infectious diseases. In the Lundby Study, which assessed both incidence and prevalence of disease in the general population, Hagnell (1966) found that increased vulnerability to infectious disease, as evidenced by a record of numerous illnesses, was a statistically significant predictor of mental disorder.

The results of a study of 50 patients with chronic anxiety and a control group of asthmatics have recently been published by Studt (1977). Working at the Psychosomatic Clinic at Mannheim, he found that the data disclosed an unanticipated correlation between neurotic anxiety, accidents, and infectious diseases. Studt concludes that patients with unstable personalities (evidencing schizoid and hysterical features) are susceptible to accidents, suicide, neurosis, mental illness, and somatic disease; whereas those who are more stable (tending to show depressive and compulsive traits) are more likely to have had multiple surgical experiences.

Seemingly inexplicable relations also exist between established mental illness and infectious disease. In particular, for years observers have recognized that chronically ill patients in mental hospitals sometimes improve dramatically after they have recovered from a serious infectious disease. Jaspers (1972) notes that as early as 1912, Friedlander reported that a few severe, chronic, catatonic patients who had been inert for years became psychically healthy following an attack of typhus. But, usually the improvement in a mental illness that occurs coincident with the development of a serious infectious disease is transitory. Although we do not know the mechanisms that account for such changes in disease processes, they arouse our scientific curiosity.

Finally, we need to be ever mindful of the complex, pervasive effects of the infectious diseases on the human being whether the organisms invade the central nervous system directly or whether it is affected by toxins produced by microorganisms in the lungs, kidneys, or other parts of the body. As we have seen in this review of psychiatric disorders associated with infectious diseases, further attention to this neglected, somewhat unglamorous topic is urgently needed. The conquest of infectious diseases is not complete. The classic epidemiologic triad—host, agent, and environment—no longer provides a sufficient conceptualization of even the well-defined infectious disease processes. In his recent article, "The Illusion of Simplicity: The Medical Model Revisited," Herbert Weiner (1978) joins others who have insisted for more than a decade that the classic infectious disease model of the pathogenesis of disease is outmoded and insufficient. Based on the new biology of viral infections, Weiner outlines a disease model that is complex, nonlinear, and broad. In summary form, the major components of the model are:

1. Most infectious diseases are endemic, and there are predisposed persons as well as carriers in every population.
2. The person's age at the time of infection and the method of infection influence the course of the illness or the carrier state.
3. A specific infectious agent can "give rise to multiple disease forms, which are determined by the characteristics of the agent in interaction with the host." (Weiner, 1978: p. 31)
4. Adaptation that depends mainly on the immune response to the agent varies quantitatively and qualitatively so far as the individual or the group is concerned.
5. Differing adaptive responses determine, at least in part, the course of the disease and its clinical form.
6. The social setting in which all diseases arise, and the cultural factors shaping the character of the individual's life influence the nature and extent of the infectious diseases, and in turn, the individual and the community are reciprocally affected by infectious diseases.
7. Infectious diseases can be transmitted horizontally—from person to person—and also vertically—from generation to generation.

Weiner concludes: "A modern, biological model of disease contains elements with which psychiatrists have often concerned themselves and is broad enough to accommodate diverse points of view from the molecular to the evolutionary level" (p. 32).

On his deathbed, Pasteur is reputed to have said: "Ce n'est pas le microbe, c'est le terrain." ("It is not the microbe, it is the soil.") (Source unknown)

ACKNOWLEDGMENTS

The author wishes to gratefully acknowledge the research and editorial contributions of his research publications editor, Helen M. Russell.

REFERENCES

Bigelow, L., Bird, R. M., Cancro, R., Cohen, G., Gjessing, L. R., Goldstein, A., Kety, S., Lipton, M., and Werthessen, N. Etiological considerations, in *The Biology of the Schizophrenic Process*. S. Wolf, ed. Plenum Press, New York (1975), pp. 134–150.

Blocker, W. W., Kastl, A. J., and Darnoff, R. D. The psychiatric manifestations of cerebral malaria. *Am. J. Psychiat.* 125:192 (1968).

Chacon, C., Monro, M., and Harper, I. A. Viral infection and psychiatric disorders, *ACTA Psychiat. Scand.* 51:2:101–103 (1975).

Chess, S. Behavior and learning of school-age rubella children. *Final Report: Congenital Rubella–Behavioral Studies (CRBS)*. Project No. MC-R-360183-03-0 (December 1974).

Infective agents implicated in two senile dementias. *Clin. Psychiat. News.* 6:8:33 (1978).

Dale, A.J.D. Organic brain syndromes associated with infections, in *Comprehensive Textbook of Psychiatry II*, 2nd ed., Vol. 1. A. M. Freedman, H. I. Kaplan, and B. J. Sadock, eds. Williams & Wilkins, Baltimore, Maryland (1975), pp. 1121–1131.

Dauer, C. C., Korms, R. F., and Schuman, L. M. *Infectious Diseases*. Harvard Univ. Press, Cambridge, Massachusetts (1968).

Fog, J. P., Black, F. L., and Kogon, A. Measles and readiness for reading and learning: 5. Evaluative comparison of the studies and overall conclusions. *Am. J. Epidem.* 88:359–367 (1968).

Hagnell, O. *A Prospective Study of the Incidence of Mental Disorder*. Scandinavian University Books, Lund Sweden (1966).

Harvey, A. M., Johns, R. J., Owens, A. H. Jr., and Ross, R. S. *The Principles and Practice of Medicine*, 19th ed. Appleton-Century-Crofts, New York (1976).

Hendler, N., and Leahy, W. Psychiatric and neurologic sequelae of infectious mononucleosis, *Am. J. Psychiat.* 135:7:842–844 (1978).

Hoeprich, P. D., ed. *Infectious Diseases: A Modern Treatise of Infectious Processes*, 2nd ed., Medical Dept., Harper and Row, New York (1977), p. 123.

Jaspers, K. *General Psychopathology*. J. Hoenig and M. W. Hamilton, trans. The University of Chicago Press, Chicago, Illinois (1972).

Makita, K. Contemporary concept of autism and autismus infantum, *ACTA Paedopsychiat. (Basel)* 41:4:5:162–169 (1975).

Moore, D. P. Rapid treatment of delirium in critically ill patients, *Am. J. Psychiat.* 134:12:1431–1432 (1977).

Nikolovski, O. T., and Fernandez, J. B. Capgras syndrome as an aftermath of chicken pox encephalitis, *Psychiat. Opin.* 15:2:39–43 (1978).

Panum, P. L. *Observations Made During the Epidemic of Measles on the Faroe Islands in the Year 1946*. Delta Omega Society, Cleveland, Ohio (1940).

Raskind, M. A., and Eisdorfer, C. Screening for syphilis in an aged psychiatrically impaired population. *West. J. Med.* 125:5:361–363 (1976).

Rimon, R., and Halonen, P. Antibody levels to viruses in psychiatric illness, in *The Impact of Biology on Modern Psychiatry*. E. Gershon, ed. Plenum Press, New York (1977), pp. 105–112.

Shelokov, A. Epidemic neuromyasthenia, in *Infectious Diseases: A Modern Treatise of Infectious Processes*, 2nd ed. P. D. Hoeprich, ed. Medical Dept., Harper and Row, New York (1977), pp. 1212–1214.

Stankiewicz, D., Kazubska, M. Wysocki, J. Ekiert, H., and Gogolowa, Z. Psychiatric disturbances in viral hepatitis. *Psychiat. Polska* (Warszawa) 9:4:399–405 (1975).

Stein, Z. A., and Susser, M. The epidemiology of mental retardation, in *American Handbook of Psychiatry,* 2nd ed., S. Arieti (ed. in chief). *Vol. 2. Child and Adolescent Psychiatry, Sociocultural and Community Psychiatry.* G. Caplan, ed., Basic Books, Inc., New York, (1974), pp. 464–491.

Studt, H. H. Partielle selbstvernichtung im gewande einer ''somatischen'' krankheit, *Zeit. Psychosomat. Med. Psychoanal.* (Gottingen) 23:3:219–232 (1977).

Torrey, E. F., and Peterson, M. R. The viral hypothesis of schizophrenia, *Schiz. Bull.* 2(1), (1976), pp. 136–146.

U.S. DHEW, *Morbidity and Mortality Weekly Report,* Vol. 27, No. 36. Center for Disease Control (1978).

Weiner, H. The illusion of simplicity: The medical model revisited, *Am. J. Psychiat.* (July Supplement) 135:27–33 (1978).

Winslow, C.-E.A. *The Conquest of Epidemic Disease: A Chapter in the History of Ideas,* Princeton Univ. Press, Princeton, New Jersey (1943).

Wolf, S., and Berle, B. B. The biology of the schizophrenic process, in *Advances in Behavioral Biology,* Vol. 19. Plenum Press, New York (1975).

Young, J. G., Caparulo, B. K., Shaywitz, B., Bennett, A., Johnson, W. T., and Cohen, D. J. Childhood autism: Cerebrospinal fluid examination and immunoglobulin levels, *J. Am. Acad. Child Psychiat.* 16:1:174–179 (1977).

Ziring, P. R. Psychiatric sequelae of the 1964–65 rubella epidemic. *Psychiat. Ann,* 8:8:57–69 (1978).

Psychiatric Presentations of Medical Illness

CHAPTER 9

Psychiatric Presentations of Endocrine Dysfunction

M.K. POPKIN, M.D.
T.B. MACKENZIE, M.D.

Psychiatric symptomatology frequently appears at some point in the course of endocrine dysfunction. This chapter will consider those psychiatric symptoms that may precede or appear simultaneously with more definitive manifestations of adult onset endocrinopathy and thereby delay the prompt recognition and treatment of the underlying disorder. Excessive or deficient concentrations of cortisol, thyroxine, parathormone, insulin, estrogen, and androgen will be reviewed. Each extreme of concentration will be further divided according to whether it arose spontaneously or was induced.

CORTISOL

Excess

Spontaneous Hypercortisolism

Hypercortisolism (Cushing's syndrome) may spontaneously result from primary dysfunction of the adrenal gland, pituitary adrenocorticotropic hormone (ACTH) hypersecretion, or ectopic ACTH-producing tumors of nonendocrine origin. The term Cushing's disease is conventionally reserved for pituitary dependent hypercortisolism, comprising more than two thirds of all spontaneous cases.

Psychiatric disturbances have been noted in hypercortisolism since Cushing's account (1932). The majority of literature detailing attendant psychopathology has not distinguished between the various forms of hypercortisolism (Sachar, 1975). Nonetheless, several clinically useful points emerge.

First, psychiatric alterations appear early in spontaneous hypercortisolism and may antedate other signs (Trethowan and Cobb, 1952; Spillane, 1951; Ross, 1966). Second, a full spectrum of psychiatric presentations has been observed. Depression is thought the most common, occurring in as many as one third of cases. Organic brain syndromes with cognitive impairment, perceptual dysfunction, and sometimes delirium have been noted in 15 percent (Whybrow and Hurwitz, 1976). Psychoses are found in 5 to 20 percent (Ettigi and Brown, 1978). Overall incidence of mental change has been reported from 40 to 84 percent (Glazer, 1953; Spillane, 1951). Recent work suggests depression is twice as frequent in Cushing's disease as in nonpituitary-dependent forms of hypercortisolism (Carroll, 1977).

Third, the literature does not satisfactorily define risk factors for psychiatric sequelae in the disorder. Nonectopic forms of hypercortisolism are four times as common in women as men and peak in the ages 35 to 50. Ectopic ACTH secretion is predominately a male disorder, occurring later in life (Besser and Edwards, 1972). It shows few of the typical features of hypercortisolism, and psychiatric features are not well explored.

In spontaneous hypercortisolism, the principal therapeutic consideration is correction of the endocrine pathology. New evidence from pituitary microsurgery supports Cushing's etiological postulate and has led to the recommendation that such intervention constitute initial therapy in Cushing's disease (Tyrell et al., 1978).

Induced Hypercortisolism

Induced hypercortisolism may result iatrogenically or factitiously from the administration of ACTH or corticosteroids, systemically or topically. Although psychiatric alterations may emerge at any point in the course of therapy, mental changes have been noted within 6 hours of the initiation of adrenocorticotropic hormone (ACTH) or corticosteroid treatment (Relkin, 1969). Goolker and Schein (1953) described a prodromal state of "cerebral excitability," characterized by irritability and mood lability, which antedated the appearance of more pronounced changes by 72 to 96 hours. Hall et al. (1979) reported the average onset of steroid psychosis to be 6 days after initiation of treatment. Alterations in mood are the most common change, with euphoria greatly exceeding depression (Prange et al., 1975). Disturbed cognition has been noted clinically in as many as one third of patients (Whybrow and Hurwitz, 1976). In any given patient, the symptomatic configuration may fluctuate during a single psychotic episode, at one moment resembling a paranoid state, in the next an acute delirium. This instability has been designated "spectrum psychosis" by Hall et al. (1979). ACTH has been suggested to be more problematic than corticoids (Truelove and Witts, 1959), but this conclusion was drawn from limited data.

The existence of risk factors for psychiatric disturbances following ACTH or steroid therapy has been debated (Hall et al., 1979) Previous steroid psychosis does not predict future reaction nor does previous tolerance assure protection (Sayers and Travis, 1970). A significant dose relationship between steroids and acute psychiatric reactions has been demonstrated (Boston Collaborative Drug Study, 1972); 18 percent of those patients receiving more than 80 mg of prednisone daily experienced major psychiatric sequelae. We know of no studies examining the incidence or nature of psychiatric sequelae in alternate day steroid protocols.

Psychiatric care will require weighing the need to maintain corticosteroids against the anticipated improvement in mental state consequent to gradual reduction of the steroid dosage. Excellent response to phenothiazines has been reported in a series of steroid psychoses (Hall et al., 1979). Tricyclics have been reported to worsen steroid-induced disturbances (Hall et al., 1978). Following removal or major reduction of steroids, spontaneous recovery has been noted to range between 2 weeks and 7 months.

Deficiency

Spontaneous Hypocortisolism

Hypocortisolism (Addison's disease) may result spontaneously from dysfunction of adrenal cortical tissue or hypothalamic-pituitary failure. In either case, it is generally insidious in onset with Addisonian crises being rare. Psychiatric concomitants of hypocortisolism, first noted by Addison (1868), have received less attention than their counterparts associated with hypercortisolism. It has been suggested that little has subsequently been added to Addison's account of the mental changes involved (Whybrow and Hurwitz, 1976).

Psychiatric alterations commonly antedate full-blown hypocortisolism (Sorkin, 1949). Such presentations incorporate mild cognitive impairment and a depressive, apathetic mood state. Early symptoms of deficiency include negativism, poverty of thought, lack of initiative, and fatigue. These may progress to a frank organic mental disorder with delirium (Ettigi and Brown, 1978). Overall incidence of mental changes has been reported to range from 64 to 84 percent (Engel and Margolin, 1941; Cleghorn, 1951). Depression in these studies ranged from 37 to 48 percent. When the disease is known to be of several years' duration, more pronounced organic deficits and euphoria have been noted to emerge (Relkin, 1969).

The psychiatric features together with symptoms such as asthenia, easy fatigability, anorexia, nausea, vomiting, syncope, hiccough, paresthesias, or lumbar pain, should alert the clinician to the possible diagnosis of hypocortisolism (Drake, 1957). Hypotension, adverse reaction to analgesics and sedatives, electrolyte disturbance, pigmentation changes, low voltage in the cardiogram, eosinophilia, or lymphocytosis may be useful in suggesting the disorder is present.

Hypocortisolism is often accompanied by EEG abnormalities and perceptual alterations, including reduced sensory thresholds (Henkin, 1970). Such changes, together with psychiatric sequelae, are reversed only with adequate glucocorticoid replacement, not electrolyte correction alone (Ettigi and Brown, 1978). The use of psychotropics has been reported to exacerbate hypotension (Thompson, 1973) in hypocortisolism; indeed, this problem may initially suggest the unrecognized diagnosis.

Induced Hypocortisolism

Hypocortisolism may occur iatrogenically following adrenalectomy, removal of an adrenal tumor, the administration of thyroid or insulin to a patient with pituitary cachexia, inadequate corticoid replacement, or removal of corticoid replacement. Any one of these may evoke adrenal crisis in which confusion and marked organicity will likely constitute the psychiatric picture. The psychiatric literature has not to date addressed induced hypocortisolism as yielding constellations that differ from those discussed in the spontaneous group.

THYROXINE

Excess

Spontaneous Hyperthyroidism

Although hyperthyroidism encompasses multiple conditions in which the gland spontaneously becomes overactive, the psychiatric literature has largely concerned itself with thyrotoxicosis. This condition is "almost invariably associated with mental changes," (Ettigi and Brown, 1978: p. 120). Nervousness (manifested as a feeling of apprehension, restlessness, and inability to concentrate), emotional lability, and hyperkinesia characterize the thyrotoxic patient (Sachar, 1975). Psychoses are rare (Smith et al., 1972), possibly restricted to the exacerbations of pre-existing disorders (Sachar, 1975). Depression is seen with apathetic hyperthyroidism, in which muscular weakness precludes hyperkinesia (Sachar, 1975). Whybrow et al. (1969) have shown that organic impairment accompanies hyperthyroidism, though it is lesser in degree than with deficiency states. Delirium may signal the onset of thyroid storm (Ettigi and Brown, 1978).

Thyrotoxicosis displays a striking female preponderance of 7:1. It is most common in ages 20 to 30 and must be differentiated from other disturbances, particularly neurasthenia. In this regard, several points are useful. In thyroid dysfunction sleeping pulse will remain accelerated; sedated pulse will exceed 80 (Crown et al., 1966); palms will be dry and warm, not cool and clammy (Sachar, 1975); fatigue will be accompanied by a desire to be active; and cognitive dysfunction is more prominent than in neurasthenia. Early thyrotoxicosis may go unrecognized by an unwary physician.

As regards treatment, Whybrow et al. (1969) suggested that the restoration of a euthyroid condition was accompanied by little residual (cognitively or affectively) in hyperthyroid subjects. However, organic deficits may persist in a minority of patients (Ettigi and Brown, 1978), and correction of hyperthyroidism alone may not always suffice from a psychiatric perspective (Deutsch, 1968). Phenothiazines have been shown useful in thyrotoxic patients, but they may intensify tachycardia (Shader et al., 1970). Tricyclics and MAO inhibitors are usually not warranted, as hyperthyroid patients may show increased sensitivity to their toxic properties (Shader et al., 1970). Use of adrenergic blockers must be tempered by their psychiatric side effects (Jefferson, 1974). Correction of the thyrotoxic state is the primary treatment consideration.

Induced Hyperthyroidism

Induced hyperthyroidism may result iatrogenically. More problematic is thyrotoxicosis factitia, a disorder usually encountered in women. The diagnosis is made from the combination of typical thyrotoxic signs (save infiltrative ophthalmopathy) together with hypofunction of thyroid hormones and can be confused with rare cases of thyrotoxicosis involving ectopic thyroid tissue.

Deficiency

Spontaneous Hypothyroidism

Since early descriptions of advanced hypothyroidism, psychiatric disturbances have been recognized as an integral part of the thyroid deficiency state. Almost every type of psychiatric reaction has been delineated in hypothyroid patients (Gibson, 1962); organic deficits (especially mental slowing and intellectual impairment) are frequently mentioned in most reports.

Psychiatric presentations may be the first sign of spontaneous hypothyroidism (Logothetis, 1963; Pitts and Guze, 1961; Pomeranze and King, 1966). Gibson (1962) noted that the diagnosis may be missed "unless the physical signs are gross" (p. 197). Most often the hypothyroid patient will show progressive cognitive impairment (Gibson, 1962) exceeding that in hyperthyroid states (Whybrow et al., 1969). The incidence of cognitive change has been observed to be as much as 93 percent (Smith et al., 1972). Affective disturbances are also common (Whybrow and Hurwitz, 1976). Psychoses occur infrequently in spontaneous hypothyroidism; reported cases of myxedematous madness (combined etiologies) are said to number 150 (Olivarius and Röder, 1970). When encountered, psychosis is organic in form, resembling organic paranoid states of epilepsy rather than delirium (*British Medical Journal,* 1977). The electroencephalogram shows slowing in severe cases proportional to the depression of metabolic rate (Ettigi and Brown, 1978).

Spontaneous hypothyroidism is predominately encountered in women, ages 40 to 60; its manifestations may be protean (Butts, 1970). They include asthenia, decreased libido, cerebellar signs, peripheral neuropathies, pseudomyotonic reflexes, paresthesias, deafness, slowed speech, facial edema, large tongue, hoarseness, decreased sweating, skin and hair changes, cold intolerance, and slowed pulse. This partial list reflects the necessity for careful review of systems and neurological examination when confronted with the aforementioned organic psychiatric presentations. Risk factors for changes in hypothyroidism are not well clarified.

Many authors have reported total remission of psychiatric disturbances with the introduction of replacement hormone. Chronic deficiency appears to leave residua (Whybrow and Hurwitz, 1976), but reversibility has been reported after an interval of 4 years (Röder and Olivarius, 1970). According to Tonks (1964), replacement appears more likely to suffice psychiatrically if patients are older than 50, have less than 2 years of deficiency, and present in an organic mode. Easson (1966) noted replacement alone worked well in spontaneous cases (but not always in induced ones). Both ECT and tricyclics have been successfully used conjointly with hormone replacement (Pitts and Guze, 1961; Pomeranze and King, 1966; Easson, 1966). Phenothiazines have precipitated hypothermic coma in advanced hypothyroidism (Jones and Meade, 1964), and minor tranquilizers may obscure thyroid function studies (Shader et al., 1970). If possible, full psychiatric intervention should await the restoration of a euthyroid condition.

Induced Hypothyroidism

Surgical removal, radioactive ablation, or the introduction of antithyroid medications, including lithium carbonate, may iatrogenically result in hypothyroidism. Most commonly, the induced deficiency becomes manifest within months of the precipitating intervention, but the cumulative incidence increases over time (Ingbar and Woeber, 1974). Few articles in the psychiatric literature explore induced hypothyroidism separately; most often this group is combined with the spontaneous. Replacement therapy, particularly in this group, has been noted to precipitate or aggravate a psychotic constellation (Easson, 1966). Whiting (1969) has suggested this occurrence may be more common when replacement is begun abruptly in larger than usual dosages.

PARATHORMONE

Excess

Spontaneous and Induced Hyperparathyroidism

In 80 percent of cases, spontaneous primary hyperparathyroidism results from adenomatous neoplasia of one of the parathyroid glands (Potts, 1977). Renal tumors and squamous cell carcinomas of the lung can produce a substance that has parathormone-like activity. Nonspecific signs such as pain, lassitude, constipation, weakness, fatigue, and anorexia, or signs of affective disturbance, such as loss of initiative and dysphoria, develop insidiously in 30 to 50 percent of cases and may predate the diagnosis by years (Granville-Grossman, 1971; Peterson, 1968; Eliasson, 1971). Psychotic disturbances with prominent paranoid and organic features may be the presenting features when the serum calcium has risen precipitously, such as in the case of parathyroid crisis (Granville-Grossman, 1971). Peterson (1968) demonstrated that affective disturbance is associated with less severe hypercalcemia (12 to 16mg%),whereas organic mental disorders predominate when the calcium exceeds16mg%. In general, correction of the hypercalcemia leads to prompt resolution of symptoms (Peterson, 1968; Agras and Oliveau, 1964).

Deficiency

Spontaneous and Induced Hypoparathyroidism

Spontaneous idiopathic hypoparathyroidism is a rare disease. The most common cause of hypoparathyroidism is accidental damage to or removal of parathyroid tissue during thyroidectomy (Potts, 1977). Postoperative symptoms may develop days or even years later. In a review of over 300 cases, Denko and Kaelbling (1962) noted that although intellectual impairment was common in idiopathic hypoparathyroidism, it was unusual in postoperative hypoparathyroidism. The same authors speculated that the diagnosis and treatment of postoperative hypoparathyroidism, given a history of neck surgery, was made before intellectual impairment could develop. The incidence of psychiatric manifestations in both idiopathic and surgical hypoparathyroidism runs between 30 to 50 percent (Smith et al., 1972; Denko and Kaelbling, 1962). Presenting psychiatric symptoms range from organic mental disorders to nonspecific symptoms, such as weakness, fatigue, irritability, and nervousness (Smith et al., 1972). It is especially important to note that hypoparathyroidism results in a lowered threshold to the occurrence of symptomatic hyperventilation (Fonseca and Calverley, 1967) and to an increased sensitivity to the acute dystonias induced by phenothiazines (Schaff and Payne, 1966). Unusual attacks of rigidity and mutism resembling catatonia have been reported as the primary manifestation of hypoparathyroidism (Fonseca and Calverley, 1967). With the exception of impaired intellect, normalization of serum calcium causes symptomatic improvement (Sachar, 1975).

INSULIN

Excess

Spontaneous Hyperinsulinism

Spontaneous hyperinsulinism can occur in either a fasting or postprandial (reactive) state. Excessive insulin concentration in a fasting state generally indicates that a pancreatic beta cell adenoma, or less commonly a carcinoma, is present. In addition, there are a few reports of nonpancreatic tumors releasing an insulin-like substance (Megyesi et al., 1974). The presenting symptoms of fasting hyperinsulinism almost invariably have a psychiatric component. The resulting symptomatology reflects hyperepinephrinemia and cerebral glucopenia. As the plasma glucose falls, the putative hypothalamic glucose thermostat causes an outpouring of epinephrine that mobilizes existing hepatic stores of glucose, promotes gluconeogenesis and reduces non-central nervous system (CNS) consumption of glucose. This state of hyperepinephrinemia mimics the central and peripheral signs of anxiety. Thus, the patient may appear nervous, pale, diaphoretic and tremulous. The pupils may be dilated, blood pressure and pulse elevated, and the patient may complain of a throbbing headache, weakness, palpitation, respiratory difficulty, and apprehension (Innes and Nickerson, 1975). If the hyperepinephrinemia is not successful in preventing the blood glucose level from falling beneath 30 to 40 mg%, signs of neuronal dysfunction may appear secondary to cerebral glucopenia. The spectrum of symptomatology then ranges from seizures, focal neurological signs and coma to paranoid thinking, hallucinations, and delirium. Episodes of fasting hyperinsulinism usually occur prior to breakfast when the period of fasting has been the longest. However, they can appear several hours after meals and thus resemble reactive hyperinsulinism. Exercise, pregnancy, fever, or alcohol consumption can hasten the onset of symptoms. The attacks themselves are usually stereotypic in a given patient, but differ from person to person. Although the symptomatology is intermittent, repeated episodes can cause sufficient neuronal damage to give a picture of dementia, depression, or schizophrenia (Martin et al., 1977).

The diagnosis of fasting hyperinsulinism depends upon demonstrating an excessively elevated plasma insulin during a period of hypoglycemia (Fajans, 1977). Thus, it is wise to collect a blood sample for determination of the plasma concentration of immunoreactive insulin (IRI) at the same time as a plasma glucose is drawn. If the latter is pathologically reduced, then the IRI sample is sent for analysis.

The first priority in the treatment of spontaneous hyperinsulinism is the correction of hypoglycemia. This is accomplished via the ingestion of carbohydrate-rich substances or the intravenous administration of glucose. Especially in the case of a beta cell carcinoma, glucose may need to be given constantly until the source of insulin secretion can be controlled.

Postprandial or reactive hypoglycemias are generally due to asynchrony of the factors that control glucose homeostasis and not to absolute hyperinsulinism. Only the reactive hypoglycemias secondary to gastrectomy (Hofeldt et al., 1974), intestinal hypermotility (Freinkel and Metzger, 1969), or accelerated intestinal glucose absorption (Permutt et al., 1973) seem to involve an excessive release of insulin. The clinical picture of reactive hyperinsulinism is usually characterized by brief episodes of hyperepinephrinemia occurring 2 to 4 hours after meals. There is seldom evidence of cerebral glucopenia, as in fasting hyperinsulinemia. However, Hafken et al. (1975) have described organic mental dysfunction in several patients with postgastrectomy hypoglycemia.

Treatment of the reactive hypoglycemias secondary to hyperinsulinism involves regulation of the rate at which glucose arrives at, and is absorbed by, the intestinal mucosa. This has been accomplished through multiple, low carbohydrate feedings, anticholinergics (Fajans, 1977), and agents that retard intestinal absorption of glucose, such as phenformin (Permutt et al., 1973).

Induced Hyperinsulinism

Induced hyperinsulinism is not an uncommon occurrence in the management of diabetes mellitus. Evidence of hyperepinephrinemia may be masked by autonomic insufficiency so that the signs of cerebral glucopenia may predominate.

Perhaps more than any other hormone, insulin has been used factitiously to induce symptoms. Typically, the patient is a single young women who has had personal, familial, or professional exposure to the use of insulin (Burnam et al., 1973). These patients exhibit histrionic features and frequently terminate hospitalization if factitious illness is discovered (Moore et al., 1973). A recently developed assay for C-peptide, which is released in equimolar concentrations to insulin, has made it possible to distinguish exogenous from endogenous insulin once the diagnosis of hyperinsulinism is made (Scarlett et al., 1977).

Deficiency

Spontaneous Hypoinsulinism

A spontaneous deficiency of insulin occurs in diabetes mellitus. The earliest manifestations of diabetes, such as fatigue, anorexia, polyuria, and blurred vision, may be mistaken for neurasthenia or hypochondriasis. Alternatively, diabetes may present explosively as ketoacidosis or hyperosmolar coma. The attendant acute organic mental disorder is usually responsive to correction of the metabolic disorder. In a small percentage of cases, impotence may be the earliest presentation of diabetes (Cooper, 1972). Thus, a workup of protracted impotence should include a glucose tolerance test. Premature atherosclerosis and the cumulative effects of recurrent ketoacidosis or hyperosmolar coma can produce an organic mental disorder that may resemble depression or schizophrenia. In these cases, treatment is symptomatic and supportive.

Induced Hypoinsulinism

A factitious deficiency of insulin may occur if a diabetic patient discontinues his or her treatment for either self-destructive and/or attention-seeking purposes. Such a situation is an indication for initiation of a dialogue about the patient's emotional concerns.

ESTROGEN

Excess

Spontaneous and Induced Hyperestrogenemia

Estrogen secreting tumors in males have been reported to diminish both libido and potency. Spontaneous hyperestrogenemia occurs in women during pregnancy and secondary to certain neoplasms. Iatrogenic hyperestrogenemia accompanies chemotherapy of prostatic carcinoma in males and feminization of male transsexuals. Psychiatric sequelae are not well described in these populations. Factitious hyperestrogenemia has not received detailed attention.

The iatrogenically induced hyperestrogenemic state that has received greatest attention is the use of birth control pills. In total, depressive symptomatology arises in some 10 percent of users (Ettigi and Brown, 1978). Women with prior psychiatric history, those with more frequent menstrual symptomatology, and those with highest expectations of adverse effects are at greater risk for depressive constellations upon taking oral contraceptives (Weissman and Klerman, 1977). There is some evidence that these depressions may relate more to the progestin action of the drugs than to the effects of estrogen (Glick and Bennett, 1972). Estrogen in oral contraceptives has reportedly given rise to a pyridoxine-sensitive depressive state (Adams et al., 1973). Struve et al. (1976) showed a significant relationship between paroxysmal EEG activity and symptomatic pill use, perhaps reflecting the CNS excitant role of estrogen.

Deficiency

Spontaneous Hypoestrogenemia

Hypoestrogenemia arises spontaneously in females attendant to ovarian failure, hypothalamic-pituitary failure, or gonadal dysgenesis (e.g., Turner's syndrome). In addition, states of relative hypoestrogenemia are encountered within the menstrual cycle and following child bearing. An estrogen-deficiency syndrome is not known in men. Psychiatric correlates of estrogen deficiency are poorly understood. The role of androgens and progesterone confound the clinical picture.

In Turner's syndrome, patients have congenitally low estrogen levels; they frequently exhibit mild mental retardation, immature personality patterns, friendliness, passivity, and low sex drive. No cases of severe antisocial behavior in Turner's syndrome have been reported (Christodorescu et al., 1970). Estrogen replacement restores sex drive in this group (Ettigi and Brown, 1978).

The withdrawal or reduction of estrogens produces physical change, vasomotor phenomena, and depressive symptomatology; these features are thought common to menopause, hypopituitarism, and clomiphene (anti-estrogen) therapy (Ettigi and Brown, 1978). Yet, Winokur (1973) found no greater risk for depression during the menopause than at other times of the life span. Neither is there evidence that depressions in the menopause have a distinct clinical pattern of presentation (Weissman and Klerman, 1977). The increased risk of endometrial carcinoma in users of conjugated estrogens (Ziel and Finkle, 1975) has tempered the prior enthusiasm for replacement therapy.

Smith (1975) has estimated that one third to three fifths of women experience negative, affective change during the late luteal phase of the menstrual cycle, when estrogen and progesterone begin to fall rapidly from the postovulatory peak. This premenstrual tension syndrome, including irritability, depression, fluid retention, headache, and lethargy, has been the subject of much debate and conjecture. Smith (1975) believes it to be a real phenomenon, though probably not a unitary one. No one sex hormone can be implicated (Weissman and Klerman, 1977), and the role of psychosocial factors should not be overlooked. There is agreement that the premenstruum represents a time of higher risk for recurrently psychotic women (Smith, 1975), irrespective of the nature of the disorder.

Abrupt reductions of estrogen and progesterone levels introduce the postpartum period, the time of highest risk for psychiatric disturbance, particularly depression, in women. The spectrum of change spans mild dysphoria to psychosis; the risk period extends several months. Postpartum blues, a nearly ubiquitous phenomenon, appears within 10 days of delivery and resolves spontaneously (Yalom et al., 1968). The appearance of vegetative signs and feelings of guilt and inadequacy 3 to 4 weeks following delivery suggests a postpartum depression. This carries a more favorable prognosis than does postpartum psychosis of a schizophrenic form. The treatment of postpartum disturbances has included most known psychotropic agents with variable success. Postpartum disorders, appearing coincident with or subsequent to rapid hormonal variation, suggest that a critical relationship exists between the levels of estrogen and progesterone and psychiatric disturbances. One recent theory holds estriol withdrawal as central to postpartum disorders (Smith, 1975). It seems prudent to recall that postadoption psychoses, nearly identical to those found in puerperal psychotic patients, have been described (Victoroff, 1952; Tetlow, 1955). Hence, efforts to implicate relative hypoestrogenemia in the etiology of psychiatric disorders remain speculative at present.

Induced Hypoestrogenemia

Iatrogenic hypoestrogenemia may follow oophorectomy or clomiphene therapy. We have no reason, at present, to distinguish psychiatric aspects of the former from spontaneously arising ovarian failure as with menopause. Psychiatric accounts of the sequelae of clomiphene are at present anecdotal; the drug is suggested to augment male libido and has been utilized in the management of impotence in patients with renal failure. Iatrogenic hypoestrogenemia in males is not known.

ANDROGEN

Excess

Spontaneous Hyperandrogenemia

Spontaneous hyperandrogenemia arises in males secondary to testicular or adrenal neoplasms and in females secondary to ovarian or adrenal neoplasms. Excess androgen in males may cause insomnia or irritability but does not lead to a consistent alteration in libido (Martin et al., 1977; Brown, 1975). In contrast, increased or even excessive libido may be the presenting manifestation of hyperandrogenemia in females (Williams et al., 1977). Since the incidence of androgen-secreting tumors in both sexes is low, a characteristic psychiatric presentation has not been identified in either case. A role for androgens in aggressive or violent behavior in males has been sought. Although these behaviors, particularly if they occur in adolescence, may be positively correlated with androgen levels, there is insufficient evidence to causally link violence and aggression to pathological elevations of androgen (Rose, 1975).

Induced Hyperandrogenemia

Induced hyperandrogenemia may occur during treatment of males for hypogonadal states, or in females during antitumor therapy. Males may complain of insomnia or irritability, whereas females may notice an increased libido. Sands and Chamberlain (1952) noted that adolescent males with character disorders and prominent aggressivity were made worse and appeared overstimulated when given dehydroisoandrosterone. Wilson et al. (1974) reported the appearance of paranoid delusions in four of five depressed males given imipramine and methyltestosterone simultaneously. Thus, in males with pretreatment psychopathology, the incidence and severity of psychiatric complications attendant to androgen therapy appears to be increased.

Deficiency

Spontaneous Hypoandrogenemia

Spontaneous hypoandrogenemia in males may be secondary to either testicular or pituitary failure. Once established, male libido and potency are relatively insensitive to changes in plasma androgen levels (Martin et al., 1977; Cooper, 1972). However, hypoandrogenemia in adult males has been associated with psychiatric symptomatology in three conditions. First, subnormal intelligence and personality disorder with passive aggressive or schizoid features are common manifestations of Klinefelter's syndrome (Swanson and Stipes, 1969). Isolated reports in these patients cover the entire range of psychopathology (Wakeling, 1972). Testosterone replacement in older males with Klinefelter's syndrome appears to be of little value in the treatment of either impotence, or the mental disturbances (Sachar, 1975). In contrast, younger subjects seem to respond more favorably to androgen replacement (Johnson et al., 1970). Second, diminished libido and impotence may be the presenting manifestations of insidious hypopituitarism (Daughaday, 1974). Third, is the syndrome described in males of variable age known as the male climacteric. In addition to alteration in sexual drive, the presenting manifestations may include vasomotor instability, irritability, inability to concentrate, and episodic depression (Feldman et al., 1976). Several uncontrolled studies report prompt reversal of these symptoms following treatment with intramuscular testosterone (Heller and Myers, 1944; Feldman et al., 1976). Other authors dispute the existence of the syndrome (Brown, 1975; Cooper, 1970). If there is a history of scrotal or inguinal surgery, an atrophy of the testes, or biochemical evidence of testicular failure (decreased testosterone, elevated LH), in a patient who complains of loss of libido and impotence, the possibility of the male climacteric should be considered.

Induced Hypoandrogenemia

Induced androgen deficiency may arise in males as a complication of irradiation or surgical procedures involving the testis, scrotum, inguinal area, or pituitary. The symptoms, similar to those associated with the male climacteric, respond to testosterone enanthate. In females, adrenal androgens appear to be necessary for the maintenance of normal libido and sex drive. Thus, adrenalectomy or hypophysectomy results in a loss of libido, which can be restored with with testosterone (Brown, 1975).

CONCLUSION

We consider the psychiatric syndromes consequent to endocrine disease to be examples of organic mental disorders. Although this designation suggests that defects in arousal, attention, cognition, or perception will be prominent, this is not always the case. The preceding discussion reflects the varied nature of the psychiatric symptomatology that may antedate or accompany endocrine dysfunction. Unless physical signs are gross, the presence of an endocrinopathy may not be suspected. To minimize this likelihood, we suggest that the clinician confronted with psychiatric disturbance attend to the following points.

First, careful attention must be given to the patient's age, sex, and personal or family history of psychiatric illness. Are these consistent with known patterns of onset and genetic features of psychiatric illness? Any initial psychiatric presentation arising beyond age 35 should suggest underlying medical illness, particularly in the absence of a family history of psychiatric illness.

Second, in obtaining a history, special attention should be given to the temporal sequence of symptom emergence, past endocrine and medical problems, and current and prior medications. The presence of situational factors does not exclude a concurrent medical illness.

Third, a detailed review of systems is imperative. Discrete symptoms of endocrinopathy such as syncope, impotence, temperature intolerance, menstrual irregularity, or skin and hair change may be obscured by a neurasthenic history and appearance.

Fourth, clinical examination must include special attention to alterations in temperature, heart rate, respiration, and blood pressure, careful inspection for known concomitants of endocrine dysfucntion, and a rigorous neurological and mental state exam. Consideration should be given to obtaining neuropsychological testing, electroencephalography, and blood determinations directly or indirectly indicative of endocrine functions.

Fifth, a corroborative history is often indispensible in correctly identifying the presence of behavioral abnormalities indicative of organic mental disorder.

In a given individual, the presenting psychiatric manifestations of an endocrine dysfunction may resemble any psychopathological entity. In practice, however, certain presentations are more common than others. Symptoms of affective disturbance and/or cognitive dysfunction account for most of the psychiatric manifestations of endocrine disorder. The affective disturbances may be either acute or insidious in onset and may have prominent paranoid features. Cognitive dysfunction, evidenced clinically by disorientation, incomprehension, dysmnesia, and hallucinations, tends to be discernible in severe endocrinopathy. Cognitive dysfunction, which develops insidiously, may be disguised by compensatory responses.

In conclusion, it is important to recognize that endocrinopathies and the attendant behavioral manifestations are generally reversible. The likelihood of reversibility is favored by early recognition and intervention. The first priority of treatment is correction of the underlying endocrine dysfunction. Full psychiatric intervention should, if possible, await such correction.

REFERENCES

Adams, P. W., Rose, D. P., Folkard, J., Wynn, V., Seed, M., and Strong, R. Effect of pyridoxine hydrochloride (vitamin B_6) upon depression associated with oral contraception. *Lancet*. 1:897–904 (1973).

Addison, T. Disease of the supra-renal capsules, in *Collection of the Published Writings of the Late Thomas Addison*. MDA, New Sydenham Society, London, England (1868) pp. 209–239.

Agras, S., and Oliveau, D. Primary hyperparathyroidism and psychosis. *Canad. Med. Assn. J.* 91:1366–1367 (1964).

Besser, G. M., and Edwards, C.R.W. Cushing's syndrome. *Clin. Endocrinol. Metabol.* 1:451–489 (1972).

Boston Collaborative Drug Surveillance Program: Acute adverse reaction to prednisone in relation to dosage. *Clin. Pharm.* 13:694–697 (1972).

Brit. Med. J., edit. The thyroid and the psychiatrist. 1:931–932 (1977).

Brown, G. M. Psychiatric and neurologic aspects of endocrine disease. *Hosp. Pract.* 10:2:71–79 (1975).

Burnam, K. D., Cunningham, E. J., Klachko, D. M., Bazzoui, W. E., and Burns, T. W. Factitious hypoglycemia. *Am. J. Med. Sci.* 266:23–30 (1973).

Butts, H. F. Psychiatric aspects of myxedema. *J. Nat. Med. Assn.* 62:134–138 (1970).

Carroll, B. J. Mood disturbances and pituitary-adrenal diseases. *Psychosom. Med.* 39:54 (1977).

Christodorescu, D., Collino, S., Zellingher, R., and Tauta, C. Psychiatric disturbances in Turner's syndrome. *Psychiat. Clin.* 3:114–124 (1970).

Cleghorn, R. A. Adrenal cortical insufficiency: Psychological and neurological observations. *Canad. Med. Assn. J.* 65:449–454 (1951).

Cooper, A. Diagnosis and management of endocrine impotence. *Brit. Med. J.* 2:34–36 (1972).

Cooper, A. Guide to treatment and short term prognosis of male potency disorders in hospital and general practice. *Brit. Med. J.* 1:157–159 (1970).

Crown, S., Crisp. A. H., and Ellis, J. P. Some aspects of the diagnosis of thyrotoxicosis. *J. Psychosom. Res.* 10:209–14 (1966).

Cushing, H. The basophil adenomas of the pituitary body and their clinical manifestations (pituitary basophilism). *Bull. Johns Hopkins Hosp.* 50:137–*195 (1932)*.

Daughaday, W. H. The adenohypophysis, in Textbook of Endocrinology, 5th ed., R. H. Williams, ed. W. B. Saunders Company, Philadelphia, Pennsylvania (1974), pp. 31–79.

Denko, J.D., and Kaelbling, R. Psychiatric aspects of hypoparathyroidism. *Acta Psychiat. Scand.* (Supp). 164:38:7–70 (1962).

Deutsch, S. F. Recent contributions in psychoendocrinology. *Psychosom.* 9:127–34 (1968).

Drake, F. R. Neuropsychiatric-like symptomatology of Addison's disease: A review. *Am. J. Med. Sci.* 234:106–113 (1957).

Easson, W. M. Myxedema with psychosis. *Arch. Gen. Psychiat.* 14:277–283 (1966).

Eliasson, S. Disorders of the nervous system in diabetes. *Med. Clin. N. Am.* 55:1001–1006 (1971).

Engel, G. L., and Margolin, S. G. Neuropsychiatric disturbances in Addison's disease and the role of impaired carbohydrate metabolism in production of abnormal cerebral function. *Arch. Neurol. Psychiat.* 45:881–884 (1941).

Ettigi, P. G., and Brown, G. M. Brain disorders associated with endocrine dysfunction, in *The Psychiatric Clinics of North America Symposium on Brain Disorders: Clinical diagnosis and management*. H. C. Hendrie, ed. W. B. Saunders Company, Philadelphia, Pennsylvania (1978), pp. 117–136.

Fajans, S. S. Hyperinsulinism, hypoglycemia, and glucagon secretion, in *Harrison's Principles of Internal Medicine*. G. W. Thorn, R. D. Adams, E. Braunwald, W. Isselbacher, and R. G. Petersdorf, eds. McGraw-Hill Book Co., New York (1977), pp. 586–595.

Feldman, J., Postlethwaite, R., and Glenn, J. Hot flashes and sweats in men with testicular insufficiency. *Arch. Intern. Med.* 136:606–608 (1976).

Fonseca, O., and Calverley, J. Neurological manifestations in hypoparathyroidism. *Arch. Intern. Med.* 120:202–206 (1967).

Freinkel, N. and Metzger, B. Oral glucose tolerance curve and hypoglycemia in the fed state. *N. Eng. J. Med.* 280:820–828 (1969).

Gibson, J. G. Emotions and the thyroid gland: A critical appraisal. *J. Psychosom. Res.* 6:93–116 (1962).

Glaser, G. H. Psychotic reactions induced by corticotropin (ACTH) and cortisone. *Psychosom. Med.* 15:280–291 (1953).

Glick, I. D., and Bennett, S. E. Psychiatric effects of progesterone and oral contraceptives, in *Psychiatric Complications of Medical Drugs*. R. I. Shader, ed. Raven Press, New York (1972), pp. 295–331.

Goolker, P., and Schein, J. Psychic effects of ACTH and cortisone. *Psychosom. Med.* 15:589–613 (1953).

Granville-Grossman, K. *Recent Advances in Clinical Psychiatry*. Churchill, London, England (1971), pp. 191–239.

Hafken, L., Leichter, S., and Reich, T. Organic brain dysfunction as a possible consequence of postgastrectomy hypoglycemia. *Am. J. Psychiat.* 132:1321–1324 (1975).

Hall, R.C.W., Popkin, M. K., and Kirkpatrick, B. Tricyclic exacerbation of steroid psychosis. *J. Nerv. Ment. Dis.* 166:738–742 (1978).

Hall, R.C.W., Popkin, M. K., Stickney, S. K., and Gardner, E. Presentation of the "steroid psychoses." *J. Nerv. Ment. Dis.* 167:229–236 (1979).

Heller, C. G., and Myers, G. B. The male climacteric, its symptomatology, diagnosis, and treatment. *J.A.M.A.* 126:472–476 (1944).

Henkin, R. I. The neuroendocrine control of perception, in *Perception and Its Disorders*. D. Hamburg, ed., Williams & Wilkins, Baltimore, Maryland (1970), p. 54.

Hofeldt, F. D., Lufkin, E. G., Hagler, L., Block, M. B., Dippe, S. E., Davis, J. W., Levin, S. R., Forsham, P. H., and Herman, R. H. Are abnormalities in insulin secretion responsible for reactive hypoglycemia? *Diab.* 23:589–596 (1974).

Ingbar, S. H., and Woeber, K. A., in *Textbook of Endocrinology*, 5th ed. R. H. Williams, ed. W. B. Saunders Company, Philadelphia, Pennsylvania (1974), pp. 95–232.

Innes, I. R., and Nickerson, M. Norepinephrine, epinephrine, and the sympathomimetic amines, in *The Pharmacological Basis of Therapeutics*, 5th ed. L. S. Goodman and A. Gilman, eds., MacMillan, New York (1975), pp. 447–513.

Jefferson, J. W. Beta-adrenergic receptor blocking drugs in psychiatry. *Arch. Gen. Psychiat.* 31:681–689 (1974).

Johnson, H. R., Myhre, S. A., Ruvalcaba, R. H., Thaline, H. D., and Kelly, V. C. Effects of testosterone on body image and behavior in Klinefelter's syndrome—a pilot study. *Develop. Med. Child Neurol.* 12:454–460 (1970).

Jones, J. H., and Meade, T. W. Hypothermia following chlorpromazine therapy in myxedematous

patients. *Geront. Clin.* (Basel) 6:252–256 (1964).
Logothetis, J. Psychotic behavior as the intial indicator of adult myxedema. *J. Nerv. Ment. Dis.* 136:561–568 (1963).
Martin, J. B., Reichlin, S., and Brown, G. M. *Clinical Neuroendocrinology*. F. A. Davis, Philadelphia, Pennsylvania (1977), pp. 275–303.
Megyesi, K., Kahn, C. R., Roth, J., and Gorden, P. Hypoglycemia in association with extrapancreatic tumors: Demonstration of elevated plasma NSILA-s by new radioreceptor assay. *J. Clin. Endocrinol. Metabol.* 38:931–934 (1974).
Moore, G. L., McBurney, P. L., and Service, F. J. Self-induced hypoglycemia: A review of psychiatric aspects and report of three cases. *Psychiat. Med.* 4:301–311 (1973).
Olivarius, B. D., and Röder, E. Reversible psychosis and dementia in myxedema. *Acta Psychiat. Scand.* 46:1–13 (1970).
Permutt, M., Kelly, J., Bernstein, R., Alpers, D., Siegal, B., and Kipnis, D. Alimentary hypoglycemia in the absence of gastrointestinal surgery. *N. Eng. J. Med.* 288:1206–1210 (1973).
Peterson, P. Psychiatric disorders in primary hyperparathyroidism. *J. Clin. Endocrin. and Metabol.* 28:1491–1495 (1968).
Pitts, F. N., and Guze, S. B. Psychiatric disorders and myxedema. *Am. J. Psychiat.* 118:142–147 (1961).
Pomeranze, J., and King, E. J. Psychosis as first sign of thyroid dysfunction. *Geriat.* 21:211–212 (1966).
Potts, J. T. Disorders of parathyroid glands, in *Harrison's Principles of Internal Medicine, 8th ed. G. W. Thorn, R. D. Adams, E. Braunwald, K. J. Isselbacher, and R. G. Petersdorf, eds. McGraw-Hill Book Co., New York (1977), pp. 2014*–2025.
Prange, A. J., Breese, G. R., Wilson, J. C., and Lipson, M. A. Pituitary and suprapituitary hormones: Brain-behavioral effects, in *Topics in Psychoendocrinology*. E. J. Sachar, ed. Grune and Stratton, New York (1975), pp. 105–120.
Relkin, R. Effect of endocrines on central nervous system. Part 1. *N.Y. St. J. Med.* 69:2133–2145 (1969).
Röder, E., and Olivarius, B. D. Reversible organic psychosyndrome in hypothyroidism. *Acta Neurol. Scand.* (Supp.) 46:43:81–82 (1970).
Rose, R. M. Testosterone, aggression and homosexuality, in *Topics in Neuroendocrinology*. E. J. Sachar, ed. Grune and Stratton, New York (1975), pp. 83–103.
Ross, E. J., Marshall-Jones, P., and Friedman, M. Cushing's syndrome diagnostic criteria. *Quart. J. Med.* 35:149–192 (1966).
Sachar, E. Psychiatric disturbances associated with endocrine disorders, in *American Handbook of Psychiatry,* Vol. 4. S. Arieti and M. Reiser, eds. Basic Books, Inc., New York (1975), pp. 299–313.
Sands, D. E., and Chamberlain, G. H. Treatment of inadequate personality in juveniles by dehydroisoandrosterone. *Brit. Med. J.* 2:66–68 (1952).
Sayers, G., and Travis, R. H. Adrenocorticotropic hormone; adrenocortical steroids and their synthetic analogs, in *The Pharmacological Basis of Therapeutics,* 4th ed. J. S. Goodman and A. Gilman, eds., MacMillan, New York (1970), pp. 1604–1642.
Scarlett, J. A., Mako, M. Rubenstein, A. H., Blix, P. M., Goldman, J., Horwitz, D. L., Tager, H., Jaspan, J. B., Stjernholm, M. R., and Olefsky, J. M. Factitious hypoglycemia. *N. Eng. J. Med.* 297:1029–1032 (1977).
Schaff, M., and Payne, C. Dystonic reactions to prochlorperazine in hypoparathyroidism. *N. Eng. J. Med.* 275:991–994 (1966).
Shader, R. I., Belfer, M. L., and DiMascio, A. Thyroid function, in *Psychotropic Drug Side Effects: Clinical and Theoretical Perspectives*. R. I. Shader and A. DiMascio, eds. Williams & Wilkins, Baltimore, Maryland (1970), pp. 25–45.

Smith, C. K., Barish, J., Correa, J., and Williams, R. H. Psychiatric disturbance in endocrinologic disease. *Psychosom. Med.* 34:69–86 (1972).

Smith, S. L. Mood and the menstrual cycle, in *Topics in Psychoendocrinology*. E. J. Sachar, ed. Grune and Stratton, New York (1975), pp. 19–58.

Sorkin, S. A. Addison's disease. *Med.* 28:371–425 (1949).

Spillane, J. D. Nervous and mental disorders in Cushing's syndrome. *Brain* 74:72–94 (1951).

Struve, F. A., Saraf, K. R., Arko, R. S., Klein, D. F., and Becka, D. R. EEG correlates of oral contraceptive use in psychiatric patients. *Arch. Gen. Psychiat.* 33:741–745 (1976).

Swanson, D. W., and Stipes, A. H. Psychiatric aspects of Klinefelter's syndrome. *Am. J. Psychiat.* 126:814–822 (1969).

Tetlow, C. Psychoses of childbearing. *J. Ment. Sci.* 101:629–639 (1955).

Thompson, W. F. Psychiatric aspects of Addison's Disease: Report of a case. *Med. Ann. D. C.* 42:62–64 (1973).

Tonks, C. M. Mental illness in hypothyroid patients. *Brit. J. Psychiat.* 110:706–710 (1964).

Trethowan, W. H., and Cobb, S. Neuropsychiatric aspects of Cushing's syndrome. *Arch. Neurol Psychiat.* 67:283–309 (1952).

Truelove, S. C., and Witts, L. J. Cortisone and corticotrophin in ulcerative colitis. *Brit. Med. J.* 1:387–393 (1959).

Tyrell, J. B., Brooks, R. M., Fitzgerald, P. A., Cofoid, P. B., Forsham, P. H., and Wilson, C. B. Cushing's disease: Selective trans-sphenoidal resection of pituitary microadenomas. *N. Eng. J. Med.* 298:753–758 (1978).

Victoroff, V. M. Dynamics and management of parapartum neuropathic reactions. *Dis. Nerv. Syst.* 13:291–298 (1952).

Wakeling, A. Comparative study of psychiatric patients with Klinefelter's syndrome and hypogonadism. *Psychol. Med.* 3:139–154 (1972).

Weissman, M. M., and Klerman, G. L. Sex differences and the epidemiology of depression. *Arch. Gen. Psychiat.* 34:98–111 (1977).

Whiting, E. G. Thyroid delirial states. *Southwest. Med.* 50:179–181 (1969).

Whybrow, P. C., and Hurwitz, T. Psychological disturbance associated with endocrine disease and hormone therapy, in *Hormones, Behavior, and Psychopathology*. E. J. Sachar, ed., Raven Press, New York (1976), pp. 125–143.

Whybrow, P. C., Prange, A. J., and Treadway, C. R. Mental changes accompanying thyroid gland dysfunction. *Arch. Gen. Psychiat.* 20:48–63 (1969).

Williams, G. H., Dluhy, R. G., and Thorn, G. W. Diseases of the adrenal cortex, in *Harrison's Principles of Internal Medicine,* 8th ed. G. W. Thorn, R. D. Adams, E. Braunwald, K. J. Isselbacher, and R. G. Petersdorf, eds. McGraw-Hill Book Co., New York, (1977), pp. 520–557.

Wilson, I. C., Prange, A. J., and Lara, P. P. L-Triiodothyronine alone and with imipramine in the treatment of depressed women, in *The Thyroid Axis, Drugs, and Behavior*. A. J. Prange, ed. Raven Press, New York (1974), pp. 49–64.

Winokur, G. Depression in the menopause. *Am. J. Psychiat.* 130:92–93 (1973).

Yalom, I. D., Lunde, D. T., Moos, R. H., and Hamburg, D. A. Postpartum blues syndrome. *Arch. Gen. Psychiat.* 18:16–27 (1968).

Ziel, H. K., and Finkle, W. D. Increased risk of endomentrial carcinoma among users of conjugated estrogens. *N. Eng. J. Med.* 293:1167–1170 (1975).

Psychiatric Presentations of Medical Illness

CHAPTER 10

Psychiatric Presentations of Cardiovascular Disease

ROBERT W. GUYNN, M.D.

INTRODUCTION

> ". . . The cause of madness is seated primarily in the blood vessels of the brain, and . . . depends upon the same kind of morbid and irregular actions that constitute other arterial diseases."
>
> Benjamin Rush (1812)

The idea that the heart, blood vessels, and blood are the sources of life and emotion (and by extension of madness) is surely as old as symbolic thought. Even an occasional modern investigator has hypothesized that cardiovascular abberrations may underlie certain so-called functional psychiatric illnesses. Labile blood pressure has been linked to juvenile delinquency (Mawson, 1977); altered cardiac function, or decreased regional cerebral blood flow, to schizophrenia (Schneider, 1969; Ingvar, 1974; Ingvar and Franzén, 1974), and hypertension to paranoia (Seidel, 1977). Such ideas of an important role for cardiovascular dysfunction in functional psychiatric illness is, of course, very much a minority opinion. At the same time, it is hardly necessary to point out that disturbances in the cardiovascular system can produce a variety of organically based behavioral changes ranging from personality disturbances to psychosis to coma. The study of such organically based mental changes resulting from cardiovascular and cerebrovascular disease (in particular) would seem to be especially important. The correlation of specific focal lesions with resulting behavioral changes would carry the potential for gaining some general insight into the mental organization of the brain. Such studies are worthwhile, even though simple cause and effect relationships will be difficult or impossible to establish—in part because personality functions are not strictly located in isolated areas, and in part because it is difficult to control for other factors that may be influencing a mental reaction to an organic lesion in a given patient.

Ideally, for anatomical/psychological correlation, one would like to be able to exclude premorbid personality factors as well as psychological responses to illness itself. Unfortunately, such exclusions are difficult and perhaps impossible to achieve absolutely. Much of the literature on the psychiatric manifestations of cardiovascular disease is anecdotal. The premorbid personality is rarely ever taken into account, even though the basic personality influences the type and extent of behavior and personality change in response to an organic assault. (The schizoid individual is probably more susceptible to organic derangements of personality than, say, the rigidly obsessive person.) Likewise, early behavioral change in response to organicity is typically an extension of the individual personality. To the extent, then, that certain personality types are at increased risk from cardiovascular diseases (Jenkins, 1978; Hurst et al., 1976), a potential bias is introduced into the form of the mental presentation of cardiovascular disease.

Likewise, it is often difficult to sort out whether a behavioral change (especially anxiety and depression) is a manifestation of an organic compromise of the central nervous system or a reaction to illness, since these emotional disturbances can be manifestations of either. For example, overt depression following stroke has been frequently observed clinically (Adams, 1963; Bell, 1966) and has usually been assumed to be reactive in response to the realization of physical impairment. Folstein et al. (1977) have tried to address the question by matching stroke patients with patients with similar physical disabilities, not of central origin. The Hamilton Rating Scale and other psychometric tests were administered to both sets of patients with the conclusion that: (1) the increased rate of depression following stroke cannot be accounted for simply by disability, implying that there is a central organic mechanism, and (2) stroke in the nondominant hemisphere is more likely to lead to depression. Unfortunately, Robins (1976), working independently and using a similar experimental design has come to the opposite conclusion: that the depression following stroke is reactive rather than organic. Presumably, either more extensive studies or increased numbers of patients will eventually resolve the issue. In spite of the lack of resolution, at least the proper questions have been asked and addressed experimentally. Unfortunately, interpretation of much of the rest of the literature is complicated by the fact that the need to distinguish between reactive and organic emotional disturbances is sometimes not even recognized.

Another problem with the literature arises simply out of diagnostic confusion. Psychotic patients may be called "schizophrenic," with little or no justification from diagnostic criteria; obtunded or demented patients may be called "depressed,'' simply because of decreased motor behavior and withdrawal from the environment. For example, Thompson (1970) reports a case of hemorrhage from an aneurysm simulating schizophrenia. This particular patient seems to mimic (albeit incompletely) certain motor aspects of catatonic schizophrenia. However, no other criteria for the diagnosis were employed, and, in fact, the patient is probably simply a case of akinetic mutism seen with such lesions, and not to be confused with schizophrenia. Even depression may not be as fool-proof a diagnosis as one might think. Take for example, the following case history:

> The patient was a 53-year-old married woman without previous psychiatric history. Carcinoma of the colon was diagnosed and the patient successfully underwent an abdominal peroneal resection soon after her hospitalization. Before surgery, she expressed considerable concern to the staff about having cancer and about the surgery. After surgery, the patient seemed withdrawn and depressed. She showed little interest in her surroundings and seemed to pay little attention to visitors. One evening her husband came to visit, and while talking with the patient, suffered a stroke and was himself hospitalized. After this event, the patient seemed even more withdrawn and depressed. She showed marked psychomotor retardation and no interest in learning about self care of her colostomy. Nevertheless, she did well medically and was scheduled for discharge. The actual discharge, however, was delayed until she could be seen in consultation for her depression.
>
> On examination, the patient presented as a pleasant individual with slow mentation. She gave only short, simple, and superficial answers to questions about how she felt. She specifically denied being depressed or anxious. She also denied particular concern about her operation or about her husband. Her affect would be better described as blunted rather than depressed. Though she superficially seemed reasonably alert, when questioned directly she did not know the name of the hospital or the city. She not only did not know the date but also did not know the year, month, or even the season.

Even though this patient has sufficient reasons to develop a reactive depression—having cancer, a colostomy, and a seriously ill husband—her problem, in fact, was an organic blunting of affect, superficially mimicking the motor and attention components of depression. Therefore, it is with some reservation that one accepts diagnostic labels or even descriptive terms in the literature unless criteria for use of the terms are explicitly stated, up to and including formal psychological testing.

Therefore, because of the absence or rarity of prospective studies taking into account the premorbid personality, because of the general absence of suitable controls, because of the poverty of rigorous diagnostic or research criteria for personality change, and because of the difficulty of separating reactive from organic components, it is almost impossible at this point in time to deal with any but the most severe disruptions of personality—disruptions so major as to overshadow uncertainties of premorbid personality, reactivity, and diagnostic criteria. The discussion to follow, therefore, will be restricted to major disorders and will leave the question of the organic basis of milder behavioral disturbances for the most part to future work.

There should, perhaps, be a clarification of terms. Whether functional psychiatric symptomatology is reproduced by physical lesions, or merely mimicked by them, is unresolved. Philosophically, the mind-body duality has become progressively untenable, but the alternate view that all mental activity and personality must have a biological basis is seldom confronted directly at a clinical level. A unified, psychobiological view of mental activity would require that not only the personality of each individual be a unique summation of his experience but, necessarily, also his brain biology. Experience and mental activity would alter neurochemistry, which in turn would modulate future behavior and reaction. Neurological development and psychological development in a unified view would be seen as mutually interdependent aspects of the same process. Likewise, a complete loss of the concept of a mind-body duality would dissolve the boundary between behavioral changes on an "organic" basis and behavioral changes on a "functional" basis. And, of course, there are many patients who do seem to straddle the boundary. Amphetamine can induce a paranoid psychosis in the absence of intellectual function deficits (Kalant, 1966), and extremely disorganized schizophrenic or manic individuals can show disorientation and other clear-cut "organic" symptoms. Nevertheless, in spite of significant reservations about the exclusiveness of the terms, it would seem wise to still retain "organic" and "functional" as a kind of shorthand. For the current discussion, since the subtlely and internal consistency of functional disorders is infrequently matched by organic brain syndromes, "organic" will be used to denote disturbances in mentation due to more or less gross externally imposed metabolic derangements of central nervous system physiology. "Functional" will be used to denote disturbances in mentation which seem to arise as a part of a longitudinal evolution and development of the individual in the absence of demonstrable physical pathology.

CARDIOVASCULAR DISORDERS AS CAUSES OF MENTAL DISTURBANCES

Simply, any cardiovascular disease or process that interferes with the blood supply to the brain has the potential to produce neurologic and psychiatric symptoms. To exhaustively list the various cardiovascular diseases and discuss the psychiatric manifestations reported with each would be a lengthy exercise to no great purpose. Such an approach would put too much emphasis on individual diseases and would tend to imply that individual diseases may have distinctive mental presentations. It is in fact, however, the extent, localization, rapidity of onset, and reversibility of the organic assault which are more important than the specific disease process. For example, cardiovascular problems that produce global compromises of brain function are indistinguishable from each other and from a wide variety of toxic and metabolic problems. All such illnesses produce nonspecific organic brain syndromes as have been described in other chapters. It is the focal cerebrovascular problems, however, that offer some special interest. The study of thromboses, emboli, hemorrhages, A-V malformations, aneurysms, and localized functional deficits of blood supply offers some insights into the mental structure of the brain. It is these localized lesions that will be the subject of the remaining discussion. The discussion has been organized along the general lines of the mental status exam (Table 1), beginning with behavioral changes that are extensive, or that may be mistaken for functional disorders.

TABLE 1. MENTAL STATUS EXAMINATION

DISORDERS OF BEHAVIOR

- Personality change
- Altered states of consciousness

DISORDERS OF AFFECT AND MOOD

- Anxiety/fear
- Depression/mania
- Inappropriate affect
  - pathological laughing
  - pathological crying
- Pacifity/rage

DISORDERS OF COMMUNICATION AND THOUGHT

- Aphasias (and the related agraphias and apraxias)
- Hallucinations
- Delusions
  - Reduplication

DISORDERS OF INTELLECTUAL FUNCTION

- Memory
- Abstracting ability
- Judgement
- Calculating

Disorders of Behavior

The patient with chronic diffuse vascular disease can present with a wide variety of often vague complaints including headaches, sleep disturbance, hypochondriasis, mood lability, and decreased concentration. Deterioration of intellectual function is part of the process, but may not be obvious initially. The symptoms of a typical organic brain syndrome eventually evolve. There are few studies attempting to correlate focal pathology with individual symptoms. The discrete ischemic (lunar) infarcts usually associated with hypertension may produce similar personality changes in combination with signs of bilateral motor involvement (increased deep tendon reflexes, extensor plantar responses, etc.) and pseudobulbar palsy. To the casual observer, the personality changes of patients with diffuse vascular disease may be seen as a wide variety of neurotic symptoms, especially since early personality changes tend to be quantitative rather than qualitative. The behavioral changes are extensions or exaggerations of the patients's normal personality.

More discrete or localized vascular lesions may also produce clinical presentations that superficially mimic functional psychiatric disease of all sorts. For example, the *thalamic syndrome* (usually resulting from occlusion of the thalamogeniculate branch of the posterior cerebral artery) produces pain and unpleasant sensations over one side or part of the body. This isolated symptom may erroneously be dismissed as hysterical. Another example would be the syndrome of *akinetic mutism* seen with infarctions in the brainstem of the hypothalamus (especially caudally) and with bilateral lesions of the thalamus (injury to the reticular activating system is presumed, Cravioto et al., 1960). The patient may follow the observer with his eyes but is unresponsive to command and has no voluntary movement. The syndrome may be confused with psychosis (catatonic schizophrenia, psychotic depression). The *syndrome of neglect* is another peculiar behavioral change that arises especially from lesions of the non-dominant parietal lobe, but may also be seen with infarction of the dominant lobe, anterior cingulate gyrus, and frontal lobe. Patients with this syndrome often show a peculiar lack of concern about their stroke or may even manifest a euphoria. They may deny that anything is wrong (anosognosia) or even that the affected limb is theirs. The patient seems to ignore sensory input to the affected side especially if simultaneous stimulation is presented on both sides. There may be an actual or functional hemianopsia with the patient demonstrating strange behavior, such as reading halves of sentences, combing one side of his head, putting on one shoe, or shaving one side of the face. Such neglect of one side of the body can take place even in the absence of paralysis. A patient referred to by Jewesbury (1969) was a conductor who, after a right parietal vascular accident, ignored the musicians on his left. Other more common psychiatric presentations of vascular disease that deserve separate mention are the *frontal lobe syndromes* and the *disturbances of consciousness*.

Frontal Lobe Syndrome

The so-called frontal lobe syndrome is especially associated with bilateral prefrontal and basiiar cortex lesions, but may arise with pathology in other areas.

The patient manifests altered behavior with a release of inhibitions and decline of social graces and moral restraint. He is inappropriate and disorderly and may manifest a wide variety of sometimes severe affective changes (irritibility, jocularity, euphoria, depression). There is a general loss of initiative with apathy and little interest in the future. Associated symptoms may include impairments in orientation, attention, learning, abstract thinking, perception, and memory, although overall intelligence on testing need not be below normal (Feuchtwanger, 1923; Kleist, 1934; Brickner, 1936; Rylander, 1939).

Altered States of Consciousness

The global disruptions of consciousness of delirium and coma occur frequently in general encephalopathies on an infectious, toxic, or metabolic basis. However, focal lesions can also produce such symptomatology. Torpor, pathological sleep, and coma result from pathology of subcortical structures, in particular the brain stem (reticular activating system). Acute confusional states (delirium) are conceptualized by Chédru and Geschwind (1972) as having an erratic shifting of attention as the basic deficit. Attention may be broken into tonic and phasic components. The tonic process sets the threshold a stimulus must reach to attain consciousness; the phasic process is essentially selective attention. Focal infarcts in the dimesencephalon markedly impair the tonic process (Segarra, 1970). It is likely that selective attention is, in part, a cortical function (Mesulam et al., 1976), and acute delerium has been reported with infarctions in the distribution of the anterior, middle, and posterior cerebral arteries (Hyland, 1933; Amyes and Nielsen, 1955; Horenstein et al., 1967; Medina et al., 1974; Mesulam et al., 1976). In general, lesions of the reticular formation; subcortical structures like the thalamus; and the parietal, temporal, and occipital cortices are especially indicted in disturbances of attention. It is worth noting that defects of attention are also found in functional psychiatric illness (Meldman, 1964; Venables, 1964; Orzack and Kornetsky, 1966). For example, the schizophrenic patient has defects in selective attention and may actually verbalize that he feels overwhelmed by a flood of sensory stimulation from the environment and from within. He is unable to sort out the important from the unimportant; everything seems to be equal.

DISORDERS OF AFFECT AND MOOD

Various affective disturbances are associated with generalized organic brain disease, including widespread vascular lesions such as arteriosclerosis. Lability of affect is probably most classic. At times, an interviewer may find himself unable to reflect or empathize with the patient's emotional state because it is shifting so rapidly. More persistent affective disturbances have also been associated with general brain disease, including depression, euphoria, jocularity (Witzelsucht), anxiety, and blunting. Focal brain disease such as bilateral thalamic lesions may also produce lability of affect.

Localized lesions that produce emotional and affective disturbances almost always impinge upon or interfere with the function of the limbic system, which includes the hypothalamus, cingulate gyrus, anterior thalamic nuclei, fornix, and hippocampus (Papez, 1937). Though particular types of affective disturbances are associated to some extent with certain areas of the limbic system, there is considerable overlap of territory, and the individual's premorbid personality probably plays an important role in the clinical manifestations. A very good review of the general subject of emotion and brain disease is that of Poeck (1969).

Anxiety and Fear

Though anxiety can be produced experimentally by stimulation of parts of the limbic system (Penfield and Jasper, 1954; Mullan and Penfield, 1959) and can be part of an epileptic attack, relatively little information is available about the effect of discrete lesions, in particular cerebrovascular disease, on this emotion. Anxiety and fear can be part of organic brain syndromes from multiple causes, and it is exceedingly difficult to decide in a given patient whether the affective disturbance is primary, or a reaction to disorientation and impaired intellectual function. It would seem premature, therefore, to try to relate specific cerebrovascular lesions to so basic an emotion as anxiety.

Depression and Mania

Depression has been associated with temporal lobe tumors especially on the nondominant side (Pia, 1953). In fact, depression is more common in tumors of the temporal lobe than in any other type of tumor (Fischer-Brügge, 1950). Folstein et al. (1977) have made a similar association between stroke in the nondominant hemisphere and depression, but, as previously mentioned, there is not agreement among investigators (Robins, 1976). Posterior fossa masses, including unruptured aneurysm, have also presented with depression (Yaskin and Alpers, 1944; Duvoisin and Yahr, 1965; Morley, 1967), and depression may be associated with frontal lobe or basal ganglia disease. Therefore, depression as a symptom probably has relatively little localizing value. Lesions of the temporal lobe (Tönnis and Schürmann, 1949), or of the hypothalamus, pons, or midbrain (Förster and Gagel, 1939), have rarely produced (or been associated with) manic-like states of euphoria.

Inappropriate Affect—Pathological Laughing and Crying

In these syndromes, the affective components of emotion are provoked by nonspecific stimuli, are generally unassociated with the corresponding mood, are out of voluntary control, and do not fatigue. The syndrome is seen in bilateral lesions affecting the pyramidal tracts together with accompanying extrapyramidal fibers, with lesions to the substantia nigra, the cerebral peduncles and caudal hypothalamus, the interal capsule and basal ganglia, and perhaps with bilateral thalamic lesions (Poeck, 1969). *Fou rire prodomique* is the very rare eruption of pathological laughter as the prodromal symptom of an impending stroke (Féré, 1903; Andersen, 1936; Baadt, 1927).

Pacifity and Aggression

A diminution of drive and emotional responsiveness implies bilateral lesions of the limbic system, particularly of the anterior cingulate gyrus and medial temporal lobe. Placidity as part of a Klüver-Bucy syndrome can arise in human patients from acute bitemporal infarctions. Bilateral involvement of Ammon's horn is probably essential. This syndrome, which was originally experimentally induced and studied in monkeys, consists of visual agnosia, hypermetamorphosis (touching and examining everything in environment), oral investigation (examining things by placing in mouth), placidity, hypersexuality, and changes in dietary habit (Klüver, 1958). The syndrome is seen only with acute lesions or acute phases of more chronic illnesses and is only variably complete in human patients (Pilleri, 1967; Poeck, 1969). The syndrome has been associated with arteriosclerosis (Pilleri, 1967).

Pathological rage arises from lesions in the anterior midline and has been reported with aneurysm of the posterior communicating artery (Poeck, 1969). The regions of the septum pellucidum, the hypothalamus, and medial temporal lobes are often the sites of the pathology. Except in some cases of epilepsy, the rage reactions are undirected. Occasionally, like pathological laughing and crying, rage may be provoked by neutral stimulations and be so stereotyped as to suggest so-called "sham-rage", seen in experimental animals. More often, however, the patient experiences the buildup of emotion until it forces itself to expression. Organically based paranoid ideas may be the stimulus in some instances.

Disorders of Communication and Thought

Acute major cerebral infarction by thrombosis, hemorrhage, or embolism may lead to the sudden disruptions and disorganizations of thought characteristic of acute delirium. Smaller, repetitive assaults and infarctions typically result in a gradual impoverishment of both the content and stream of thought. The patient becomes more concrete and literal, and the structure of sentences and the vocabulary become less complicated. Speech becomes circumstantial, and ideas perseverate. Evasiveness and defensiveness intrude themselves if the patient's declining intellectual capacity is challenged. Dementia becomes the final evolution. Occasional patients with transient ischemic episodes without infarction will show such disturbances in thought rapidly alternating with normal behavior within the space of a single interview.

A number of disturbances of communication and thought can also be produced by localized vascular lesions or infarctions which, in the absence of motor deficits, may be confused with functional disturbances. The rapid output of abnormal speech (logorrhea) which may be seen in fluent aphasias may be misdiagnosed as psychosis, as may the halting telegraphic speech of the nonfluent aphasias. Decreased verbalization may be misinterpreted as the mutism of catatonia, hysteria, or psychotic depression. Body image distortions or indifference resulting from parietal lesions may be labeled hysterical. Hallucinations, paranoid delusions, jargon aphasia (in which the patient responds with nonsense words), anosognosia (denial of illness), and apraxia add to the strangeness that may be part of presentation of an individual with a vascular lesion.

Aphasias

Compromise or infarction of specific areas of either the dominant or nondominant cortex can produce more or less discreet defects of language (Goodglass and Kaplan, 1972; Heilman, 1974; Brain, 1961). Most of these lesions result from infarction in the distribution of the middle cerebral artery.

Pure word deafness resulting from destruction of the primary auditory area of the temporal lobe, or the connections of this area with the posterior superior temporal region (Wernicke's area), produce a syndrome in which the patient has normal spoken language, writing, and reading comprehension but is unable to interpret speech. Destruction of Wernicke's area itself results in more severe disturbances (*Wernicke's aphasia*). The patient not only has impaired comprehension but also expression. He can neither understand nor repeat speech. He may manifest logorrhea, paraphrasia and jargon aphasia, sometimes of a severe degree. In the latter case, the patient may respond to all questions only with a perseveration of nonsense words or syllables. Visual as well as auditory comprehension is compromised and the patients are often unaware of their deficits (anosognosia).

Broca's aphasia (expressive or motor aphasia) is a nonfluent aphasia (often accompanied by hemiplegia) that results from damage to the posterior portion of the third frontal gyrus and the frontal operculum. The language of such patients is telegraphic, impoverished, and agrammatical. Articles, prepositions, and normal punctuation may be omitted. What little speech is produced is done slowly and with great effort. In extreme cases, the patient neither speaks nor writes. The patient is aware of the deficit and may manifest affective excess. Series speech such as reciting the alphabet or singing may be well preserved, however. There is often an associated inability to write spontaneously (agraphia), or to copy (acopia).

Conduction aphasia arises when only the connections between Wernicke's and Bronca's areas are damaged, but the areas themselves are spared. The lesion is usually deep in the parietal lobe above the sylvian fissure. Although speech comprehension is intact, repetition, naming, and writing are poor. Repetition of short words seems to be especially difficult. Reading comprehension and spontaneous speech are variably affected.

Global aphasia resulting in both receptive and expressive defects arises from massive lesions destroying both Wernicke's and Broca's areas. The patient neither comprehends nor speaks, and there is typically a severe hemiplegia.

Nominal aphasia arises with lesions in the angular gyrus, or between the angular gyrus and the posterior part of the superior temporal gyrus of the dominant parietal lobe. In mild forms, a difficulty in naming familiar objects is also seen in diffuse brain disease, or with fatigue or anxiety. This difficulty with naming results in certain circumlocutions in speech.

Amnesic aphasia arises from lesions in the region of the angular gyrus and sometimes from diffuse lesions such as arteriosclerosis. The patient has poor speech impulse and limited vocabulary and seems to be unable to find the right words. He is aware of the deficit.

Infarction of the corpus collosum (supplied by anterior cerebral artery) results in an inability to name stimuli received only in the nondominant hemisphere (Geschwind, 1967).

Infarctions of the medial dominant hemisphere (in the distribution of the anterior cerebral artery) produce a usually transient aphasia (*transcortical aphasia*) resembling that of Broca, except that repetition and series speech are sometimes preserved (Heilman, 1974).

Agraphia

Though inability to write correctly often accompanies aphasia, agraphia can arise as an isolated phenomenon if motor memory areas of either parietal lobe are infarcted. *Gurstmann's syndrome,* arising from infarction of the dominant parietal lobe, consists of agraphia, difficulty with calculations, confusion of right and left, and difficulty naming one's own fingers.

Apraxia

The nondominant parietal lobe seems to be important for visual-spatial function, whereas the dominant parietal lobe is involved in language function (Liepmann, 1914; Nielson, 1941; Walsh and Hoyt, 1969; Jewesbury, 1969; Heilman, 1974). Patients with nondominant parietal lobe infarctions, therefore, may manifest a loss of depth perception and a *constructional apraxia* (inability to assemble pieces into a whole or to draw or copy three-dimensional objects). Such patients may also have difficulty drawing maps and recognizing familiar people. Constructional apraxia is also seen with dominant parietal lobe lesions, but there is improvement in the tasks with practice. Infarction of the visual association areas 18 and 19 of Brodmann, or the posterior parietal cortex, produces the deficit. Another type of apraxia arises with infarction of the submarginal gyrus of the parietal lobe. The patient is not able to understand a request or to initiate a plan of movement even for simple tasks.

Ideomotor apraxia is the most common type of apraxia and is seen with diffuse brain disease including arteriosclerosis. The patient is able to understand a request but is unable to carry out the task. He may, however, be able to carry out the same task automatically. For example, an individual may not be able to tie his shoe laces on command but may be observed doing so automatically. Upon a command, movements may be transferred to inappropriate parts of the body, may become amorphous or may be simply omitted. In the related *ideational apraxia,* individual movements may be correct but cannot be assembled into a plan of action to accomplish a task.

Limbokinetic apraxia may be difficult to distinguish from paresis. The patient is able to initiate movement, but there is an awkwardness and clumsiness to the actions. Fine movements such as buttoning are impaired. Parietal lobe lesions are implicated.

Dressing apraxia may be a mixture of constructional and ideational apraxias but is worth mentioning separately because of the strange presentation of the patient. Clothes may be put on backwards, upside down, inside out, or on the wrong limbs. Superficially, such patients are reminiscent of the bizarre appearance of severe chronic schizophrenics.

Delusions

Paranoid delusions are commonly associated with organic brain syndromes of all types. Acutely, the delusions are likely to be restricted to the immediate environment and lack the expansive, global, or universal qualities seen with functional paranoid disorders. That is, the patient is more likely to worry about a plot by the hospital staff than by the FBI or martians. Chronic, organically based paranoid delusions may become more expansive but, in the presence of concommittent intellectual function deficits, are unlikely to have the elaboration and internal consistency seen with functional disorders. Maintaining a well-integrated, well-systematized, and internally consistent delusion requires attention, concentration, and a certain amount of intact intellectual capacity—qualities often compromised in the organic patient. There seems to be little evidence for localization of paranoid delusional ideation, and this form of thought distortion can be observed in all cerebrovascular and other central nervous system lesions.

Hallucinations

The presence of visual hallucinations and illusions are commonly seen in delirious states and diffuse brain disease of multiple etiologies. Typically, the patient will tend to report his hallucination in the context of his environment. He will report faces *at the window,* bugs *on the wall,* etc. In contrast, the schizophrenic patient with visual hallucinations is likely to ignore the environment, or say that it fades. There is also evidence that more focal lesions of the temporal, parietal, and occipital lobes can produce these phenomena.

Unlike the aphasias, which are produced by destructive lesions, visual hallucinations and misperceptions tend to arise from irritative lesions. Therefore, the literature deals predominantly with epilepsy, tumors, and trauma. However *ischemia* (presumably usually without infarction) can also produce visual phenomena (Williams, 1969). Decreased blood flow in the vertebrobasilar system and ischemia of the occipital lobe often produce unformed visual hallucinations (Williams and Wilson, 1962). The patient sees black or white spots, irregular lines, or colored patches obscuring vision. Such visual phenomena have been reported with vascular insufficiency due to arteriosclerosis, aneurysm, basilar artery insufficiency, migraine, and compression of the vertebral arteries in cervical spondylosis. Ischemia of the temporal lobe may intermittently produce elaborate visual distortions reminiscent of the psychedelic phenomena seen in hysteria, schizophrenia, or with drugs like mescaline. Lines and surfaces may appear wavy, and there may be color hallucinations.

Though Weinberger and Grant (1940) have concluded that visual hallucinations are of no localizing value, it would seem that the majority opinion would not agree, but would hold that formed visual hallucinations are more likely to arise from the temporal lobe than from elsewhere. Again, irritative lesions are especially indicted, including ischemia. For example, Hart (1967) has reported two cases of formed visual hallucinations with *temporal arteritis,* presumably involving the temporal lobe. Undoubtedly, the premorbid personality of the patient has bearing on the particular formed hallucination "chosen".

Other visual misperceptions that may occur with vascular lesions include *paliopsia, macropsia, micropsia,* and *monocular polyopia.* Any of these may be mistaken for hysterical symptoms. Paliopsia (visual perseveration) is recurring visual after-image. The image may simply persist or recur in the visual field after the object viewed is out of sight. Illusory visual spread is a related visual misperception of an extension of the image beyond the boundaries of the object. *Metamorphosia* (distortion of form perception) may appear in a variety of conditions (Van Bogaert, 1934; Critchley, 1949; Geyer, 1963; Gassel, 1969), including such disparate lesions as thrombosis of the right middle cerebral artery and aneurysm projecting into the hypothalamus. Disturbances in perception of the size of an object—being either too large (macropsia) or too small (micropsia)—may arise from peripheral lesions in the visual system or from lesions in the cortical, subcortical, and association systems (Wilson, 1916; Gassel, 1969; Walsh and Hoyt, 1969). Ischemia of the occipital lobe may be etiologic in some cases, but the symptoms of the macropsia and micropsia seem to have little localizing value (Walsh and Hoyt, 1969) and may occur in delirium as well.

Reduplication

Reduplication (Weinstein et al., 1954; Lukianowicz, 1967; Weinstein, 1969) is a peculiar phenomenon that may be seen with ruptured circle of Willis aneurysms; lesions of the third ventricle; and lesions of the frontal, parietal, or temporal lobes, which interrupt cortical-limbic reticular connections. This is basically a delusional phenomenon in which the patient perceives a duplication of himself or some aspect of his environment. He may be able to name the hospital he is in but qualify his answer by saying he is not in the actual hospital but a perfect replica of it. He may refer to another individual as if he were either twins or two different people; he may think he has multiple limbs or heads; may transform his house or other object into multiple objects; may say he has had multiple operations (instead of one); or may see his own double carrying out actions. These reduplication phenomena encompass delusion, illusion, and hallucination and are also seen in functional disorders. Reduplication of person has some resemblance to *Capgras syndrome*, a rare functional disorder in which the patient denies that certain individuals in his environment are who they appear to be. In both functional and organic reduplication, the premorbid personality and symbolism seem to play a role in the selection of what is to be reduplicated. For example, Todd and Dewhurst (1957) have suggested that narcissistic individuals are more likely to reduplicate the self.

Disorders of Intellectual Function

Memory

Deterioration of recent memory with relative preservation of remote memory is commonly associated with diffuse brain diseases of all sorts, and is usually accompanied by deficits in other intellectual functions, such as orientation, calculation, judgment, abstraction, etc. Isolated memory deficits are a relatively uncommon but very interesting group of illnesses brought about by focal disease, often vascular in origin. *Korsakow's syndrome* is probably the best known of the focal memory deficits. The patient demonstrates the classic triad of: (1) continuous anterograde amnesia, (2) confabulations, and (3) disorientation. The patient is unable to retain new memories. Though the information is taken in, it is not processed further into memory. The patient fills in the memory gaps by creating a generally possible (as opposed to bizarre) reconstruction of events. Though remote memory is relatively intact, the patient with Korsakoff's syndrome demonstrates a peculiar dislocation of memories. He will have trouble giving a longitudinal history before the illness and will transpose events out of temporal sequence even though the individual events themselves may be well remembered. Korsakoff's syndrome is commonly associated with chronic alcoholism (and presumably thiamine deficiency) and infarction of the mammillary bodies. Besides the mammillary bodies, this syndrome has been described in lesions of the mamillothalamic tract (Benedek and Juba, 1941; Conrad and Ule, 1951), the hippocampus (Glees and Griffith, 1952; Környey and Saethre, 1937; Smith and Smith, 1966; Victor et al., 1961), the dorsomedial thalamus (Orchinik et al., 1955; Brierley, 1961), the floor of the third ventricle and aqueduct (Williams and Pennybacker, 1954; Förster and Gagel, 1934; Adams 1959), in aneurysms of the anterior communicating artery (Talland et al., 1967), and with diffuse damage in subarachnoid hemorrhage (Walton, 1953).

Hippocampal amnesia is clinically the type of common recent memory deficit seen with almost any diffuse cerebrovascular or other disease; however, bilateral lesions on the medial surface of the temporal lobes may be sufficient to produce the syndrome. The deficit is in registration. Unlike Korsakoff's syndrome, these patients have neither confabulations nor distortion of remote memories. Memory deficits from frontal lobe lesions are not specific and are generally, but not inevitably, part of a frontal lobe syndrome.

Other intellectual function deficits

Disturbances of complex mental functions such as *judgement* and *abstraction* have been associated with frontal lobe lesions; and specific deficits such as *acalculia,* with parietal lobe lesions. However it seems likely that these functions as well as orientation and intelligence are exceedingly complex, requiring integration of multiple areas of the brain. As such, they are subject to disruption at multiple sites and a variety of pathologies. For example, even the so-called *frontal lobe syndrome* is not restricted to frontal lobe lesions (Bleuler, 1951). It seems clear that more clinical material is needed before trying to define anatomically higher mental activity. Therefore, it would seem to be at least premature to try to localize intellectual function; and, perhaps, such localization would prove to be a vain quest.

COMMENT

The above has been a very condensed overview of a complex subject. The hope is that two purposes have been served: (1) to remind the clinician that the presentation of brain disease can draw from a large repertoire of behavioral manifestations, and (2) to encourage the researcher to systemically approach the question of the mental organization of the brain. In spite of the fact that pathoanatomical correlations of mental disorders go back at least to the time of Morgagni in the eighteenth century, our state of knowledge remains very incomplete. The literature is largely anecdotal, and case studies reported are often of the unusual. Exceedingly few studies have tried to correlate specific lesions with behavioral changes while controlling for: (1) the premorbid personality of the patient, (2) the incidence of the particular behavior on a matched control population, or (3) the psychologic reaction of the patient to his illness. The literature of the last decade, in fact, has been rather sparse, at least from the vantage point of cardiovascular and cerebrovascular disease. This fact is unfortunate. It would seem that a systematic and scientific study of these diseases would offer potential insight into the mental organization of man and be of considerable importance to the clinician.

REFERENCES

Adams, G. F. Mental barriers to recovery from strokes. *Lancet*. 2:533–537 (1963).

Adams, R. D. Nutritional diseases of the nervous system in the alcoholic patient. *Trans. Am. Clin. Climat. Assn*. 71:59–93 (1959).

Amyes, E. W., and Nielsen, J. M. Clinicopathological study of vascular lesions of the anterior cingulate region. *Bull. L. A. Neurol. Soc*. 20:112–130 (1955).

Andersen, C. Crise de rire spasmodique avant décès. Hémorragie thalamique double. *J. Belge. Neurol*. 36:223–227 (1936).

Baadt, B. Lachen als erstes Symptom eines apoplektischen Insultes. *Z. Ges. Neurol. Psychiat*. 10:297–300 (1927).

Bell, D. S. Psychiatric aspects of cerebral vascular disease. *Med. J. Aust*. 2:829–833 (1966).

Benedek, L., and Juba, A. Korsakow-Syndrom bei den Geschwülsten des Zwischenhirns. *Arch. Psychiat. Nervenkeilk* 114:366–376 (1941).

Bleuler, M. Psychiatry of cerebral diseases. *Brit. Med. J*. 2:1233–1238 (1951).

Brain, W. R. *Speech Disorders. Aphasia, Apraxia, and Agnosia*. Butterworth and Co., Toronto, Canada (1961).

Brickner, R. M. *The Intellectual Functions of the Frontal Lobes*. Macmillan, New York (1936).

Brierley, J. B. Clinico-pathological correlations in amnesia. *Geront. Clin. (Basel)* 3:97–109 (1961).

Chédru, F., and Geschwind, N. Disorders of higher cortical functions in acute confusional states. *Cort*. 8:395–411 (1972).

Conrad, K., and Ule, G. Ein Fall von Korsakow Psychose mit anatomischen Befund und klinischen Betrachtungen. *Deut. Z. Nervenheilk* 165:430–445 (1951).

Cravioto, H., Silberman, J., and Feingen, I. A clinical pathological study of akinetic mutism. *Neurol*. 10:10–21 (1960).

Critchley, M. Types of visual perseveration: "Paliopsia" and "illusory visual spread." *Brain*. 74:267–299 (1951b).

Critchley, M. Visual perseveration. *Trans. Ophthal. Soc. U.K*. 71:91–96 (1951a).

Critchley, M. Metamorphosia of central origin. *Trans. Ophthal. Soc. U.K*. 69:111–121 (1949).

Duvoisin, R. G., and Yahr, M. D. Posterior fossa aneurysms. *Neurol*. 15:231–241 (1965).

Féré, M. C. Le fou rire prodromique. *Rev. Neurol*. 11:353–358 (1903).

Feuchtwanger, E. *Die Funktionen des Stirnhirns, ihre Pathologie und Psychologie*. Springer, Berlin, Germany (1923).

Fischer-Brügge, E. Ein psychisches Syndrom bie Schläflappenprozessen. *Zbl. Neurochir.* 10:253–264 (1950).

Folstein, M. F., Maiberger, R., and McHugh, P. R. Mood disorder as a specific complication of stroke. *J. Neurol. Neurosurg. Psychiat.* 40:1018–1020 (1977).

Förster, O., and Gagel, O. Ein Fall von Ependymcyste des III Ventrikels. *Z. Neurol. Psychiat.* 149:312–344 (1934).

Förster, O., Gagel, O., and Mahoney, W. Die encephalen Tumoren des verlängerten Markes, der Brücke und des Mittelhirns. *Arch. Psychiat.* 110:1–74 (1939).

Gassel, M. M. Occipital lobe syndromes (excluding hemianopia), in *Handbook of Clinical Neurology, Vol. 2, Localization on Clinical Neurology*, P. J. Vinken and G. W. Bruyn, eds. John Wiley and Sons, New York (1969), pp. 700–724.

Geschwind, N. The varieties of naming errors. *Cort.* 3:97–112 (1967).

Geyer, K. H. Zentrale Störungen des Formensehens: zur Pathogenese der Metamorphopsie. *Deut. Z. Nervenheilk* 184:378–387 (1963).

Glees, P., and Griffith, H. B. Bilateral destruction of hippocampus (cornu ammonis) in case of dementia. *Mschr. Psychiat. Neurol.* 123:193–205 (1952).

Goodglass, H., and Kaplan, E. *The Assessment of Aphasia and Related Disorders*. Lea and Febiger, Philadelphia, Pennsylvania (1972).

Hart, C. T. Formed visual hallucinations: A symptom of cranial arteritis. *Brit. Med. J.* 3:643–644 (1967).

Heilman, K. M. Neuropsychologic changes in the stroke patient. *Geriat.* 2:153–160 (1974).

Horenstein, S., Chamberlain, W., and Conomy, J. Infarctions of the fusiform and calcarine regions with agitated delerium and hemianopsia. *Trans. Am. Neurol. Assn.* 92:85–89 (1967).

Hurst, M. W., Jenkins, C. D., and Rose, R. M. The relation of psychological stress to onset of medical illness. *Ann. Rev. Med.* 27:301–312 (1976).

Hyland, H. H. Thrombosis of intracranial arteries. *Arch. Neurol. Psychiat.* 30:342–356 (1933).

Ingvar, D. H. rCBF in presenile dementia and in chronic schizophrenia, in *Cerebral Vascular Disease*. J. S. Meyer, H. Lechner, and M. Reivich, eds. C. V. Mosby Co., Saint Louis, Missouri (1974), pp. 66–75.

Ingvar, D. H., and Franzén, G. Abnormalities of regional blood flow distribution in patients with chronic schizophrenia. *ACTA Psychiat. Scand.* 50:425–462 (1974).

Jenkins, C. D. Behavioral risk factors in corony artery disease. *Ann. Rev. Med.* 29:543–562 (1978).

Jewesbury, E.C.O. Parietal lobe syndromes, in *Handbook of Clinical Neurology, Vol. 2, Localization in Clinical Neurology*. P. J. Vinken, and G. W. Bruyn, eds. John Wiley and Sons, New York (1969), pp. 680–699.

Kalant, O. J. *The Amphetamines: Toxicity and Addiction*. University of Toronto Press, Toronto, Canada (1966).

Kleist, K. *Girhirn Pathologie*, Barth, Leipzig, Germany (1934).

Klüver, H. The temporal lobe syndrome produced by bilateral ablations, in *Ciba Foundation Symposium on the Neurological Basis of Behavior*. G.E.W. Wolstenholme, C. M. O'Connor, eds. Little, Brown and Co., Boston, Massachusetts (1958), pp. 175–182.

Környey, S., and Saethre, H. Die hypothalamische Lokalisation der histologischen Befunde in Korsakowfälen. *ACTA Psychiat Neurol.* 12:491–498 (1937).

Liepmann, H. Bemerkungen zu Von Monakow's Kapitel 'Die Lokalisation der Apraxie' in seinem Buch: Die Lokalisation im Grosshirn (1914). *Mschr. Psychiat. Neurol.* 35:490–516 (1914).

Lukianowicz, N. "Body image" disturbances in psychiatric disorders. *Brit. J. Psychiat.* 113:31–47 (1967).

Mawson, A. R. Hypertension, blood pressure variability, and juvenile delinquency. *S. Med. J.* 70:160–164 (1977).

Medina, J. L., Rubino, F. A., and Ross, E. Agitated delirium caused by infarctions of the hippocampal formation and fusiform and lingual gyri. *Neurol.* 24:1181–1183 (1974).

Meldman, M. J. A nosology of the attentional diseases. *Am. J. Psychiat.* 121:377–379 (1964).
Mesulam, M-M., Waxman, S. G., Geschwind, N., and Sabin, T. D. Acute confusional states with right middle cerebral artery infarctions. *J. Neurol. Neurosurg. Psychiat.* 39:84–89 (1976).
Morley, J. B. Unruptured vertebro-basilar aneurysms. *Med. J. Aust.* 2:1024–1027 (1967).
Mullan, S., and Penfield, W. Illusions of comparative interpretation and emotion. *Arch. Neurol. Psychiat.* 81:269–284 (1959).
Nielsen, J. M. The unresolved problems of apraxia and some solutions. *Bull. L. A. Neurol. Soc.* 6:1–20 (1941).
Orchinik, C. W., Spiegel, A., Wycis, H. T., and Freed, H. The thalamus and temporal orientation. *Sci.* 121:771–772 (1955).
Orzack, M. H., and Kornetsky, C. Attention dysfunction in chronic schizophrenia. *Arch. Gen. Psychiat.* 14:323–326 (1966).
Papez, J. W. A proposed mechanism of emotion. *Arch. Neurol. Psychiat.* 38:725–743 (1937).
Penfield, W., and Jasper, H. *Epilepsy and the Functional Anatomy of the Human Brain.* Little, Brown and Co., Boston, Massachusetts (1954).
Pia, H. W. Klinik und Syndrome der Schläfenlappengeschwülste. *Fortschr. Neurol. Psychiat.* 21:555–595 (1953).
Pilleri, G. The Klüver-Bucy-syndrome in man. *Psychiat. Neurol.* (Basel) 152:65–103 (1967).
Pilleri, G. Orale Einstellung nach Art des Klüver-Bucy-Syndroms bei hirnatrophischen Prozessen. *Schweiz. Arch. Neurol. Psychiat.* 87:286–298 (1961).
Poeck, K. Pathophysiology of emotional disorders associated with brain damage, in *Handbook of Clinical Neurology, Vol. 3, Disorders of Higher Nervous Activity.* P. J. Vinken, and G. W. Bruyn, eds. John Wiley and Sons, New York (1969), pp. 343–367.
Poeck, K., and Pilleri, G. Pathologisches Lachen und Weinen. *Schweiz. Arch. Neurol. Psychiat.* 92:323–370 (1963).
Poeck, K., and Pilleri, G. Wutverhalten und pathologischer Schlaf bie Tumor den vorderen Mittellinie. *Arch. Psychiat. Nervenkr.* 201:593–604 (1961).
Robins, A. H. Are stroke patients more depressed than other disabled subjects? *J. Chron. Dis.* 29:479–482 (1976).
Rush, B. *Medical Inquiries and Observations upon the Diseases of the Mind.* Grigg and Elliott, Philadelphia, Pennsylvania (1812), p. 11.
Rylander, G. Personality changes after operation on the frontal lobes. *ACTA Psychiat. Neurol.* (Supp). 20:1–327 (1939).
Schneider, D. E. Anxiety preceding a heart attack—effect of person (the heart as a potential hallucinogenic pump.) *Cond. Ref.* 4:169–186 (1969).
Segarra, J. M. Cerebral vascular disease and behavior. *Arch. Neurol.* 22:408–418 (1970).
Seidel, U. P. Hypertension and paranoid states. *Lancet.* 1:906 (1977).
Smith, R. A., and Smith, W. A. Loss of recent memory as a sign of focal temporal lobe disorder. *J. Neurosurg.* 24:91–95 (1966).
Talland, G. A., Sweet, W. H., and Ballantine, H. T. Amnesic syndrome with anterior communicating artery aneurysm. *J. Nerv. Ment. Dis.* 145:179–192 (1967).
Thompson, G. N. Cerebral lesions simulating schizophrenia: Three case reports. *Biol. Psychiat.* 2:59–64 (1970).
Todd, J., and Dewhurst, K. The double: Psychopathology and physiology. *J. Nerv. Ment. Dis.* 122:47–54 (1957).
Tönnis, W., and Schürmann, K. Depressive Verstimmungszustände bei Schläfenlappengeschwülsten. *Allg. Z. Psychiat.* 125:239–246 (1949).
Van Bogaert, L. Sur des changements métrique et formels de l'image visuelle dan les affections cérébrales (micropsies, macropsies, métamorphosies, téléopsies). *J. Belge. Neurol. Psychiat.* 34:717–726 (1934).
Venables, P. H. Input dysfunction in schizophrenia, in *Progress in Experimental Personality Research.* B. A. Maher, ed. Academic Press, New York and London, England (1964), pp. 1–47.

Victor, M., Angevine, J. B., Jr., Mancall, E. L., and Fisher, C. M. Memory loss with lesions of hippocampal formation. *Arch. Neurol.* 5:26–45 (1961).

Walsh, F. B. *Clinical Neuro-Ophthalmology,* 2nd ed. Williams and Wilkins, Baltimore, Maryland (1957), p. 72.

Walsh, F. B. *Clinical Neuro-Ophthalmology,* 2nd ed. Baltimore, Maryland (1957), p. 72.

Walsh, F. B., and Hoyt, W. F. The visual sensory system: Anatomy, physiology, and topographic diagnosis, in *Handbook of Clinical Neurology, Vol. 2, Localization in Clinical Neurology.* P. J. Vinken, and G. W. Bruyn, eds. John Wiley and Sons, New York (1969), pp. 506–639.

Walton, J. N. The Korsakov syndrome in spontaneous subarachnoid haemorrhage. *J. Ment. Sci.* 99:521–530 (1953).

Weinberger, L. M., and Grant, F. C. Visual hallucinations and their neuro-optical correlates (review). *Arch. Ophthal.* 23:166–199 (1940).

Weinstein, E. A. Patterns of reduplication in organic brain disease, in *Handbook of Clinical Neurology, Vol. 3, Disorders of Higher Nervous Activity.* P. J. Vinken, and G. W. Bruyn, eds. John Wiley and Sons, New York (1969), pp. 251–257.

Weinstein, E. A., Kahn, R. L., Malitz, S., and Rozanski, J. Delusional reduplication of parts of body. *Brain.* 77:45–60 (1954).

Williams, D. Temporal lobe syndromes, in *Handbook of Clinical Neurology, Vol. 2, Localization in Clinical Neurology.* P. J. Vinken, and G. W. Bruyn, eds. John Wiley and Sons, New York (1969), pp. 700–724.

Williams, D., and Wilson, T. G. The major tumour syndromes of basilar insufficiency. *Brain.* 85:741–774 (1962).

Williams, M., and Pennybacker, J. Memory disturbances on third ventricle tumours. *J. Neurol. Neurosurg. Psychiat.* 17:115–123 (1954).

Wilson, S.A.K. Dysmetropsia and its pathogenesis. *Trans Ophthal. Soc. U.K.* 36:412–444 (1916).

Yaskin, H. E., and Alpert, B. J. Aneurysm of the vertebral artery. Report of a case in which the aneurysm simulated a tumour of the posterior fossa. *Arch. Neurol. Psychiat.* 51:271–281 (1944).

Psychiatric Presentations of Medical Illness

CHAPTER 11

Psychiatric Presentations of Pulmonary Disorders

JOHN PETRICH, M.D.
THOMAS H. HOLMES, M.D.

INTRODUCTION

The relationship between respiratory function and psychological states is well known. The frequency and severity of acute respiratory symptoms often include emotional states and psychiatric illness. Optimal rehabilitation involves attention to the patient's psychosocial environment. Primary psychiatric illness in patients with chronic obstructive airway disease (COAD) presents challenging diagnostic and treatment problems.

This chapter will present some of the research into the relationship of emotion to respiratory function in such a way as to permit practical treatment of patients. Specific treatment techniques, including psychotherapy and medication, will be discussed.

PULMONARY SYNDROMES AND SYMPTOMS

COAD includes three syndromes: asthma (intrinsic and extrinsic types), chronic bronchitis, and emphysema. Asthma is characterized by intermittent attacks of reversible airway obstruction. The course of the illness may involve months to years, and is associated with a variable and fluctuating level of disability. Chronic bronchitis is a disease with a cough productive of sputum for at least 3 months of the year for 2 consecutive years in the absence of other diseases to account for the symptoms. Emphysema is characterized by some degree of irreversible airway obstruction with dyspnea, inappropriate for age and level of functioning. Little disability may be found early in the course of the disease, but severe disability is associated with progression (Hodgkin et al., 1975).

Dyspnea, the cardinal symptom of COAD, is best described as the subjective judgment by the patient of air hunger, inability to obtain sufficient air, and labor in respiration. Dyspnea is not necessarily associated with structural damage to the pulmonary apparatus or abnormalities in respiration or blood gases (Dudley et al., 1969a: pp. 225–227).

PSYCHOPHYSIOLOGY OF RESPIRATION

The respiratory apparatus is a system of organs that conducts, conditions, and exchanges the respiratory gases. The lungs, the respiratory mucous membranes, the nose, and lacrimal glands are important elements of the system. The functions of all these organs change with emotions in a logical and understandable pattern. Sir Charles Bell (1847), in one of the first scientific investigations of the psychology of respiration, described sighing, decreased respiratory rate, and decreased tidal volume as associated with grief and depression. Anger was associated with increased tidal volume and nasal dilation. His, and the observations of others, suggest a biological utility in respiratory changes associated with emotion.

Organ Function

Changes in organ function associated with emotion can occur in the absence of respiratory disease. Experimentally induced feelings, using simple discussion, hypnosis, or noxious stimuli, can produce changes in the respiratory pattern (Stevenson and Ripley, 1952). Increased respiratory rate, depth of breathing, and sighing are associated with anxiety, as well as with anger and resentment. Decreased respiratory rate and decreased tidal volume are seen in patients who are feeling sad and dejected. Irregularity is associated with suppressed anger, guilt, weeping, and indecision. Stevenson and Wolff (1949) and Holmes et al. (1950a) have studied the association of feeling states to mucous production and nasal secretions, respectively. With both naturally occurring and experimentally induced depression, nasal secretions were decreased and became more viscous. Tension and conflict, on the other hand, tended to produce mucous membrane hyperfunction. Conflict-induced nasal hyperfunction was found experimentally to contribute to the vulnerability of the nasal mucous membrane to pollen and manifestations of hay fever rhinitis (Holmes et al., 1950b). Conflicts involving interpersonal and social adjustment were observed to produce sustained alterations of nasal function. These emotion-related pathological changes, when combined with pollution or infection, can result in significant morbidity. Lacrimal gland function is also involved in reactions of the upper airway. The feeling of helplessness, present in a range of emotions, is most specifically associated with crying and hypersecretion. Psychosocial factors, including age, sex, and situation, are significant modifiers of crying behavior.

Pulmonary Function

Changes in pulmonary function are associated with emotional changes. In a study of experimentally induced acute emotional reactions, Dudley et al. (1964), noted changes in respiratory rate, minute ventilation, and oxygen consumption. Alterations in alveolar carbon dioxide production were found in chronic, naturally occurring emotional states. States of anxiety, irritability, restlessness, desire to act, hostility, tension, or panic—so-called action-oriented emotions—are associated with hyperventilation with increased minute ventilation and oxygen consumption. Hyperventilation was the predominant response to noxious stimuli (Dudley et al., 1965). Hypoventilation was associated with nonaction-oriented emotions—feelings of despair, withdrawal, apathy, sadness, or helplessness. In these states, alveolar ventilation and oxygen consumption were reduced. The respiratory changes with action-oriented emotional states were similar to those occurring with exercise. Respiratory changes occurring with nonaction-oriented states were similar to those occurring with sleep.

In the intact individual, respiratory changes correspond to activity changes and permit optimal functioning of the organism. With COAD, respiratory response may no longer be adequate for metabolic needs and symptoms may result. Respiratory changes and metabolic demand are linked to emotional as well as physical activity areas. Significant respiratory symptoms can result with any discrepancy between respiratory and metabolic needs. The COAD patient may become acutely hypoxic in response to stimuli that provoke action behaviors or action-oriented emotional responses. Nonaction-oriented emotions or behaviors are associated with serious hypoxia and hypercarbia, because some patients decrease ventilation in excess of metabolic changes.

A clinically significant result of respiratory symptoms is the experience of anxiety by the patient. This secondary or symptom-related anxiety, when superimposed upon the pre-existing action or nonaction-oriented behavior, is associated with increased metabolic demand, and results in increased dyspnea, hypoxia, and hypercarbia. The resultant positive feedback cycle increases respiratory inadequacy and symptoms and represents a significant complication in the management of pulmonary patients.

Symptoms

Respiratory symptoms depend upon past experiences and on the attention the patient pays to his or her body, not solely on the degree of respiratory disability.

Most commonly, symptoms result from an awareness of increased breathing and are linked to the patient's perception of the real or symbolic importance of breathing to the organism. Wheezing reflects the degree of bronchial narrowing and secretion of mucous, and the patient's patterns of expiration. The symptoms of constriction are derived from the sense of increased muscle tension and spasm of the intercostal muscles and the diaphragm. Irregularities of respiration are associated with conflict between feelings and preparation for action or inaction.

Dyspnea is perceived by patients as the feeling of air hunger. Experimental studies of dyspnea demonstrated an association to both emotional and physiological changes (Dudley et al., 1968). Dyspnea was not limited to patients with pulmonary disease. It was observed both in hypo- and hyper-ventilatory states. The phenomenon was explained by a decrease in the functional capacity of the respiratory system, by an increase in the demand on the system, or both. Yet, changes in respiratory variables were not associated with dyspnea in all people. The lack of a consistent relationship between physiological variables and symptoms of dyspnea has prompted thinking that dyspnea reflects past conditioning. Breath-holding, weeping, and allergic episodes may lead to the association of physiologic change with the emotional state in which dyspnea is produced. Some patients then respond to relatively minimal physiological changes with marked disability.

THE PSYCHOSOCIAL CHARACTERISTICS OF COAD PATIENTS

Certain observations regarding the psychosocial characteristics of COAD patients have clinical relevance. Respiratory patients are frequently seen as anxiety-ridden and potentially reactive to environmental events, while simultaneously constricted in social experiences. These patients are seen to avoid emotionally laden social stimuli to protect themselves from symptom-producing physiologic changes (Dudley et al., 1969b). Patients with the greatest range of adaptation and coping assets have been found to respond best to medications and rehabilitation therapies. Their counterparts with fewer such skills respond less well and demonstrate increased morbidity and mortality (Agle, 1977).

ASTHMA

Psychobiologic factors are significant in the onset and maintenance of asthma symptoms (deAraujo et al., 1973). Asthma attacks tend to develop in a setting of emotional conflict or follow an intense emotional experience. Any intense emotion, especially fear or anger, accompanied by frustration, frequently coincides with or is followed by asthma.

Treuting and Ripley (1948) studied the psychosocial attitudes of 51 patients. Depression was identified as a predominant mood at the time of an attack. The depression was not always discernible early in the contact with the patient, but became clear after extended examinations, or over the course of treatment. The depression often involved overdependence on others and difficulty in functioning as an independent individual. The dependency was often ambivalent and mixed with guilt.

The relationship of asthma and crying has received some attention (Greenacre, 1945). In naturally occurring cases and experimentally induced attacks, the suppression of crying behavior resulted in wheezing and dyspnea.

EMPHYSEMA

As a group, these patients have been found to use denial, repression, and isolation as defense mechanisms. The resultant behavior protects the patient from incoming stimuli that may produce emotional change and associated respiratory distress. Anxiety and depression follow an exacerbation of dyspnea, producing additional emotional change and additional dyspnea. This positive feedback cycle is very disabling.

Pulmonary patients are responsive to treatment programs aimed at respiratory rehabilitation (Lustig et al., 1972; Baum et al., 1973; Haas and Luczak, 1963). Programs directed at teaching improved respiratory functioning and social and work skills are considered more effective than psychotherapy alone. Improvements in self-esteem and functioning are sometimes short-lived unless continued psychosocial support is provided (Haas and Luczak, 1963).

Death

Observations of dying emphysema patients indicate that death in itself is not necessarily uncomfortable or threatening (Dudley et al., 1969b). Some patients view death as a natural consequence of living and may regard the experience as comfortable and even pleasant. It appears that the patient's interactions with the environment are a prime cause of discomfort. They relate to the inability of those around the patient to come to terms with the patient's death. Patients seem to need human contact while dying as they do while living. Staff finds it difficult to know how to interact with dying patients. Patients prefer to relate to staff on a "business as usual" basis. They have complaints and questions regarding their management up until the time of death. They are interested in pain relief, sleep, and the multitude of small details concerned with daily living. One lawyer, dying with emphysema, telephoned his office and engaged in last minute business arrangements until 3 days before his death. His continued interest in work-related activities was his method of occupying time and coping with his impending death. Patients do worry about resuscitation procedures. Power struggles between the patient who insists on dying and the medical staff and family who refuse to allow the patient to die or even talk about death are common. For the severely ill patient, death may be problem-solving (Holmes, 1978).

PRINCIPLES OF MANAGEMENT

Psychiatric treatment of the COAD patient must be tailored to the individual patient's unique needs. The principal tools of the psychiatric therapist are: (1) a supportive relationship and the opportunity for free expression, (2) offering advice, (3) reassurance, (4) support, and (5) drug therapy. These strategies are as much the repertoire of the internist and general practitioner as they are of the psychiatrist.

PSYCHOTHERAPY

Treatment must be individualized, especially when one remembers the importance of activating and nonactivating emotional states with respiratory symptoms. Understanding the patient's unique emotional reactions comes only slowly and must be built on a feeling of mutual understanding and confidence—the supportive therapeutic relationship.

Treatment Approaches

The doctor-patient relationship is the bedrock on which all therapy is based. The physician should listen to the patient and not attempt to question the patient too soon or too intensely, thus avoiding the image of an inquisitor. Relevant information invariably comes forth in the context of an ongoing relationship and a few thoughtful questions. A diary of symptoms can help identify psychosocial variables of a patient's illness.

In view of the disastrous effects on pulmonary function of situations that produce anxiety and other emotions, strategies designed to minimize anxiety or remove emotional symptoms are preferred over those that induce anxiety, force abreaction, or demand "working through." The therapist is verbal and responsive with the COAD patient. Passivity and silence on the therapist's part are intended to instill patient-anxiety and promote the exposure of a patient's defenses, and these techniques are generally avoided with pulmonary patients. Isolation, repression, and denial are defenses important in protecting the organism from the deleterious effects of stimuli. These patient defenses may need active support by a physician with no attempt at removing them.

Experience has not confirmed the assertion that psychiatric symptom substitution follows simple removal of the symptoms. Patients appear to receive substantial and permanent benefit from the treatment of depression, anxiety, and other symptoms. With proper counseling, symptom removal results in a change in life style and reduction of the risk of relapse.

Reports are contradictory regarding the efficacy of group therapy. Rehabilitation programs can be viewed as a type of activity group treatment and have proven beneficial (Agle, 1977). Conventional group psychotherapy was reported by Dudley et al. (1969a:p. 303) to be associated with increased respiratory symptoms in pulmonary patients. Critical aspects of the positive group therapy experience are the group therapist's ability to promote a sense of comfort and well-being in the patient and the maintenance of a one-to-one supportive relationship with a physician. Group therapy can function as an important source of emotional support and a laboratory for teaching and reinforcing coping and adaptive abilities, if it is coupled with a strong relationship with the physician.

Managing Life Change

Management of life change and psychosocial assets is an important content issue in the psychotherapy of all patients with chronic illness. A body of empirical research has demonstrated that life change is associated with increased risk of illness (Rahe et al., 1964). Life change, regardless of the psychological significance to the patient, necessitates readjustment of his coping style. These changes in equilibrium appear to affect internal homeostasis in such a way as to make the organism more susceptible to illness. This effect is most pronounced in the natural history of chronic diseases and explains, in part, the timing and onset of symptoms. The ability to quantify psychosocial variables has permitted the documentation of life change (Holmes and Rahe, 1967). Seriousness of illness and life-change magnitude are linearly correlated (Wyler et al., 1971). The basic principle of management is to help patients to understand the role and impact of life change on their illness. Such mechanisms as planning ahead, delaying decisions, and anticipating alternate coping strategies permit patients to reduce their life changes and minimize the impact of these changes on their lives.

Maximizing Psychosocial Assets

Another line of empirical research has demonstrated that the prognosis of patients with chronic disease varies directly with the patient's psychosocial assets (Berle et al., 1952). COAD patients exist in dynamic equilibrium with their environments. As long as their psychosocial assets are not exceeded by environmental demands (life change, infection), they continue to function well and are relatively symptom-free. To the degree that their assets are insufficient to deal effectively with the environment, these patients experience symptoms and may fall ill. The physician should promote or maximize the patient's psychosocial assets. But what are these assets? The ability to deal with the environment can be roughly divided into three general categories: social support, coping ability, and adaptive ability.

Social support is that milieu in which the patient lives. It is comprised of the elements of a mutual defense system against the problems of living. Essential ingredients are those people who help the patient feel loved and respected. The most highly valued social support in our culture is the "family." Spouse, children, relatives, or other "family," such as roommates, close friends, or work associates, are significant. Work is important both for the human relationship that it brings and for the associated self-esteem and role identification. The supportive value of such relationships varies among patients and may fluctuate over time with individual patients as the life style and communication patterns change. The extent and quality of social support are modifiable by direct educational approaches, psychotherapy, and by environmental manipulation. The physician must identify the most important social supports for each patient and involve them in the management of the patient's illness. Special attention should be given to maintain the patient's work role.

Coping ability is a distinct set of skills that reflect the patient's ability to modify the environment to meet his or her individual needs. Resources such as creativity, flexibility, energy, and independence are personal attributes positively correlated with successful coping. Coping usually requires an active response on the part of the patient, although the impact on the environment may be direct or indirect. The patient's coping strategies may be problem-solving and deal with environmental problems in such a way as to remove them from further impact. Successful problem-solving results in social learning and enhances the individual's abilities to cope with related problems in the future. Some coping strategies may not be problem-solving, but instead may be misdirected or incomplete solutions to the existing problem. The problem is likely to recur some time in the future. The effectiveness of these partial solutions is short term and does not contribute to the patient's overall assets. Effective coping strategies should be reinforced. Ineffective ones should be pointed out to the patient and alternatives explored.

Adaptive ability includes those skills that allow the patient to adjust to his or her life style in the existing environment. This ability is distinct from coping strategies, for the target of change is the organism rather than the environment. Both are similar in that they require activity and may be direct or indirect. The ability to delay reward, to control one's emotions, and to find alternative sources of gratification or sense of self worth are characteristics of patients with good adaptive abilities. The physician can help patients adapt. Relaxation therapy or physical conditioning programs are common examples. Supportive psychotherapy is another useful technique.

The Chronic Disease Model

COAD patients are confronted with chronic disability and recurrent acute symptoms. This is a frightening and discomforting experience. Patients with chronic disability cannot always become independent and self-reliant following acute attacks. Supportive psychotherapy is useful in the long-term maintenance of COAD patients and reduces the magnitude of disability. The patient should be allowed to express freely his or her feelings. The physician should be sympathetic and supportive. The behavioral medicine techniques have much to offer. The patient should be encouraged to report current or past patterns of emotional reactions and keep a diary with emphasis on the circumstances surrounding the attacks. The physician should review the diary or reports for precipitants of attacks as well as reinforcements for illness behavior in the patient's social environment.

Once such behavior patterns are identified, steps can be taken with the patient to restructure his or her reactions to minimize illness-causing behavior. Lack of awareness of the relationship between symptoms and life events is common in the initial stages of treatment. Many times, this relationship has to be demonstrated repeatedly to the patient. In the context of a warm and supportive relationship, some understanding will usually follow.

Choosing the optimal intervention requires judgment on the part of the treating physician. Interventions appropriate for one stage of the natural history of the disease may be inappropriate for another. The enhancement of coping skills may be fruitful in the early management of the employed COAD patient. Some adjustments of his or her environment may allow the patient to continue working and maintain accustomed activities with little disability. The same patient, confronted with significant pulmonary insufficiency later in life, may have to change his or life style to adapt to the demands of the environment. Emphasis on social support and adaptive skills may yield the greatest dividends in terms of reducing the patient's morbidity. Those patients with the greatest capacity to recognize alternate or different life patterns have the best prognosis. Patients should not only be seen during times of crisis, but also during well periods. This is important to sustain improvement and to avoid inadvertently becoming an unwitting reinforcer for illness behavior.

MEDICATION

Antianxiety Agents

The patient's appeal to the physician for his magic in the form of a pill, coupled with the physician's awareness of the pathologic influences of anxiety in respiratory functioning, tempt the physician to overuse these agents. The main advantage of antianxiety agents is the prompt and short-lived reduction of anxiety and the increased sense of well-being. The main disadvantages are long-term habituation and dysphoric effects, such as depression and paradoxical rage. Medications may be a poor substitute for an educational and psychotherapeutic regimen directed at altering the patient's life style. Antianxiety agents, however, are especially useful as adjuncts in the management of patients with short-lived acute episodes of anxiety or for those patients suffering from true anxiety neurosis with recurrent severe panic attacks. Medication is administered for short periods, a few days to a few weeks, in adequate doses to control the most disabling anxiety symptoms. The benzodiazepines are generally preferred for their high antianxiety to central nervous system depression ratio. The medication should be discontinued at the earliest date and saved for the next episode. Most patients can be trained to use sedatives in this fashion. Limited prescriptions coupled with frequent follow-up examinations discourage inappropriate and prolonged use of these medications. Sedative agents are useful in the form of narcotherapy in the treatment of acute dyspnea. An effective method of ameliorating attacks is 100 to 500 mg of intravenous amobarbital administered slowly, combined with relaxation and the suggestion of feelings of security and well-being.

Antidepressants

Antidepressants are the preferred agents for treatment of clinical depression. Depression is associated with pulmonary disease and is often produced by it. Subclinical and masked forms are difficult to recognize. The classic syndromes present little diagnostic ambiguity. Subclinical depression consists of chronic anedonia, emotional blunting, behavior inhibition, and hypoactivity combined with sleep disturbance. Manifest depressive complaints with or without death wishes frequently herald, or appear simultaneously with, the onset or with acute respiratory decompensation. Masked depression consists of the appearance of typical signs of depression—psychomotor retardation, sleep disturbance, weight loss, and apathy in a patient who denies any depressive affect by the patient. Denial and the fear of experiencing depression with its accompanying respiratory alterations effectively hide depressive symptoms from the physician. In suspected cases of subclinical or masked depression, a trial of antidepressants is indicated, combined with supportive psychotherapy and optimal medical management.

Conventional guidelines for the indications and dosage are usually satisfactory for pulmonary patients. The rule of thumb for reducing dosage and using caution when increasing dosage, in direct relationship to the patient's age and disability, should be followed. Clinical trial is sometimes necessary to identify the most effective drug and dosage. An amphetamine trial can help in the choice of antidepressant medication (Fawcett and Siomopoulos, 1971). This technique can result in prompt, temporary relief from depressive symptoms and can replace the trial-and-error process sometimes necessary in the selection of tricyclics. Awareness of a drug's specific sedating or activating effects is necessary for proper treatment planning. Sedating antidepressants, such as amitriptyline hydrochloride and doxepin hydrochloride, should be prescribed as single doses at night, when sleep disturbance is prominent. Relief is usually rapid and dramatic and is seen by patients as a tangible sign of improvement. The more activating agents, such as protriptyline hydrochloride and desipramine hydrochloride, are most properly administered in the morning to take advantage of the patient's sleep-awake cycle. Significant antianxiety effects of some of these agents may result in an immediate and dramatic improvement of the patient's functioning. This should not be confused with a true antidepressant effect, which may follow only after 1 to 3 weeks of drug therapy. Tricyclic blood levels are increasingly available and are sometimes useful in patient management. Data regarding the relationship of blood levels to efficacy in pulmonary patients are not yet available.

Tricyclic antidepressants potentiate the action of steroids and are compatible with or augment bronchodilators. The anticholinergic effects of these agents are not thought to contribute to patient morbidity, provided good pulmonary toilet and adequate hydration are employed. Dry mouth and thickened mucous may indicate the usage of desipramine hydrochloride with its reduced anticholinergic activity (Snyder and Yamamura, 1977).

Antipsychotic Agents

The primary indication for this class of drugs is the treatment of psychoses—psychotic depression, mania, schizophrenia, and dementia with agitation as a prominent symptom. These conditions are present in a small percentage of COAD patients, yet effective management of the respiratory symptoms in such cases is possible only after adequate treatment of the psychosis. The management of psychosis in the debilitated COAD patient can be life-saving.

Haloperidol is the drug of choice in patients with cardiac and pulmonary disease. Its antipsychotic potency, combined with low peripheral autonomic activity, is an important characteristic of this useful agent. Dudley and Rowlett (1978) in one study, and Cassem and Sos (1978) in another, have reported on the efficacy and safety of haloperidol by the intravenous route in severely ill patients. Ayd (1978) has reviewed the world's literature on the use of intravenous haloperidol. The agent is effective and complications are few. Fauman (1978) has reported on the usefulness of intramuscular haloperidol in the treatment of toxic delirium, a common condition in respiratory, intensive-care-unit patients. Centrally mediated hyperthermia with haloperidol is sometimes seen in pulmonary patients who are also expending much energy in the work of breathing. This effect is usually mild, and usual treatment methods such as a cooling blanket and hydration are useful in its management. Occasionally, small doses of a peripheral alpha-blocking agent, such as 5 to 15 mg of chlorpromazine intravenously, are necessary to control the hyperthermia.

Chlorpromazine is a second-line antipsychotic drug commonly available and useful especially for its sedative effects. Mild to moderate hypotension secondary to its peripheral alpha-blocking effect is common. The beta-stimulating effect of epinephrine and related compounds can aggravate the hypotension. Hypo- and hyper-thermia are seen as well. Simple measures, such as recumbency and attention to fluid balance, are sufficient to combat the hypotension in mild to moderate cases. The addition of an alpha-stimulating agent, such as dopamine or norepinephrine, may be necessary in unusually severe cases of hypotension.

Extraparamidal side effects—dystonia and/or Parkinsonism—are especially worrisome in COAD patients where these symptoms can severely impair respiratory movements. Patients should be screened at regular intervals for such side effects. Cogwheel rigidity, micrographia, and bradykinesia are common signs. Symptoms of extraparamidal effects should be treated with intravenous or intramuscular benztropine mesylate or diphenhydramine hydrochloride. Maintenance therapy with any of the standard anti-Parkinsonism agents can then be instituted.

Low-dose antipsychotic agents, such as haloperidol ½ to 1 mg twice a day, or chlorpromazine 25 mg twice a day, are useful adjuncts in the management of acute anxiety of the panic type associated with severe exacerbation of respiratory symptoms (Winkelman, 1971). Variable patient acceptance and the risk of precipitating tardive dyskinesia argue against long-term treatment of anxiety with these agents.

REFERENCES

Agle, D. P. Psychological aspects of chronic obstructive pulmonary disease. *Med. Clin. N. Am.* 61:749–758 (1977).

Ayd, F. T., Jr. Intravenous haloperidol therapy. *Int. Drug. Ther. Newsletter*. 13:6:20–23 (1978).

Baum, G. L., Agle, D. P., Chester, E. H., Schey, G., Anteda, E., Buch, P., Bahler, R., and Wendt, M. Multidiscipline treatment of chronic pulmonary insufficiency: Functional status at one-year followup, in *Pulmonary Care*. R. F. Johnson, ed. Grune and Stratton, New York (1973).

Bell, Sir C. *The Anatomy and Philosophy of Expression,* 4th ed. John Murray, London, England (1847).

Berle, B. B., Pinsky, R. H., Wolf, S., and Wolff, H. G. A clinical guide to prognosis in stress diseases. *J.A.M.A.* 194:1624–1638 (1952).

Cassem, N., and Sos, J. Intravenous use of haloperidol for acute delirium in intensive care settings. Scientific Proceedings, 131st Annual Meeting, American Psychiatric Association, p. 204 (May 1978).

deAraujo, G., Van Arsdel, P. P., Jr., Holmes, T. H., and Dudley, D. L. Life change, coping ability, and chronic intrinsic asthma. *J. Psychosom. Res.* 17:359–363 (1973).

Dudley, D. L., and Rowlett, D. Emergency use of intravenous haloperidol. Scientific Proceedings, 131st Annual Meeting, American Psychiatric Association, p. 59 (May 1978).

Dudley, D. L., Martin, C. J., and Holmes, T. H. Psychophysiologic studies of pulmonary ventilation. *Psychosom. Med.* 26:645–660 (1964).

Dudley, D. L., Martin, C. J., and Holmes, T. H. Dyspnea: Psychologic and physiologic observations. *J. Psychosom. Res.* 11:325–339 (1968).

Dudley, D. L., Martin, C. J., Masuda, M., Ripley, H. S., and Holmes, T. H. *Psychophysiology of Respiration in Health and Disease.* Appleton-Century-Crofts, New York (1969a).

Dudley, D. L., Masuda, M., Martin, C. J., and Holmes, T. H.: Psychophysiologic studies of experimental action oriented behavior. *J. Psychosom. Res.* 9:209–221 (1965).

Dudley, D. L., Verhey, J. W., Masuda, M., Martin. C. J., and Holmes, T. H. Long term adjustment, prognosis and death in irreversible diffuse obstructive pulmonary syndromes. *Psychosom. Med.* 31:310–325 (1969b).

Fauman, M. A. Treatment of the agitated patient with an organic brain disorder. *J.A.M.A.* 240:380–382 (1978).

Fawcett, J., and Siomopoulos, V. Dextroamphetamine response as a possible predictor of improvement with tricyclic therapy in depression. *Arch. Gen. Psychiat.* 25:247–255 (1971).

Greenacre, P. Pathological weeping. *Psychoanal. Quart.* 14:62 (1945).

Haas, A., and Luczak, A. *The Application of Physical Medicine and Rehabilitation to Emphysema Patients*. Rehabilitation Monograph XXII, Institute of Rehabilitation Medicine, New York University Medical Center, New York (1963).

Hodgkin, J. E., Blachum, O. J., Kass, I., Glaser, E. M., Miller, W. F., Haas, A., Shaw, D. B., Kimbel, P., and Petty, T. L. Chronic obstructive airway diseases, current concepts in diagnosis and comprehensive care. *J.A.M.A.* 232:1243–1260 (1975).

Holmes, T. H. Death and dying, in *Aging: The Process and the People*. G. Usdin and C. K. Hofling, eds. Brunner Mazel, Inc., New York (1978), pp. 166–183.

Holmes, T. H., and Rahe, R. H. The Social Readjustment Rating Scale. *J. Psychosom. Res.* 11:213–218 (1967).

Holmes, T. H., Goodell, H., Wolf, S., and Wolff, H. G. *The Nose: An Experimental Study of Reactions Within the Nose in Human Subjects During Varying Life Experiences*. Charles C. Thomas, Springfield, Ill. (1950).

Holmes, T. H., Treuting, T., and Wolff, H. G. Life situations, emotions, and nasal disease: Evidence on summative effects exhibited in patients with "hayfever." *Res. Pub. Assn. Res. Nerv. Ment. Dis.* 29:545–565 (1950).

Lustig, F. M., Haas, A., and Castillo, R. Clinical and rehabilitation regime in patients with COPD. *Arch. Phys. Med. Rehab.* 53:315–322 (1972).

Rahe, R. H., Meyer, M., Smith, M., Kjaer, G., and Holmes, T. H. Social stress and illness onset. *J. Psychosom. Res.* 8:35–44 (1964).

Snyder, S. H., and Yamamura, H. I. Antidepressants and the muscarinic acetylcholine receptor. *Arch. Gen. Psychiat.* 34:236–239 (1977).

Stevenson, I. P., and Ripley, H.S. Variations in respiration and in respiratory symptoms during changes in emotion. *Psychosom. Med.* 14:476–490 (1952).

Stevenson, I. P., and Wolff, H. G. Life situations, emotions, and bronchial mucous. *Psychosom. Med.* 11:223–227 (1949).

Treuting, T. F., and Ripley, H. S. Life situations, emotions, and bronchial asthma. *J. Nerv. Ment. Dis.* 108:380–398 (1948).

Winkelman, N. W., Jr. Haloperidol as a treatment of anxiety in psychoneurotic patients. *Curr. Ther. Res.* 13:451–456 (1971).

Wyler, A. R., Masuda, M., and Holmes, T. H. Magnitude of life events and seriousness of illness. *Psychosom. Med.* 33:115–122 (1971).

Psychiatric Presentations of Medical Illness

CHAPTER 12

Psychiatric Manifestations of Gastrointestinal Disorders

MARVIN M. SCHUSTER, M.D.

"For this is the great error of our day—that physicians separate the soul from the body."

Plato

INTRODUCTION

Just as functional disease cannot exist without disordered physiology, no illness is completely devoid of an emotional component. As with patients with other disorders, successful treatment of patients with gastrointestinal disorders demands consideration and management of emotional response to illness as well as the response of illness to emotions. The inter-relationship between patient, illness, environment, and treatment is a dynamic one, with each factor influencing another factor, thereby altering it so that it is no longer the same as before. Each altered factor then continues to interact with each of the altered factors, maintaining a dynamic interchange (Schuster, 1967).

Physical illness is a major cause of psychiatric morbidity; the severity of physical and psychiatric illnesses need not necessarily correlate. Physical illness may produce psychologic disturbances by: (1) impairing brain function, (2) impairing the patient's capacity to achieve his goals, (3) interfering with the patient's capacity to meet social, sexual, and economic needs, (4) altering body image, (5) disrupting normal sleep-wakefulness pattern, or (6) arousing inner conflicts that are determined by the meaning and significance of the illness to the patient (Lipowski, 1975). Thus, the psychological manifestations of physical illness can be influenced by the nature of the illness, the patient's personality, and his life experiences.

Because of the importance of psychosocial and interpersonal factors, the physician needs to be familiar with the patient's family constellation, his job situation, his attitude towards stressful situations, and the inter-relationship between family members (Kolb, 1977).

Psychosomatic symptoms may be of three types:

1. Physical expressions of emotional disorders. These are "functional" disorders in which no physical disease is present.
2. Physical diseases produced by emotional causes ultimately resulting in pathological changes, which may or may not be irreversible.
3. Emotional components of physical disorders. These may be biochemically or electrophysiologically determined as a result of the illness, or may represent the patients emotional response to the illness (Kolb, 1977).

PSYCHIATRIC SYMPTOMS OF GASTROINTESTINAL DISORDERS

Psychiatric symptoms of gastrointestinal disturbances have been categorized among three major headings: (1) affective, (2) disturbances of thought process, and (3) organic brain syndrome (McKeghy, 1977). Affective symptoms are further divided into anxiety, depression, and anger. Anxiety may be experienced and expressed as fear, or panic or may be recognized objectively on the basis of psychomotor agitation. This symptom is commonly seen in early stages of portosystemic encephalopathy associated with hepatic insufficiency and is also encountered in alcohol withdrawal (Peterson and Martin, 1973). Anxiety may also be a manifestation of carcinoid syndrome associated with high circulating levels of serotonin and bradykinin.

Depression is experienced as feeling "blue," "down in the dumps," or "hopeless". The objective appearance is a sad affect. Depression often results in a lowered level of self-esteem but may also result from a feeling of low esteem, as for example when patients respond to surgery (e.g., ostomy surgery) with feelings of self-depreciation. Depression may also accompany the malaise, weakness, and fatigue which result from debilitating chronic disturbances, such as inflammatory bowel disease or from poorly understood or poorly managed chronic gastrointestinal pain. Nutritional deficiencies and anemia due to gastrointestinal blood loss may produce symptoms of depression, or some of the above disorders may mimic depression and produce a vicious cycle as the patient becomes more depressed because of feeling depressed. It is often difficult to differentiate the somatic equivalants of depression from the clinical symptoms with which they intermingle.

Medications used to treat gastrointestinal disorders may produce psychiatric symptoms. Anticholinergic medications can produce a toxic delirium. Azulfidine may induce a dissociative state, and steroids are known to be responsible for hyperkinesis, acute brain syndrome, and psychosis in some patients. Drug addiction may follow injudicious use of narcotics by patients with painful gastrointestinal syndromes such as chronic relapsing pancreatitis or functional bowel disease. Depression may be the earliest detectable symptom of carcinoma of the pancreas and may antidate other symptoms by one or more years (Fras et al., 1967).

Anger that represents another affective expression may be appropriate or inappropriate. Although often difficult to determine, the basis for anger should be identified in order to appropriately manage this symptom. When the patient's anger concerning his predicament is projected to family or medical personnel, this may evoke a defensive hostility from the family and the treatment team. Demands for medicine may represent the need for continuous expression of the physician's commitment to the patient's comfort and continued survival. The patient who trusts and respects his physician often tends to get good effects from medication; whereas distrustful, angry patients have a higher incidence of side effects and poor results (Freedman et al., 1976).

Disturbances of thought processes are often manifested by accelerated or retarded speech and thought, which may be logical and coherent or illogical and incoherent, and which are seen in organic brain syndromes such as hepatic encephalopathy, alcohol intoxication, and alcohol withdrawal syndrome. Cognitive and intellectual disturbances may be associated with disorientation, impaired concentration, memory impairment, and disturbed abstract thinking. Severe disturbances are manifested by delusions and hallucinations, which may require management by psychopharmacologic agents, reality orientation, and by maintaining a familiar environment and familiar people in the environment (Fras et al., 1967).

Organic brain syndromes, whether acute or chronic, are usually characterized by: (1) the patient's awareness of a change in his ability to think clearly, (2) the physician's observation of impaired sensorium, memory, and ability to communicate, or (3) a history from a third party of change in the patient's personality. Examples of this type of disorder are hepatic insufficiency, toxic states such as toxic megacolon, alcohol withdrawal, and acute pancreatitis (Schuster and Iber, 1965). Acute brain syndrome responds to successful treatment of the underlying organic disorder, whereas chronic brain syndromes may be irreversible and may require psychiatric treatment directed toward reality orientation, ego support, and interpersonal and environmental manipulation (Lipowski, 1975; Cadoret and King, 1974).

Cognitive impairment and emotional problems are more commonly encountered than recognized in medical patients. This was demonstrated by a Mini Mental State Examination and General Health Questionnaire that detected cognitive impairment in 33 percent of patients on a medical ward, and emotional problems in 46 percent. The cognitive impairment was unrecognized by physicians in 37 percent of instances and by nurses in 55 percent. Emotional disorders went unrecognized by physicians in 35 percent of instances and by nurses in 70 percent. The authors concluded that doctors and nurses have acquired a technological focus that diverts them from the recognition of their patient's suffering and cognitive impairment (Knights and Folstein, 1977).

PSYCHIATRIC MANIFESTATIONS OF SOME SPECIFIC GASTROINTESTINAL DISORDERS

Peptic Ulcer

Much has been written about the role of emotions in the possible pathogenesis of peptic ulcer but little about the effect of peptic ulcer on the emotional state and psychologic well-being of the patient. Engel (1976) has utilized the peptic ulcer paradigm as an example of somatopsychic-psychosomatic concepts based on the experiments of Weiner and Mirsky (1957). Their studies indicated that peptic ulcer disease is primarily an organic disorder that determines not only the disease but also contributes to the development of specific psychologic characteristics, influencing eating habits, concepts, and attitudes, which, in turn influence ulcerogenesis (Weiner and Mirsky, 1957; Mirsky, 1958). The authors demonstrated that high serum pepsinogen identifies an ulcer-susceptible population, high pepsinogen being present at a very early age and persisting throughout life. The pepsinogen level appears to be in part determined by inherited characteristics related to parietal cell mass and remains high even after ulcer healing and during asymptomatic stages, suggesting that gastric hypersecretion is essential, but not the sole determinant in ulcer development.

Therefore, three parameters appear to contribute to the onset of duodenal ulcer: (1) a physiological parameter (hypersecretion), which determines the susceptibility to duodenal ulceration; (2) a psychological parameter, which determines the relatively specific conflict that induces psychic tension; and (3) a social parameter, which determines environmental events that will prove noxious to the particular individual. Accordingly, a duodenal ulcer should develop in an individual who has gastric hypersecretion, an intrapsychic conflict, and exposure to an environmental situation that mobilizes the conflict and induces psychic tension. It follows that psychotherapy cannot be expected to eliminate the underlying somatic determinants (life-long hypersecretion, absence of mucosal resistance); nor can psychotherapy protect the individual completely from the stresses of life. However, improved modes of adapting to external stresses can be learned as well as better means for dealing with internal conflicts. The concept that emotional stress can induce ulcer formation is so widespread in the general population that the presence of an ulcer itself is enough to produce anxiety, worry, and concern, which in turn may retard healing or predispose to recurrence.

It is generally held that duodenal ulcers tend to occur in highly motivated, driving, obsessive compulsive persons with high aspirations, who often respond to their illnesses by further obsessive compulsive maneuvers. Such people become preoccupied with concerns over their ulcer as well as concerns over dietary and emotional factors that might be aggravating it. These concerns are to some degree reinforced by the necessity of maintaining fairly rigid eating and medication schedules (Weiner, 1971).

Peptic Ulcer with Hyperparathyroidism

Hyperparathyroidism may be associated with hypercalcemia, gastric hypersecretion, and peptic ulceration. Females with this disorder outnumber males 3:1 in contrast to the usual duodenal ulcer ratio of 4 males to 1 female. The age prevalence of 40 to 60 is also higher than the usual duodenal age incidence. The medical symptoms are those of weakness, anorexia, fractures, and biliary and renal calculi. Psychiatric manifestations include hyperactivity, anxiety, and irritability; or in some instances, depression, apathy, and withdrawal. Anorexia, malaise, and listlessness may represent systemic manifestations that are mistaken for psychologic reactions. These symptoms progress to apathy, nausea, vomiting, and weakness. Performance is impaired and confusion, disorientation, and a toxic psychosis may ensue. The anorexia and fatigue may mimic involutional depression. The diagnosis is suggested by concomitant, renal, or biliary calculi in association with peptic ulcer, and is established on the basis of hypercalcemia and hypophosphatemia. Successful treatment involves surgical resection (Reilly and Wilson, 1965).

Pancreatic Carcinoma

Cancer of the pancreas is seen more often in males than in females (3:1) and is more common from the age of 50 to 70. Medical symptoms are those of weight loss, abdominal pain, weakness, and jaundice. Psychiatric symptoms are those of depression, a sense of imminent doom (but without severe guilt), impaired performance, loss of drive, and motivation. Diagnosis may be difficult, since the age range and symptoms are those of involutional depression. In 10 to 20 percent of patients with carcinoma of the pancreas, psychologic symptoms may antedate the discovery of the carcinoma by ½ to 4 years. The insomnia that accompanies depression in this disorder is often resistant to the usual hypnotic medication (Fras et al., 1967; Yaskin, 1931; Cliffton, 1956; Ulett and Parsons, 1948; Savage and Nobel, 1954).

Pancreatitis

A prospective medical and psychiatric evaluation of patients during an acute exacerbation of pancreatitis demonstrated this disorder to be associated with an acute toxic psychosis in 53 percent of patients, manifested primarily by transient hallucinations. This complication therefore occurred more frequently than any of the commonly accepted complications of pancreatitis, such as diabetes (30 percent), pancreatic insufficiency (34 percent), and pancreatic calcification (17 percent). Other psychiatric manifestations included memory deficit (29 percent), agitation (23 percent), disorientation (25 percent), impairment of concentration (26 percent), and confabulation (19 percent). Although the majority of patients were alcoholics, one patient who was not an alcoholic developed hallucinations during pancreatitis, and in 10 percent it could be ascertained that pancreatitis was not associated with recent alcoholic intake and therefore not associated with alcoholic withdrawal. Furthermore comparison with a group of severe alcoholics with a nonpancreatic febrile illness (pneumonia) revealed that only 13 percent of this control group developed hallucinations (Schuster and Iber, 1965). Other instances of psychosis with pancreatitis have been reported (Doubilet et al., 1959; Tulley and Lowenthall, 1958; Bauer, 1954; Rothermich and von Hamm, 1941; Savage et al., 1952). Anxiety, depression, insomnia, and narcotic addiction have also been described in association with pancreatitis (Lawton and Phillips, 1955; Rickels, 1945).

Constipation

Children who suffer from episodic constipation from a variety of causes have been described by their parents as developing marked irritability as each episode of constipation progresses (Schuster, 1977). Irritability disappears after evacuation and reappears during subsequent episodes of constipation. Not infrequently, constipation has its origin in painful fissures; and under these circumstances the anticipated pain induces a sense of fright and sometimes panic, especially in children, with the result that the child refuses to defecate in a sitting position on the toilet and often has his movement standing with the legs tensely straightened.

Encopresis may be secondary to constipation as a paradoxical overflow phenomenon. This type of encopresis may be associated with bizarre behavior manifested by the hiding of soiled underclothing in closets, shoe boxes, or rafters; and behavior can be so abnormal that etiological significance is ascribed to a personality disturbance. However, complete disappearance of the bizarre behavior can occur within a few weeks following a successful bowel training program. Parents usually report a "miraculous change" in the child's personality. Psychotherapy is not required for this group in contrast with children in whom psychological disturbance appears to be primary in the etiology of constipation.

Proctalgia Fugax

Proctalgia fugax is a disorder of undetermined origin consisting of fleeting and often severe rectal pain occurring episodically without demonstrable organic cause. A psychogenic etiology has been deduced from the finding that these patients are anxious and perfectionist and tend to focus on pain and to somatize emotional conflicts to the gastrointestinal tract (Pilling et al., 1965). However, it could also be inferred that these traits were a result, rather than a cause, of this syndrome. Some patients who report sexual intercourse as a precipitating factor tend to avoid intercourse for fear of initiating the syndrome.

Inflammatory Bowel Disease

Although there is vast (but poorly controlled) literature on the possible etiologic significance of various psychological factors in inflammatory bowel disease (particularly ulcerative colitis), there is little information concerning the effects of these devastating diseases on psychological, emotional, and mental well being (Karush et al., 1977; Engel, 1958, 1955; Feldman et al., 1967). It is generally accepted, but incompletely proven, that psychologic disturbances are more common with ulcerative colitis than with Crohn's disease. It is the author's clinical but uncontrolled impression that many of the psychological symptoms such as obsessive compulsiveness, strong dependence on key figures, preoccupation with bowel function, social withdrawal, anxiety, etc., that are associated with ulcerative colitis, are a consequence rather than a cause. This is because these symptoms seem to disappear after ulcerative colitis is cured by total colectomy and the patient is no longer prey to the general systemic ravages of his disease and susceptible to sudden uncontrollable urgent bowel movements, and sometimes incontinence. The rapidity with which patients with a supposed "ulcerative colitis personality" can adjust to so drastic an operation as total colectomy with ileostomy is often quite remarkable, strongly suggesting that many of the psychological symptoms that have been assigned etiologic significance in ulcerative colitis are actually effect of the disease rather than cause.

Posthepatitis Neurosis

Posthepatitis neurosis syndrome seems to be a result of ultraconservative management of hepatitis during and after World War II, when long periods of enforced bedrest were felt to be the only available treatment. A "convalescent center" was established for the purpose of gradual rehabilitation of patients over a period of weeks in convalescent hospitals after recovery from hepatitis. Many patients became fearful of liver damage if they were to overexert themselves, and a large proportion of patients complained of persistent pain in the liver area (Palmer, 1967).

Hepatic Encephalopathy

Hepatic encephalopathy is associated with liver cell failure, most often with cirrhosis. The portal hypertension that accompanies cirrhosis results in shunting of portal venous blood into the systemic venous system, thus bypassing the liver. Since the liver is essential in metabolizing many circulating substances, liver cell failure, or shunting blood around the liver into systemic circulation, prevents detoxification. Blood ammonia is thought to be one of the substances important for the production of this syndrome, which progresses from agitation to lethargy and somnolence, with asterixis (flapping tremor) to hyperkinesis and eventual coma. Blood ammonia levels are often increased, and there is associated fetor hepaticus, electroencephalogram (EEG) changes, and jaundice. Treatment consists of bowel cleansing by cathartics or enemas, lactulose, and antibiotics to alter blood flora and to decrease the breakdown of nitrogenous products to ammonia. Sodium glutamate and l-arginine are thought by some to be helpful when given intravenously.

Nutritional Encephalopathy

A variety of mental, psychological, and neurological disturbances have been described in association with vitamin-deficiency syndromes, most of which represent multiple deficiencies. In this country, chronic alcoholism is one of the major determinants of nutritional deficiency. Thiamine deficiency produces Wernicke's encephalopathy, which is manifested by apathy, progressive dementia, memory deficit, confabulation, ataxia, and ophthalmoplegia. Histologic evidence of neuronal and nerve-fiber degeneration as well as small petechiae have been described in the brain stem. Vertical and horizontal nystagmus and ophthalmoplegia characterize this syndrome. Lesser degrees of thiamine deficiency may produce symptoms indistinguishable from depression, including lack of drive, easy fatigability, irritability, and depression. Korsakoff's psychosis is similar to Wernicke's syndrome, but lacks the eye signs.

Pellagra encephalopathy is associated with nicotinic acid (niacin) deficiency or deficiency of the amino acid, tryptophan. Vague symptoms of hyperkinesis, irritability, lack of drive, mild anxiety, and mild memory defect are some of the early manifestations, which are succeeded by a syndrome of dementia, delirium with disordered sensorium, and severe memory defect. Behavior may be manic, depressed, or paranoid. Early symptoms respond to 100 mg of Niacin TID. More advanced cases may be irreversible, and when amenable to therapy, require high doses of nicotine parenterally (up to 1500 ml per day).

Cancerphobia

Cancerphobia in men often focuses upon the gastrointestinal tract, whereas women are more concerned about breast and uterine cancer. Because of its high prevalence, most people are familiar with gastrointestinal cancer, and many have had at least transient gastrointestinal symptoms, which alert them to the possibility of cancer. This is especially due to some of the signs of gastrointestinal cancer (widely publicized by the American Cancer Society) being as vague as "altered bowel habits." Management requires an evaluation that is thorough enough to convince both physician and patient that every possible avenue of investigation has been explored prior to arriving at the conclusion that cancer does not exist. The intensity of these investigations will be different for different people.

Cancer

In dealing with the patient's reaction to malignancy, the physician must determine, on the basis of his knowledge of the individual patient, exactly what the patient needs to know, what he can tolerate, and the descriptive terms that are acceptable to him. Timing is a critical feature as is the physician's attitude. Whenever possible, the attitude should be one of genuine concern, compassion, understanding, and support. A demeanor of false cheerfulness should be avoided. Alexander Solzhenitsyn, borrowing from his own experience as a cancer patient, has beautifully described in "Cancer Ward" how adept patients are in detecting the medical team's anxiety from small innuendos, such as spending a shorter amount of time at a patient's bedside after a pathology report has returned.

Obesity

A number of etiological factors interact with each other contributing to obesity (Stunkard, 1976). Some of these are:

1. Genetic factors (Seltzer and Mayer, 1964): Patterns of body build are found to be familial.
2. Developmental: Early nutritional factors influence the number of fat cells and their size. Since the number of fat cells does not change in life, childhood obesity is related to both an increased number and size of adipose cells; whereas adult onset obesity is associated with an increased size of existing adipose cells. Persons with juvenile obesity may have five times the normal number of fat cells, and may therefore find it quite difficult to lose weight.
3. Physical activity: Not only does physical activity influence obesity, but it is also influenced by the obesity and by the self image of the obese person.

Obese persons are unusually susceptible to extrinsic stimuli to eating, but have a diminished sensitivity to internal stimuli (Schacter, 1971). There seems to be a number of emotional consequences of obesity, since specific personality patterns have been noted in obese persons who often have a disturbance in their body image, feeling grotesque and self-conscious. Both obesity and emotional disturbances are more commonly encountered in lower socioeconomic strata.

Some of the therapeutic implications correlate with the observation that the prognosis is poor for juvenile obese persons, emphasizing the importance of prevention in this group. The most successful therapeutic approaches employ motivation by peers and other forms of peer pressure. There are a number of complications of weight reduction therapy. One half of patients routinely treated by family physicians experience mild anxiety and depression. A smaller number develop psychosis. Patients should therefore be cautious in initiating weight reduction programs if there is a prior history of significant emotional disturbance or a person is undergoing a particular life crisis.

PSYCHIATRIC REACTIONS TO GASTROINTESTINAL SURGERY

Postgastrectomy Syndromes

There are few postoperative conditions that are more widely studied than postgastrectomy and postostomy surgery. Reactions to gastrectomy vary from total acceptance and adaptation to psychosis; but fatigue and weakness have been reported as the most common complaints seen postoperatively, occurring in 50 percent of patients and often interfering with work and social activities. In one study, one third of postgastrectomy patients accepted jobs with less pay, alleging that they did so because of weakness and exceptional fatigue. Dumping syndromes were not found to be a major cause of disability (Roth et al., 1959).

Late postoperative results are strongly determined by the indications for surgery. Operative results were found to be more successful when the indications were definitive (for example, obstruction, bleeding, or perforation); whereas surgery for pain alone was less successful (Morgan, 1973). The incidence of continued abdominal pain and severe dumping symptoms are significantly higher when patients undergo surgery for persistent abdominal pain as opposed to operations for pyloric obstruction. This makes the important point that studies designed to compare various operative approaches to duodenal ulcer must take into account the reasons for which the operation was performed (Landau et al., 1961). These factors should also be considered when deciding the advisability of surgery.

A postoperative study of patients undergoing vagotomy and drainage for peptic ulcer reported a failure rate of 21 percent, predominantly for three basic reasons. One third of failures was due to reucrrent peptic ulcer; one third was cured of ulcer but developed postgastrectomy syndromes that rendered them as sick after the operation as before; and one third had no detectable or correctable explanation. The first two groups might respond to further corrective surgery, whereas the latter group might have been detected preoperatively by careful psychiatric screening (Alexander-Williams et al., 1977).

Indeed, an uncontrolled study has demonstrated that almost 70 percent of patients with proven peptic ulcer had detectable psychiatric disturbance upon careful preoperative assessment. Psychiatric disturbance was associated with poor postoperative result (Cay et al., 1969). The importance of preoperative evaluation was confirmed by a study using the Eysenck Personality Inventory Psychologic Interview, which was able to accurately predict the outcome of gastric surgery (McColl et al., 1971). Although it would be impractical to perform a complete preoperative psychiatric assessment on all patients, the authors suggest that psychiatric screening questionnaires such as "The General Health Questionnaire" (Goldberg, 1972) and the "Middlesex Hospital Questionnaire" (Crown and Crisp, 1966) might be suitable. Patients rated in the abnormal range would then be referred to psychiatrists.

One might add that a keen and sensitive internist and surgeon should also be able to detect clues that would alert him if his patient needs further psychiatric evaluation. Preoperative detection of severe depression or anxiety that appears unrelated to peptic ulcer should be treated psychiatrically prior to surgery, unless there are urgent surgical indications; this is because depression or anxiety may be causing the patient's symptoms of pain. Other patients with evidence of personality disturbance might possibly be helped by preoperative and postoperative psychotherapy, and in any event, should be appraised of the possible effect that psychological factors might play in their illness. Routine psychiatric screening of all patients with postgastrectomy symptoms is recommended, particularly if reoperation is contemplated.

Adjustment to Ostomy Surgery

Although ostomy surgery is more externally deforming than ulcer surgery, imposes a new mode of elimination of body wastes, and requires the wearing of prosthetic appliances, postoperative adjustment is most often gratifyingly good. This is large part due to the massive and successful efforts of self-help organizations such as the United Ostomy Association, which provides preoperative and postoperative counseling and group support; the advent of special training in enterostomal therapy; and the increasing recognition by physicians, surgeons, and nurses that care of the patient undergoing ostomy surgery requires special understanding and skills. Ileostomates tend to fare better than colostomates, in large part because of the nature of the underlying illness requiring surgery. When total colectomy and ileostomy was performed for ulcerative colitis, all but 1 of 41 patients considered themselves to be in good general health and preferred their present life to that of chronic ulcerative colitis. There was no evidence of psychosis or of symptom substitution. However, almost half of the patients experienced subjective states of discomfort and uneasiness with the ileostomy, manifested by concern over sexual function, fear of contamination by leakage, and other feelings of embarrassment. The majority felt that acceptance by key figures in their environment was extremely important (Druss et al., 1968).

By contrast, when colostomies were performed for carcinoma of the large bowel, a large percentage of patients experienced depression, shame, and helpless anger. Those patients who were successful in regaining bowel control utilized obsessional defenses during the first year, while those who were unsuccessful experienced a sense of fear, isolation, and inability to cope with everyday life (Druss et al., 1969). In this regard, ileostomates might adjust more readily to the imposed new method of elimination. This is because continence is not anticipated or expected, since an ileostomy flows almost continuously; whereas patients with a distal colostomy generally expect and are urged to try to achieve a reservoir type of continence either by daily irrigations or dietary means. They therefore strive to live up to expectations that cannot always be met. Failures result in severe disappointments, especially since they resurrect feelings of inadequacy because of societal attitudes and early childhood experiences with bowel training.

Postoperative adjustment depends in large part on preoperative preparation, appropriate timing of surgery, and proper disclosure in preparation of the patient. The optimal time for surgery depends in part on the nature and degree of illness and in part on the patient's reaction to it. Not only should the cure be better than the disease, but whenever possible, the patient should be convinced of this. Patients requiring surgery for the usual forms of ulcerative colitis have in most instances suffered intensely enough and long enough to make ileostomy more acceptable then their disease. This is less true for acute fulminant ulcerative colitis, which has allowed little time for reflection and acceptance (Schuster, 1969). One survey showed that three fourths of patients who were unable to adjust emotionally to ileostomy had undergone colectomy after having been sick for less than 4 months. Two committed suicide (Fierst, 1965). Acceptance may be quite difficult when the indications for surgery are prophylactic in the completely asymptomatic patient with familial multiple polyposis.

The more well-adjusted the patient is, the better his tolerance and acceptance of ileostomy; the more neurotic, the worse. But, no matter how well-adjusted, all patients can be expected to experience at leave five basic fears: (1) fear of death, (2) fear of pain, (3) fear of mutilation, (4) fear of loss of function, and (5) symbolic fears. The first two concerns and their management should be self-evident and are not specific for ileostomy patients. The fear of mutilation involves the cosmetic concern about noticeable bulges from appliances, odors, sounds, and accidents as well as the distortion of body image (Schuster, 1969). Concerns about functional adjustment include distorted concepts about invalidism and interferences with working, sex, and sports. The symbolic reaction can be a response to the illness, the surgery, or the ostomy in terms of their special meaning to the patient. In some instances, ostomy surgery is viewed as an assault or a punishment for wrongdoings, as the basis for rejection by family and friends;

or as symbolic castration, which makes the patient unworthy and incapable of further sexual contacts.

Because of early toilet training and socialization experiences, loss of sphincter control is often equated with loss of self-control and is frequently accompanied by a feeling of guilt or of being "dirty," undesirable, and unlovable. Preoperative and postoperative counseling of the patient, the patient's spouse, and other family members is vital to successful adjustment.

Immediate postoperative responses include embarassment, helplessness, a sense of disfigurement, a reduced sense of value; or feelings of rejection, disgust, and revulsion. Depression, regression, and denial may accompany these reactions. Depression and anxiety may be expressed as guilt and self-blame, or by somatic complaints. Severe depression may require psychiatric therapy.

Regression to a more dependent stage often has adaptive usefulness in adjusting to the hospital scene. However, some of the manifestations of regression, such as irritability, a demanding attitude, unreasonable expressions of helplessness, and inability to achieve self-care, may evoke anger and hostility in the medical staff, if the staff is not trained and prepared for this eventuality.

Denial, like regression, may serve a useful purpose in reducing anxiety and depression but may also interfere with the treatment when carried to a pathologic extreme (Schuster, 1969).

Long-term adjustment is primarily dependent on two factors: the patient's inherent strengths, and outside counseling and support. The family is particularly important in restoring social function and self-esteem. Educated and understanding physicians, nurses, enterostomal therapists, and ostomy associations also play a major role.

Postoperative sexual maladjustment may result from a number of causes:

1. Impotence may follow sympathetic nerve transection. This is more likely to occur in urostomy surgery, or when colostomies are performed for rectal carcinoma (which requires extensive pelvic dissection), than in ileostomy (which is usually performed in inflammatory bowel disease and does not require extensive dissection).
2. Debilitation from the underlying illness, or as a result of surgery, may interfere with satisfactory sexual performance, expecially if attempts are made too early postoperatively. This failure in itself may lead to a sense of impotence that perpetuates itself and is aggravated by depression. Patients may set the stage for further failures by approaching sexual performance as a test that they will pass or fail.
3. Depression may produce loss of libido, and as before, failure may perpetuate itself in a vicious cycle.
4. Feelings of humilation and embarassment may interfere with sexual functions.
5. Spouse's reaction to the ileostomy may provide a barrier to harmony and sexual relations.

Successful treatment requires some information as to which of these factors individually or in combination is responsible. Only 2 percent of ileostomates attribute breakdown of marriage to the ileostomy, while 10 percent attribute tension and unhappiness to the stoma (Burnham et al., 1977). Fewer than 10 percent of married women find that ileostomy makes intercourse difficult. One of the problems voiced by teenagers is the concern of how much information to impart to their partners, and many express concern about their acceptability to a new partner. In contrast to patients who have had gastrectomy for peptic ulcer, fewer than 10 percent of people change their employment, and 85 percent of people continue their usual social activities without difficulty (Burnham et al., 1977).

Postcholecystectomy Syndrome

Forty percent of a large series of patients (2000 patients) who underwent cholecystectomy for gall stones suffered postcholecystectomy distress, with 10 percent having dyspepsia, 24 percent having mild attacks of pain, and 3 percent having severe pain (Bodvall and Overgarrd, 1967). Symptoms are much less likely to occur after cholecystectomy, when the preoperative history has been that of typical recurrent biliary colic and especially when gall stones are found at the time of surgery. However, vague symptoms (of bloating, heartburn, flatulence, and right upper quadrant pain that may radiate to other areas of the abdomen) and associated normal cholecystograms more often result in failure to find stones and in persistent postcholecystectomy symptoms (Womack and Crider, 1974). Postoperative symptoms may be the same as those that were present preoperatively, or they may represent new symptoms related to surgery, or represent a combination of both.

There is some indication that functional postcibal abdominal pain may be related to intestinal contractions induced by cholecystokinin (Harvey and Read, 1973). Serum cholecystokinin levels are elevated after cholecystectomy, possibly due to the fact that cholecystokinin inhibitors in the gall bladder have been removed (Johnson and Marshall, 1976). It is therefore possible that functional bowel symptoms might be aggravated by increased circulating cholecystokinin levels after cholecystectomy.

Postcholecystectomy syndromes may therefore result from a number of possible causes: (1) persistence of irritable bowel syndrome unaffected by surgery, (2) emergence of irritable bowel syndrome relating to postoperative elevation of cholecystokinin levels, or (3) symptoms resulting from spasm of the remaining musculature in the common bile duct and periampullary duodenum (Collins, 1977). The possible application of these principals to therapy have been suggested by the demonstration that some patients with postcholecystectomy syndrome become asymptomatic or improved by progesterone steroids, which have a direct antagonism to the stimulating effect of cholecystokinin on smooth muscle (Bodvall and Overgarrd, 1967).

INDICATIONS FOR PSYCHIATRIC CONSULTATION

Psychiatric consultations are indicated when: (1) there is a basic underlying psychiatric disturbance that may or may not be related to the gastrointestinal tract; (2) the patient's reaction to his disease (anxiety, depression, denial, resistance, anger, guilt, psychosis, etc.) interferes with appropriate management or with the patient's effective functioning in society; (3) when psychiatric evaluation is required to determine competency; and (4) when the underlying gastrointestinal disorder leads to lasting metabolic changes that result in chronic brain syndromes such as hepatic or alcoholic encephalopathy.

IMPORTANT REFERRAL TACTICS

The patient should be given to understand that consultation with another medical colleague is indicated to assist in the diagnosis of factors that may result from a gastrointestinal illness or may be influencing the illness and the patient's ability to deal with it, and because his condition could possibly be improved by appropriate diagnosis and management of these factors. It is generally acceptable to most patients to hear that they have an illness that is aggravated by pressures, tension, and strain; or that itself is stressful enough to require expert assistance in managing some of the stressful consequences. One of the most frightening things that a physician can imply to his patient is that there is no physical (i.e., real) problem, or that it is all in the patient's head. Far more reassuring is the recognition that the illness may itself produce stressful reactions which, in turn, adversely affect the patient and his illness and require expert assistance and management.

REFERENCES

Alexander-Williams, J., Betts, T. A., and Pidd, S. Psychiatric disturbance and the effects of gastric operations. *Clin. Gastroenterol.* 6:694–698 (1977).

Bauer, H. Nervöse und psychotische störungen bei pancreatitis. *München Med. Wschr.* 96:136–137 (1954).

Bodvall, B., and Overgarrd, B. Computer analysis of postcholecystectomy in biliary tract symptoms. *Surg. Gyn. Obstet.* 124:723–732 (1967).

Burnham, W. R., Leonard-Jones, J. E., and Brooke, E. N. Sexual problems among married ileostomates. *Gut.* 18:673–677 (1977).

Cadoret, R. J., and King, L. J. *Psychiatry in Primary Care.* C. V. Mosby, St. Louis, Missouri (1974).

Cliffton, E. E. Carcinoma of pancreas. *Am. J. Med.* 21:760–780 (1956).

Collins, P. G. Functional disorders following surgery of the biliary tract. *Clin. Gastroenterol.* 6:689–694 (1977).

Crown, S., and Crisp, A. H. A short clinical diagnosis self rating scale for psychoneurotic patients. *Brit. J. Psychiat.* 112:917–923 (1966).

Doubilet, H., Raffensberger, E. C., and Brackney, E. L. What is the best treatment for acute pancreatitis. *Mod. Med.* 27:20–27 (1959).

Druss, R. G., O'Connor, J. R., Prudden, J. F., and Stern, L. O. Psychological response to colectomy II. Adjustment to a permanent colostomy. *Arch. Gen. Psychiat.* 20:419 (1969).

Druss, R.G., O'Connor, J. R., Prudden, J. F., and Stern, L. O. Psychological response to colectomy. *Arch. Gen. Psychiat.* 18:53 (1968).

Engel, G. L. Psychophysiological gastrointestinal disorders, in *Comprehensive Textbook of Psychiatry,* II A. M. Freedman, H. I. Kaplan, and B. J. Sadock, eds. (1976) p. 1638.

Engel, G. L. Studies of ulcerative colitis, V. Psychological aspects and their implications for treatment. *Am. J. Dig. Dis.* 3:315–337 (1958).

Engel, G. L. Studies of ulcerative colitis, III. The nature of the psychologic processes. *Am. J. Med.* 19:231–256 (1955).

Feldman, F., Cantor, D., Soll, S., and Bachrach, W. Psychiatric study of a consecutive series of 34 patients with ulcerative colitis. *Brit. Med. J.* 3:14–17 (1967).

Fierst, M. Complications of ileostomy. *Am. J. Gastroenterol* 44:366–369 (1965).

Fras, I. Litin, E. M., and Pearson, J. S. Comparison of psychiatric symptoms in carcinoma of the pancreas with those of some other intraabdominal neoplasms. *Am. J. Psychiat.* 123:1553–1562 (1967).

Freedman, A. M., Kaplan, H. I., and Sadock, B. J. *Modern Synopsis of Comprehensive Book of Psychiatry II.* Williams & Wilkins, Baltimore, Maryland (1976).

Goldberg, D. G. The Detection of Psychiatric Illness by Questionnaire. Maudsley Monograph. Oxford University Press, New York (1972).

Harvey, R. F., and Read, A. E. Effect of cholecystokinin on colonic motility and symptoms in patients with irritable bowel syndrome. *Lancet.* 1:1–3 (1973).

Johnson, A. G., and Marshall, C. E. the effect of cholecystectomy on serum cholecystokinin bioactivity. *Brit. J. Surg.* 63:153–154 (1976).

Karush, A., Daniels, G. E., Flood, C., and O'Connor, J. F. *Psychotherapy in Chronic Ulcerative Colitis.* W. B. Saunders Company, Philadelphia, Pennsylvania (1977).

Knights, E. B., and Folstein, M. F. Unsuspected emotional and cognitive disturbance in medical patients. *Ann. Int. Med.* 87:723–724 (1977).

Kolb, L. C. *Modern Clinical Psychiatry,* 9th ed. W. B. Saunders Company, Philadelphia, Pennsylvania (1977).

Landau, E., Sullivan, M. E., Dwight, R. W., and Donaldson, R. M. Partial gastrectomy for duodenal ulcer: Comparison of late results in relation to the indication for surgery. *N. Eng. J. Med.* 264:428–430 (1961).

Lawton, M. P., and Phillips, R. W. Psychopathological accompaniments of chronic relapsing pancreatitis. *J. Nerv. Ment. Dis.* 122:238–253 (1955).

Lipowski, Z. J. Psychiatry of somatic diseases: Epidemiology, pathogenesis, classification. *Comp. Psychiat.* 16:105–124 (1975).

McColl, I., Drinkwater, J. E., Hulme-moir, I., and Downan, S.P.B. Prediction of success or failure of gastric surgery. *Brit. J. Surg.* 58:768–771 (1971).

McKeghey, F. P. Psychiatric syndromes associated with gastrointestinal symptoms. T. P. Almy and J. F. Fielding, eds. *Clin. Gastroenterol.* 6:675–688 (1977).

Mirsky, I. A. Physiologic, psychologic, and social determinants in etiology of duodenal ulcer. *Am. J. Dig. Dis.* 3:285–314 (1958).

Morgan, D. Psychosomatic aspects of peptic ulcer disease. *Psychosom. Med.* A. Munro, ed. Churchill, Livingstone, Edinburgh, Scotland 46–52 (1973).

Palmer, E. D., ed. Post hepatitis neurosis, in *Functional Gastrointestinal Disease.* Williams & Wilkins, Baltimore, Maryland (1967), p. 119.

Peterson, H. W., and Martin, M. J. Organic disease presenting as psychiatric syndrome. *Postgrad. Med.* 54:78–82 (1973).

Pilling, L. F., Swenson, W. M., and Hill, J. R. The psychologic aspects of proctalgia fugax. *Dis. Col. and Rect.* 81:372 (1965).

Reilly, E. L., and Wilson, W. P. Mental symptoms in hyperparathyroidism. *Dis. Nerv. Syst.* 26:361–363 (1965).

Rickels, N. K. Functional symptoms as first evidence of pancreatic disease. *J. Nerv. Ment. Dis.* 101:566–571 (1945).
Roth, H. P., Cogbill, C. L., and Onufrock, H. M. Symptoms in patients' adjustment after subtotal gastrectomy. *Ann. Int. Med.* 51:23–30 (1959).
Rothermich, N. O., and von Haam, E. Pancreatic encephalopathy. *J. Clin. Endocrinol.* 1:872–881 (1941).
Savage, C., and Nobel, D. Cancer of pancreas: Two cases simulating psychogenic illness. *J. Nerv. Ment. Dis.* 120:62–65 (1954).
Savage, C., Butcher, W., and Nobel, D. Psychiatric manifestation in pancreatic disease. *J. Clin. Exp. Psychopath.* 13:9–16 (1952).
Schacter, S. Some extraordinary facts about obese humans and rats. *Am. Psychol.* 26:129 (1971).
Schuster, M. M. Constipation and anorectal disorders. *Clin. Gastroenterol.* 6:643–658 (1977).
Schuster, M. M. Ileostomy and Colostomy Management, in *Tice's Practice of Medicine,* Vol. VII, Chap. 26. Harper and Row, New York (1969).
Schuster, M. M. Functional gastrointestinal disorders. *G.P.* 35:131–139 (1967).
Schuster, M. M., and Iber, F. L. Psychosis with pancreatitis: A frequent occurrence infrequently recognized. *Arch. Int. Med.* 116:228–233 (1965).
Seltzer, C., and Mayer, J. Body build and obesity—Who are the obese? *J.A.M.A.* 189:677 (1964).
Small, W.P., Cay, E.L., Dugard, P., Sircus, W., Falconer, G.W.A. Peptic ulcer surgery: Selection for operation by "earning." *Gut.* 10:996–1003 (1969).
Stunkard, A. L. In, *Comprehensive Textbook of Psychiatry, II.* A. M. Freedman, H. I. Kaplan, and B. J. Sadock, eds. Williams & Wilkins, Baltimore, Maryland (1976), p. 1648.
Tulley, T., and Lowenthall, J. J. Diabetic coma of acute pancreatitis. *Ann. Intern Med.* 48:310–319 (1958).
Ulett, G., and Parsons, E. H. Psychiatric aspects of carcinoma of pancreas. *J. Missouri Med. Assn.* 45:490–493 (1948).
Weiner, H., ed. *Advances in Psychosomatic Medicine 6. Duodenal Ulcer.* S. Krager, Basel, Switzerland (1971).
Weiner, H., and Mirsky, I. A. Etiology of duodenal ulcer. I. Relation of specific psychological characteristics to rate of gastric secretion (serum pepsinogen). *Psychosom. Med.* 19:1–10 (1957).
Womack, A., and Crider, R. L. The persistence of symptoms following cholecystectomy. *Ann. Surg.* 126:31–55 (1974).
Yaskin, J. C. Nervous symptoms as earliest manifestations of carcinoma of pancreas. *J.A.M.A.* 96:1664–1668 (1931).

CHAPTER 13

Psychiatric Presentations of Selected Genitourinary Disorders

WILLIAM. W. LUKENSMEYER, M.D.

GENITOURINARY ORGAN SYSTEM

The genitourinary organ system serves complex and diverse functions, including excretion of fluids and wastes, homeostatic regulation of metabolism, control of blood pressure, reproduction, hormone production, and sexual activity. External and internal anatomic differences between male and female are most pronounced in this organ system.

The focus of this chapter will be to detail for the physician the psychological manifestations of disease, the psychological sequellae of treatment, and patient attitudes that affect the physician's role in treating genitourinary disorders. Attention will be given to those symptoms that are frequently dismissed as being of "psychogenic" origin.

Topics covered will be uremia, dialysis, benign prostatic hypertrophy, veneral disease, enuresis, and sexual dysfunction. Hypertension, cystitis, prostatitis, urethral stricture, nephroptosis, and pain syndromes will not be discussed. The approach to patients who "complain too much," or who suffer from character disorders or neuroses, is also beyond the scope of this chapter. Individuals with primary psychiatric disorders who present with symptoms referable to the genitourinary tract will not be approached at this time. Future volumes of this text will be directed toward topics not covered at this writing.

UREMIA

Uremia is recognized as having profound effects on behavior. From a review of the literature, Baker and Knutson (1946) noted six psychiatric presentations associated with uremia: asthenic, acute delirium, schizophrenic, depressed, manic, and paranoid. The latter four may simply reflect other psychiatric syndromes present in renal failure. Schreiner (1959), Locke et al. (1961), Tyler (1975), and Teschan and Gin (1976) all give descriptions of the psychological and neurological manifestations of uremia from onset to death. Early uremic symptoms of difficulty concentrating, drowsiness, apathy, and fatigue tend to be intermittent. If headaches occur, they are often vague in location and character unless hypertension is present. Loss of appetite, memory deficits, slowing and slurring of speech, decreased sexual performance, and reduction of activity occur as uremia progresses. Irritability, restlessness, insomnia, diminished attention span, and muscle twitching are often accompanied by more profound personality changes, psychotic episodes, or delirium. Focal neurological signs of meningeal irritation and cerebellar dysfunction may progress quickly to stupor, coma, and death. Clinical suspicion of uremia is easily confirmed by laboratory measurement of blood urea nitrogen or serum creatinine. When patients present with symptoms involving both the central nervous system (CNS) and musculoskeletal system, they should not be dismissed as "psychogenic." It is extremely difficult to distinguish uremia and depression because of the similarity of symptoms and because the conditions often co-exist. As will be noted in the following section on dialysis, depressive symptoms and delirium due to uremia remit after the institution of hemodialysis or renal transplantation.

DIALYSIS

Selection of Candidates

Early studies of potential dialysis candidates focused on prediction of outcome. In part, this emphasis was related to the limited availability of dialysis equipment and personnel. Given current resources, our program rarely excludes individuals for treatment of end-stage renal disease (ESRD) except in cases where death is imminent from a co-existing disease such as terminal cancer. Emphasis is placed on which type of treatment is most appropriate as opposed to selection for or exclusion from dialysis. Current modalities of treatment include home or in-center hemodialysis, home peritoneal dialysis, and renal transplantation from a relative or cadaver. Treatment choice is based on data from three principal categories: identification of resources; identification of known problems; and patient response to information about treatment alternatives. Assessment of patient resources includes developing an understanding of the individual's response to previous illness, his coping skills, and emotional strengths. Family interviews are held to identify supportive members, potential home partners, or donor candidates for living related transplants. Financial data are collected and help is given to secure financial assistance through Medicare, Medicaid, or voluntary organizations. Vocational rehabilitation is planned for those individuals who attempt to return to work. Staff members support defenses and explore fears and expectations as treatment begins.

Specific problem areas are also sought out. Past emotional problems, history of depression, anxiety, or psychosis are explored. Marital and sexual history are reviewed and psychiatric treatment rendered when necessary.

The process of education is made more difficult by the effects of uremia on memory, concentration, and mood. Much information must be repeated, and complicated instructions are carefully written out for the patient. The merits and problems of dialysis and transplantation are discussed, including discussion of the side effects of drugs, risks of surgery, and treatment procedures. Nursing personnel in the home training unit observe patient and partner for signs of anxiety or failure to understand the dialysis procedure. Those patients and partners unable to complete home training are transferred to in-center programs.

Psychological Sequellae

Psychological sequellae of dialysis will be discussed by reviewing troublesome issues that arise in the course of treatment. Before focusing on the difficulties involved with treatment, it should be noted that dialysis patients cope remarkably well. Many continue to work; others conduct their lives with continued equanimity. Mutual support groups have been established by patients. Foster (1976) gives an eloquent description of what being a home dialysis patient is like. At the First International Conference on Psychological Factors in Hemodialysis and Transplantation held in Brooklyn, New York, a dialysis "client" commented during discussion that medical personnel focus on "problems," but patients focus on "living." With the caveat that patients cope remarkably well, the task of identifying and treating psychological sequellae of dialysis remains.

Anger and Dependence

Ellis (1974), another dialysis patient, comments, "The remarks concerning the consequences of expressing anger in the presence of unit personnel are totally accurate. So far as I am aware, few if any of the thriving patients, other than myself, have made more than tentative moves to ventilate their negative feelings to the medical staff or nurses."

Anger and dependency conflicts occur frequently in dialysis patients. Generally, suppression of anger occurs rather than direct expression of this feeling.

Anger may be inferred from a patient's statements about God, about being ill, about well family members and friends, and about restrictions and diet. When one's life literally hangs in the balance, it is not surprising to see muted anger directed to staff and family.

Dependency conflicts arise not only from suppressed anger but from treatment itself. Death will result if treatment does not occur. Ten to twelve hours each week must be spent in a sitting or supine position. Patients may feel poorly during dialysis. Physical activity cannot be carried out. Sleep becomes a frequent alternative to reading, knitting, conversation, or watching television. Many individuals have become less active and adopt a dependent style as uremia progresses prior to treatment. Early transplantation or institution of dialysis before a patient's life style becomes too constricted are helpful in diminishing dependent behaviors. Children are rendered vulnerable to dependence by mothers and fathers who care for them. Staff attempts to encourage independent activity on the part of children may be met with anger from parents. Dependency conflicts are also generated by staff and family when high expectations to continue work or remain physically active are beyond the capacity of the individual (Abram, 1974; Kaplan De-Nour et al., 1968).

Denial

Denial is a major defense mechanism utilized by patients and families. There is no doubt denial serves adaptive functions to avoid the reality of eventual death, to minimize awareness of acute complications, to decrease awareness of needle sticks, painful diagnostic procedures, and seeing one's blood in tubing outside of the body, and to minimize suffering associated with the loss of physical strength or sexual function. The maladaptive component of denial may lead to emotional isolation from family and friends, disappointment and despair, and a series of behaviors that we label "non-compliance" (Beard, 1969; Short and Wilson, 1969).

Depression

Depression occurs in dialysis patients both as a transient mood disturbance and as a physiologically significant disease process. Both Wise (1974) and Foster (1976) have addressed the difficulty of diagnosing depressive disease in the presence of renal failure. Uremia and depression produce similar symptoms. Wise's major point is that profoundly depressed patients should not be denied treatment by dialysis or transplantation. Thus, the initial approach to depression is to achieve the best medical status possible.

The cardinal signs of depression are: persistent mood disorder of blueness, sadness, a sense of loss, hopelessness, and worry or irritability, generally of at least 3 to 4 weeks duration. Additionally, several physiological signs must be present: poor appetite, weight loss, psychomotor retardation, difficulty thinking or concentrating, sleep disturbance (especially early morning awakening), fatigability, loss of energy, loss of general interest, decreased sexual drive, and alteration of diurnal rhythm. Psychological signs are the presence of guilt and thoughts of suicide or death (Feighner et al., 1972). A clear history of persistent mood change supports the diagnosis of depression. When depression is suspected, it is appropriate to start periodic psychiatric evaluation, or to begin a trial of tricyclic antidepressants.

Starting dosages of tricyclics are 50 to 75 mg given at bedtime, increasing the amount by 25 to 50 mg every other day in hospitalized patients, and weekly in outpatients. The amount is gradually increased until a therapeutic response begins or until side effects become excessive. The end point is somewhat lower in patients with ESRD—generally in the 100 to 200 mg range given in a single bedtime dose. The presence of intolerable dry mouth occurs more frequently in fluid-restricted patients and with amitriptyline because of greater anticholinergic effects. Chewing gum or eating hard candy may partially alleviate dry mouth. Orthostatic hypotension is a problem. Patients should be instructed to sit several minutes before standing when getting out of bed or after napping. Slight decreases in antihypertensive drug levels may be necessary when tricyclics are used. Guanethidine should be avoided because of decreased effectiveness when given with tricyclics. Reserpine is known to cause depression; alpha methyldopa is also reported to cause depression. Confusion and increased difficulty in thinking can be precipitated by tricyclics and warrant a decrease in dose. The elderly patient may be particularly vulnerable to urinary retention precipitated by antidepressants. The induction or aggravation of arrhythmias may preclude tricyclic use in patients with rhythm disturbance. Continuous cardiac monitoring during institution of drug therapy is useful to determine tricyclic effects on arrhythmias in individual patients.

Reports of the effects of dialysis on antidepressant blood levels suggest that there is marked variability in the amount of antidepressant removed during dialysis (Rosser, 1976). Studies are needed to clarify whether clinical monitoring of tricyclic antidepressant blood levels in dialysis patients should be undertaken routinely. Studies may also confirm the importance of a postdialysis loading dose of drug.

A literature review produced no reports of ECT in dialysis. Our program has had success with two patients by using ECT. The advantages of ECT in this population are that undesirable side effects of drugs may be avoided and a rapid response to treatment is likely. ECT was unsuccessful in two patients in whom depression was probably related to physiological deterioration and approaching death.

Other psychological sequellae of dialysis have been reported. The quality of life on dialysis has been discussed by Poznanski et al. (1978) and Wright et al. (1966). Changes in body image are noted by Kaplan De-Nour and Czaczkes

(1969, 1971) and Abram (1969). Abram (1969) and Levy (1977) have reported stages or phases of adaptation and stress during dialysis treatment.

Suicide

Suicide and suicidal behavior in dialysis patients were studied by Abram et al. (1971) who found that the incidence of actual suicide was 400 times greater in dialysis patients than in the general population. Goldstein and Reznikoff (1971) suggest that noncompliance and poor adherence to restrictions are best not viewed and interpreted to patients as suicidal, e.g., "What are you trying to do, kill yourself?" They offer the explanation that many patients actually do *not* believe that behavior such as dietary indiscretion is harmful. They state that the externally oriented individual does not believe that behavior affects his own life. McKegney and Lange (1971) suggest that patients and families be made aware early in treatment that they have an option to stop dialysis. They feel that openness of communication about this issue may actually lead to decreased morbidity and mortality by reduction of stress. Ethical dilemmas about discontinuing treatment remain the shared province of the patient, his family, and the physician. Allowing someone to stop treatment should be a fundamental human right. Patient exercise of such a right is rarely agreed to by family and physician.

Dysequilibrium Syndrome

Dysequilibrium syndrome and dialysis dementia must be recognized and distinguished from psychological aspects of dialysis. Dysequilibrium syndrome occurs during or following dialysis and presents with a variety of symptoms generally of central nervous system or muscular origin. Restlessness and headache, often followed by nausea and vomiting, are the typical symptoms. Hypertension, disorientation, tremors, and/or seizures, usually of the grand mal type, may develop in severely affected patients. Resolution of symptoms occurs in hours to days. The etiology remains unclear, but cerebral edema, delay in fall of cerebrospinal fluid urea, paradoxical acidosis of CSF, hypoglycemia and/or hyponatremia are suspected. Treatment is begun by adding osmotically active solutes, shortening dialysis periods, lowering blood flow rate or prophylactic use of anticonvulsants. Psychological intervention is of no benefit, although appropriate support should be given to patients experiencing these symptoms (Arieff and Massry, 1976).

Dialysis Dementia

Dialysis dementia was first described by Alfrey et al. (1972) and is generally regarded as a progressive syndrome with a fatal outcome. The earliest symptom is a disorder of speech. Characteristically, the speech disorder progresses and myoclonus, tremulousness, and asterixis ensue. Further deterioration of movement, memory loss, difficulty thinking and frank psychosis occur as time passes. The etiology is not known although intoxication with aluminum and other metals has been implicated. EEG changes suggest that this syndrome may be mediated through a seizure disorder (Alfrey et al., 1976; Mahurkar et al, 1973). Subdural hematoma, hyperosmolar coma, cerebral vascular accidents or emboli, diminished cardiac output, arrhythmias, excessive ultrafiltration, generalized infection, and hypoglycemia constitute only a partial list of direct medical complications of dialysis that have psychological or neurological effects on the patient. Before symptoms are dismissed as "psychogenic," a review of history, repeat physical exam, and review of laboratory findings is in order.

Summary

The discussion of uremia and dialysis has not included specific disease states, both of renal and non-renal origin, which cause uremia. There is also a long list of medical complications of uremia and dialysis, such as anemia, secondary hyperparathyroidism, and hepatitis, that in part are manifested through psychological or neurological symptoms. Indeed, many times it is impossible to determine the exact cause of weakness, lethary, or even depression when present. In relating to patients, time is often better spent in addressing known problems at home, undertaking an empirical drug trial, performing repeat examinations, or providing direct emotional support, than considering whether a symptom is psychogenic or functional. In the clinical situation, a plan to help compliance is generally superior to questioning "why" patients do not take medications or follow dietary restrictions.

BENIGN PROSTATIC HYPERTROPHY

Symptoms of prostatic hypertrophy of local origin are usually not confused with psychological problems. Nocturia, hesitancy, increased urinary frequency, dribbling, urgency, and incontinence are present to varying degrees. The constitutional symptoms of fatigability or flank pain may be misinterpreted as being of psychological origin. If obstruction occurs slowly, uremia may result. Prostatic hypertrophy is a disease of elderly males. Other debilitating disease or the presence of dementia may render the patient unable to give an accurate history. Urinary obstruction with or without infection is a common precipitant of delirium in this age group. The clinician is also reminded of the anticholinergic effects of antidepressants, which can precipitate obstruction in the individual with occult benign prostatic hypertrophy.

Postoperative delirium in patients with prostatic surgery can be treated with careful orientation, by leaving a light on in the hospital room, by allowing frequent family visits, and with small doses of Haloperidol.

VENEREAL DISEASE

Venereally transmitted diseases, in particular gonorrhea, syphilis, venereal warts, haemophilus vaginitis, trichomoniasis, and herpes genitalis, do not produce psychological manifestations directly from the disease process. Symptomatic syphilis, a late consequence of syphilitic infection, has a wide variety of psychological and neurological manifestations and will be discussed in more detail. The physician's treatment of venereal disease, however, is profoundly influenced by patient attitudes. Early symptoms of venereal disease may go unrecognized, particularly in women. This in part may be due to the nature of the lesion, a painless chancre in the urethra, absence of discharge in gonorrhea in females, or small inconspicuous warts. Embarrassment and fear contribute to delay. When gonorrhea infection progresses to the diseminated form, fever, arthralgias, and malaise may go unrecognized as venereal in origin. Likewise, the varied rash of secondary syphilis, or constitutional symptoms of weight loss, fever, and malaise may not easily be recognized.

Even after the physician suspects a venereal disease, the patient is likely to be hesitant in reporting symptoms. Patients conceal and distort information about symptoms and sexual contacts. The embarrassment that occurs can be related to extramarital sexual activity, homosexual contact, or simply to discussion with a physician. Patients frequently have irrational and exaggerated beliefs about the consequences of venereal disease. Their fears encompass these beliefs and include fear of discovery by a spouse or partner. Frequently, marital discord is an additional problem that inhibits accurate assessment.

To gain the confidence of a patient, the physician can be reassuring about the adequacy of treatment and remain nonjudgmental in approaching the problem. Patience during history-taking is helpful. Careful explanation of treatment is necessary to facilitate adherence. Since many patients stop pills when symptoms remit, followup is essential. In patients whose reliability is uncertain, particularly in emergency room settings, injectable forms of medication are preferable to dispensing oral medications.

NEUROSYPHILIS

Asymptomatic neurosyphilis, like latent syphilis, is characterized by the absence of psychological and neurological findings. The disease must be recognized from serological or cerebrospinal fluid studies. Symptomatic neurosyphilis results from meningovascular involvement and/or parenchymal involvement of the brain (general paresis) and spinal cord (tabes dorsalis). Vascular damage may produce stroke-like syndromes, or focal pupillary and reflex changes. Parenchymal neurosyphilis commonly produces profound depression, dementia, or both (Dewhurst, 1969). Specific symptomatology can mimic virtually any psychotic syndrome. Delusions and grandiosity may be present. Hooshmand (1976) reported that 24.1 percent of 282 patients with neurosyphilis had related seizure disorder. Patients presenting with depression, dementia, acute psychosis, seizures, or focal neurological signs require serologic and frequently cerebrospinal fluid examination. The Center for Disease Control Treatment Schedules for Syphilis (U.S. DHEW, 1976) indicates that treatment for neurosyphilis in symptomatic or nonresponsive patients may require doses of aqueous crystalline penicillin G up to 24 million units daily for 10 days.

ENURESIS

Enuresis or bed-wetting is classified as primary, or secondary, depending on whether the individual has ever achieved voluntary control over urination. Primary enuresis defines those who have not achieved control; secondary enuresis refers to patients who have attained a period of control for at least several months. Nocturnal enuresis further describes the group of enuretics who have difficulty only during sleep. This group encompasses 85 percent of all enuretics.

Enuresis presents in childhood and persists into adulthood with an incidence of 1 percent. Enuresis is a symptom, not a disease, and may have multiple etiologies. Current theories explaining this disorder include: (1) maturational or developmental delay; (2) habit deficiency; (3) genetic factors; (4) sleep disorders; (5) organic factors; (6) psychologic factors; and (7) environmental factors. The maturational delay hypothesis is supported by evidence of age-related improvement in this disorder. Males have an increased incidence of enuresis. Genetic factors are supported by an increased family incidence, although this could be related to training or environmental factors. Proponents of the sleep disturbance hypothesis note increased occurrence of sleep EEG disturbance in enuretics. Enuresis is generally related to the first sleep cycle in Stage 4, although enuresis also occurs during arousal from rapid eye movement (REM) sleep in some individuals. Most clinicians agree that evaluation of enuretics for infection, allergy, occult urinary tract lesions, or bladder outlet obstruction can be highly selective and undertaken when other symptoms such as pain occur, or when abnormalities of urinalysis are present. The presence of environmental and psychological factors varies. Gross psychiatric disturbance is present infrequently, but insecurity and anxiety are often noted in these children. In younger children, the parents' attitudes of embarrassment and concern may be greater than the child's.

Two major approaches to treatment are utilized: a signal alarm system, and drug therapy with imipramine. Alarm systems seem to produce better cure rates.

Disadvantages of these systems are a longer control period to achieve success and the requirement for more supervision. Imipramine dosage is 25 mg for ages 5 to 8 and 50 mg for children over 8 years of age. The main disadvantages of imipramine are its side effects and a high relapse rate when the drug is discontinued (Perlmutter, 1976; Kolvin et al., 1972).

EVALUATION OF SEXUAL DYSFUNCTION

The successful evaluation of sexual dysfunction requires careful history-taking and selective use of physical examination, laboratory data, and psychological testing. Patients' attitudes and feelings about sexual performance include embarrassment, guilt, fear of failure, and anger. These feelings greatly inhibit the exchange of information between physician and patient. Sexual dysfunction may be related to marital discord or overt homosexual activity. The degree of discomfort and conflict experienced by the patient may be outweighed by concerns about revealing sexual problems. Patients may not believe that help is possible. Thus, the physician's first task is to be alert for clues indicating sexual problems. Evaluation necessitates a discussion of sexual practices, assessment of existing relationships, and physiological screening.

Sexual Dysfunction in the Male

A useful distinction has been to classify impotence into erectile and ejaculatory dysfunction. Currently, the medical use of impotence is often restricted to disorders of erection (Kaplan, 1974).

Erectile Dysfunction

Classification of erectile dysfunction distinguishes between primary and secondary types and separates dysfunction by organic and psychogenic origins. Primary erectile dysfunction occurs in males who have never had normal erectile function. The incidence of primary dysfunction is very low. Secondary problems occur in men who have had a distinct change in ability to achieve erection.

Small (1978a) used six organic categories to identify erectile dysfunction: (1) trauma, including spinal cord injuries, genital trauma, and pelvic fracture; (2) postsurgical complications, including prostatectomy, lumbar sympathectomy, perineal resection, cystectomy, and external sphincterotomy; (3) vascular disease; (4) neurological disease, including multiple sclerosis, myelitis, hypothalmic disorders and peripheral neuropathy; (5) endocrine and metabolic disorders, including diabetes and Addison's disease; and (6) medication side effects, including antihypertensives, particularly alpha methyldopa, Reserpine, guanethidine and spironolactone, major tranquilizers, antidepressants, anticholinergic agents, estrogens, alcohol, and drugs of abuse. He groups psychogenic erectile disorders into four major groups: (1) problems related to the sexual partner; (2) stress; (3) job fatigue; and (4) psychopathological states, such as depression. It should be noted that a mixed etiology can frequently be found, and for a number of patients it may be impossible to determine how much weight to give to the variety of etiologic components that are present. Levine (1976) adds the category "ambiguous impotence" to his classification of erectile disorders. Performance anxiety is a contributing factor to almost all cases of erectile dysfunction.

Levine directs history-taking toward four major areas: (1) psychological dysfunction, i.e., problems in achieving or maintaining erection; (2) constancy of erection, i.e., masturbation, change of partners, or an erection during sleep; (3) specific details of penile tumescence; and (4) exploration of related life events.

Beutler et al. (1975) were able to discriminate psychogenic erectile dysfunction in 90 percent of 32 males by two rules: MF scale above about 60, and one or more scales with a T score of 70 or above on the MMPI. They found no significant difference in the mean MMPI scores of patients with psychogenic and organic erectile dysfunction.

The clinician who does not treat erectile disorders may best refer such patients to a sexual counselor with a brief history that includes suspected contributing factors.

Cooper (Kaplan, 1974) has concluded that short-term therapy directed toward active intervention is superior to long-term insight-oriented approaches. He also found that inclusion of a partner in therapy added to the success rates with erectile dysfunction.

Penile Prosthesis

Surgical implantation of a penile prosthesis is being utilized with widespread satisfaction for carefully screened individuals with erectile dysfunction. The best candidates demonstrate high motivation, acceptance by a female partner, and have residual penile sensation or partial loss of erectile ability. Poor candidates have a history of total loss of sensation or total loss of erectile function. Careful discussion and demonstration of the function of the device, including expected results and possible complications, are important (Furlow, 1978; Wood and Rose, 1978).

Psychological screening interviews and MMPI evaluation are useful (Osborne, 1976). Studies of penile tumescence during REM sleep are considered by Karacan et al. (1975) to identify surgical candidates with little or no nocturnal penile tumescence. Small (1978b) has had success using penile prosthesis in patients who have erectile dysfunction with predominantly psychological causes, and who do have nocturnal penile tumescence and have failed with psychiatric treatment. Most frequently, surgically treated patients have had erectile dysfunction associated with diabetes mellitus, prostatectomy, trauma, Peyronie's disease, arterial insufficiency, or neurologic dysfunction.

Two types of prosthesis are available. The Small-Carrion prosthesis is a noninflatable rod that can be inserted by a simpler and less expensive procedure. The penile dimensions are smaller and the penis remains constantly erect. The inflatable type is of greater dimension and simulates normal function. Complications with this type are more frequent and surgical insertion is more difficult..

Ejaculatory Dysfunction

Premature ejaculation can be recognized without difficulty. Erectile function is not disrupted. Most clinicians define premature ejaculation as the occurrence of orgasm before 30 to 90 seconds after vaginal entry. Kaplan (1974) has emphasized the inability to exert voluntary control over the ejaculatory reflex. Secondary premature ejaculation occurs in men with previously normal ejaculatory function. These patients require thorough medical evaluation for local prostatic disease or progressive neurological disease. Primary premature ejaculation occurs in the great majority of patients. These males have a history of never having attained adequate control of ejaculation. This group is effectively treated in as many as 95 percent of cases by the "squeeze" or "stop-start" techniques devised by Semans (1956), Masters and Johnson (1970), and Kaplan. The interested clinician can easily learn such treatment techniques which can be taught in the office setting. Otherwise, premature ejaculators identified by history should be referred for sexual counseling.

Retarded ejaculation involves inhibition of the ejaculatory reflex and inability to discharge semen. Excess alcohol or repeated intercourse may transiently cause this condition. Mellaril, other phenothiazines, and antihypertensives may inhibit ejaculation. Neurological disease and depressed androgen levels cause this condition. Psychological issues are frequently associated with this problem and are often revealed historically when a man is able to successfully masturbate to orgasm but not experience orgasm with intercourse, or when he achieves orgasm with a partner other than a spouse.

Female Sexual Dysfunction

Masters and Johnson (1970) and Kaplan (1974) report that the sexual response of women may be less vulnerable to physical problems. General debilitation from illness inhibits sexual interest. The organic causes of problems are fewer, including progressive neurological disease; genital malignancy; endocrine disorders; diseases affecting muscle contractibility; and endometriosis, which may cause excessive bleeding, dysmenorrhea and pain directly related to intercourse. Having ascertained that one of these diseases is not present, the clinician who evaluates sexual dysfunction may find Kaplan's classification of these disorders helpful.

General sexual dysfunction refers to disorders of inhibited sexual response.

Physiological components are poor vaginal lubrication, lack of vaginal expansion, little vasocongestion during sexual response, and no orgasmic platform. Subjectively, women report feeling unaroused by sexual stimulation. The term "frigidity" for this disorder is less desirable than general sexual dysfunction.

Orgasmic dysfunctions are most common and are limited to those problems in which orgasmic response is inhibited. Most women in this category report feelings of arousal and show early physiological responses of lubrication and genital engorgement, but complain of inability to achieve orgasm.

Vaginismus is a condition of involuntary muscular contraction of the muscles at the vaginal orifice. Symptoms may vary. In its most severe form, vaginal penetration cannot be achieved. Painful intercourse may frequently result from this condition.

Sexual anesthesia involves a lack of any erotic feelings. Genital contact results only in feelings of being "touched." Kaplan considers sexual anesthesia to be a neurosis and not a "true sexual dysfunction."

Specific treatments are available for these disorders but will not be discussed here.

REFERENCES

Abram, H. S. The "uncooperative" hemodialysis patient: A psychiatrist's viewpoint and a patient's commentary, in *Living or Dying: Adaptation to Hemodialysis*. N. B. Levy, ed. Charles C. Thomas, Springfield, Illinois (1974), pp. 57–61.

Abram, H. S. The psychiatrist, the treatment of chronic renal failure, and the prolongation of life: II. *Am. J. Psychiat.* 126:157–167 (1969).

Abram, H. S., Moore, G. L., and Westervelt, F. B. Suicidal behavior in chronic dialysis patients. *Am. J. Psychiat.* 127:1199–1204 (1971).

Alfrey, A. C., LeGendre, G. R., and Kaehny, W. D. The dialysis encephalopathy syndrome: Possible aluminum intoxication. *N. Eng. J. Med.* 294:184–188 (1976).

Alfrey, A. C., Mishell, J. M., Burks, J., Contiguglia, S. R., Rudolph, H., Lewin, E., and Holmes, J. H. Syndrome of dyspraxia and multifocal seizures associated with chronic hemodialysis. *Trans. Am. Soc. Artif. Int. Org.* 18:257–261 (1972).

Arieff, A. I., and Massry, S. G. Dialysis disequilibrium syndrome, in *Clinical Aspects of Uremia and Dialysis*. S. G. Massry and A. L. Sellers, eds. Charles C. Thomas, Springfield, Illinois (1976), pp. 34–52.

Baker, A. B., and Knutson, J. Psychiatric aspects of uremia. *Am. J. Psychiat.* 102:683–687 (1946).

Beard, B. H. Fear of death and fear of life. *Arch. Gen. Psychiat.* 21:373–380 (1969).

Beutler, L. E., Karacan, I., Anch, A. M., Salis, P. J., Scott, F. B., and Williams, R. L. MMPI and MIT discriminators of biogenic and psychogenic impotence. *J. Consult. Clin. Psychol.* 43:899–903 (1975).

Dewhurst, K. The neurosyphilitic psychoses today: A survey of 91 cases. *Brit. J. Psychiat.* 115:31–38 (1969).

Ellis, J. P. A patient's commentary, in *Living or Dying: Adaptation to Hemodialysis*. N. B. Levy, ed. Charles C. Thomas, Springfield, Illinois (1974), pp. 57–61.

Feighner, J. P., Robins, E., Guze, S. B., Woodruff, R. A., Winokur, G., and Munoz, R. Diagnostic criteria for use in psychiatric research. *Arch. Gen. Psychiat.* 26:57–63 (1972).

Foster, L. An account by a dialysis patient: Man and machine: Life without kidneys. *Hast. Cent. Rep.* (June, 1976), pp. 5–8.

Foster, T. A. Why patients decide to discontinue renal dialysis. *J. Am. Med. Wom. Assn.* 31:234–235 (1976).

Furlow, W. L. The current status of the inflatable penile prosthesis in the management of impotence: Mayo Clinic experience updated. *J. Urol.* 119:363–364 (1978).

Goldstein, A. M., and Reznikoff, M. Suicide in chronic hemodialysis patients from an external locus of control framework. *Am. J. Psychiat.* 127:1204–1207 (1971).

Hooshmand, H. Seizure disorders associated with neurosyphilis. *Dis. Nerv. Syst.* 37:133–136 (1976).

Kaplan De-Nour, A., and Czaczkes, J. W. Professional team opinion and personal bias—a study of a chronic hemodialysis unit team. *J. Chron. Dis.* 24:533–541 (1971).

Kaplan De-Nour, A., Shaltiel, J., and Czaczkes, J. W. Emotional reactions of patients on chronic hemodialysis. *Psychosom. Med.* 30:521–533 (1968).

Kaplan, H. S. *The New Sex Therapy: Active Treatment of Sexual Dysfunctions*. Brunner/Mazel, New York (1974).

Karacan, I., Williams, R. L., Thornby, J. I., and Salis, P. J. Sleep-related penile tumescence as a function of age. *Am. J. Psychiat.* 132:932–937 (1975).

Kolvin, I., Taunch, J., Currah, J., Garside, R. F., Nolan, J., and Shaw, W. B. Enuresis: A descriptive analysis and a controlled trial. *Develop. Med. Child. Neurol.* 14:715–726 (1972).

Levine, S. B. Marital sexual dysfunction: Erectile dysfunction. *Ann. Intern. Med.* 85:342–350 (1976).

Levy, N. B. Psychological studies at the Downstate Medical Center of patients on hemodialysis. *Med. Clin. N. Am.* 61:759–769 (1977).

Locke, S., Merrill, J. P., and Tyler, H. R. Neurologic complications of acute uremia. *Arch. Int. Med.* 108:519–530 (1961).

Mahurkar, S. K., Salta, R., Smith, E. C., Dhar, S. K., Meyers, L., and Dunea, G. Dialysis dementia. *Lancet*. 1:1412–1415 (1973).

Masters, W., and Johnson, V. *Human Sexual Inadequacy*. Little, Brown and Co., Boston, Massachusetts, (1970).

McKegney, F. P., and Lange, P. The decision to no longer live on chronic hemodialysis. *Am. J. Psychiat.* 128:267–273 (1971).

Osborne, D. Psychologic evaluation of impotent men. *Mayo Clin. Proc.* 51:363–366 (1976).

Perlmutter, A. D. Enuresis, in *Clinical Pediatric Urology*. P. P. Kelalis, L. R. King, and A. B. Belman, eds. W. B. Saunders Company, Philadelphia, Pennsylvania (1976), pp. 166–181.

Poznanski, E. O., Miller, E., Salguero, C., and Kelsh, R. C. Quality of life for long-term survivors of end-stage renal disease. *J.A.M.A.* 239:2343–2347 (1978).

Rosser, R. Depression during renal dialysis and following transplantation. *Proc. Roy. Soc. Med.* 69:832–834 (1976).

Schreiner, G. E. Mental and personality changes in the uremic syndrome. *Med. Ann. D. C.* 28:316–362 (1959).

Semans, J. Premature ejaculation, a new approach. *S. Med. J.* 49:353–358 (1956).

Short, M. J., and Wilson, W. P. Roles of denial in chronic hemodialysis. *Arch. Gen. Psychiat.* 20:433–437 (1969).

Small, M. P. Brief guide to office counseling: Differential diagnosis of impotence. *Med. Asp. Hum. Sexual.* 12:55–56 (1978).

Small, M. P. Small-Carrion penile prosthesis: A report on 160 cases and review of the literature. *J. Urol.* 119:365–368 (1978).

Teschan, P. E., and Ginn, H. E. The nervous system, in *Clinical Aspects of Uremia and Dialysis*. S. G. Massry and A. L. Sellers, eds. Charles C. Thomas, Springfield, Illinois (1976), pp. 3–33.

Tyler, H. R. Neurological aspects of uremia: An overview. *Kidney Int.* (Supp.), 188–193 (1975).

U.S. DHEW. *Recommended Treatment Schedules for Syphilis*. Public Health Service, Atlanta, Georgia (1976).

Wise, T. N. The pitfalls of diagnosing depression in chronic renal disease. *Psychosom.* 15:83–84 (1974).

Wood, R. Y., and Rose, K. Penile implants for impotence. *Am. J. Nurs.* 78:234–238 (1978).

Wright, R. G., and Sand, P., and Livingston, G. Psychological stress during hemodialysis for chronic renal failure. *Ann. Intern. Med.* 64:611–621 (1966).

Psychiatric Presentations of Medical Illness

CHAPTER 14

Psychiatric Presentations of Hematological Disorders

M. K. POPKIN, M.D.

As with any chronic or disabling illness, hematological disease often evokes psychiatric sequelae. Psychiatric presentations may also be among the early indicators of many adult onset hematological disorders, though they infrequently serve a heralding function. This chapter will review such phenomena, emphasizing clinical recognition of the hematological etiology and subsequent psychiatric management. Psychiatric presentations accompanying or heralding selected adult onset disorders of the red cell, the white cell and lymphoid tissue, hemostasis, pigment metabolism, and factitious blood disease will be considered.

RED CELL DISORDERS

Anemias

Many of the general symptoms of anemia, and especially those referable to the central nervous system (CNS), are also prominent in psychiatric disturbances. Easy fatigability, lassitude, tiredness, and generalized weakness are the most common and often earliest symptoms of anemia (De Gruchy, 1970). This symptom cluster also defines neurasthenia. Headache, vertigo, tinnitus, faintness, spots before the eyes, numbness and tingling of the extremities, drowsiness, and impaired concentration are common symptoms of anemia referable to the CNS. They likewise may be encountered in Briquet's syndrome (hysteria) or affective disturbances. Menstrual irregularities, decreased libido, anorexia, nausea, and constipation are associated with both anemia and psychiatric illness, especially depressive disorders.

Anemias are four times as common in women as men. Incidence is highest in the child-bearing years for women; for men, the peak incidence is after 60 years of age. The clinical features are the result of the anemia itself and the disorder causing the anemia. The patient's age and the rate of the development of the anemia determine the hemoglobin level at which symptomatology will become manifest (De Gruchy, 1970). For the physician confronted with the aforementioned psychiatric or anemic symptoms, a careful history and clinical examination may reveal signs of anemia or the disorder causing the anemia.

Causes of anemia include blood loss, impaired red cell formation by the marrow, and excess red cell destruction. Using these groupings, psychiatric presentations of specific anemias will be discussed.

Acute Blood Loss

A normal man can rapidly lose up to 20 percent of his total blood volume without becoming symptomatic (Hillman, 1972). When loss exceeds 20 percent, signs of cardiovascular distress appear and may include organic mental features. When the blood loss exceeds 30 percent of the original volume, there is a gradual onset of shock.

Chronic Blood Loss

Chronic blood loss resulting in iron deficiency is the most common cause of anemia seen in clinical practice. Clinical features vary with the rate and amount of loss. Onset is usually insidious, and the symptoms are those common to all anemias. Iron-deficiency anemia is an important cause of chronic fatigue and ill health in menstruating women (De Gruchy, 1970).

Young adults may manifest little psychiatric or anemic symptomatology with hemoglobin levels as low as 6 gms/dl, if the loss has been gradual and chronic. Even middle-aged and elderly patients with severe iron deficiency need not show mental abnormality (Strachan and Henderson, 1967). However, with pronounced chronic blood loss, the psychiatric presentation may include organic mental disorder with confusion, memory deficits, or delirium as a feature of cerebral hypoxia. Treatment entails correction of the disorder causing the blood loss anemia.

Impaired Red Cell Formation by the Marrow

Psychiatric presentations associated with deficiencies of vitamin B_{12} and folic acid, both essential for hematopoiesis, have been the subject of considerable speculation and controversy. The picture remains poorly clarified.

Vitamin B_{12} Deficiency. The human daily requirement of vitamin B_{12} is about 1 μg, and body stores range from 1000 to 2000 μg. Deficiency occurs due to disorders of ingestion, utilization, or malabsorption. These include Addisonian pernicious anemia, intestinal strictures, blind loops, diverticulii, ileal resection, gastrectomy, sprue, tapeworm infestation, and certain drugs. Barbiturates, antibiotics, cytotoxics, and some neuroleptics, including chlorpromazine, may transiently reduce B_{12} levels (Carney, 1969).

Clinical manifestations of B_{12} deficiency appear only when tissue stores are sharply depleted (De Gruchy, 1970). These manifestations include megaloblastic anemia, glossitis, and involvement of the nervous system (myelopathy, peripheral neuropathy or cerebral features). A common diagnostic triad includes sore tongue, weakness, and paresthesias. Other features include gastrointestinal symptoms, lemon-yellow complexion, and dorsal column signs. Less commonly encountered are visual disturbances, congestive heart failure, angina, impotence, bladder atony, and hemorrhage.

Examination of the psychiatric aspects of vitamin B_{12} deficiency has been largely confined to studies of Addisonian pernicious anemia, a disorder in which a full range of psychiatric disturbances has been reported. Onset of pernicious anemia before the age of 40 is uncommon, and the disorder predominates in people of northern European origin. However, recent work has revealed a higher than expected incidence in black women with an early age of onset (Carmel and Johnson, 1978). Patients with a family history of pernicious anemia, or with an associated auto-immune disorder, such as thyroiditis or rheumatoid arthritis, are at greater risk. The electroencephalogram (EEG) in pernicious anemia shows slowing (e.g., diffuse slow-wave activity), which generally improves after treatment with B_{12} (Samson, et al., 1951). Serum B_{12}, a sensitive parameter of deficiency (Sullivan, 1970) is decreased. Leukopenia and thrombocytopenia are usual; RBC survival is decreased. Serum LDH is increased; cholesterol and alkaline phosphatase are decreased. A Schilling test is diagnostic.

Jefferson (1977) suggested that no psychiatric presentation is pathognomonic in pernicious anemia, though organicity is perhaps most common and psychotic states occur in 4 to 16 percent of these patients. Disturbances of memory and affect are noted in most reports together with a lesser incidence of paranoid patterns, hallucinations, lack of spontaneity, and confusion (Sullivan, 1970). Roos and Willanger (1977), studying 42 gastrectomized patients with serum B_{12} levels less than 200 pg/ml, found half with intellectual impairment on formal psychological testing. There is agreement that untreated cerebral lesions in B_{12} deficiency may progress to an irreversible organic brain syndrome, thus making early recognition critical.

It has been suggested that psychiatric alterations may precede all other features of pernicious anemia (Langdon, 1905; Holmes, 1956). Strachan and Henderson (1965) described three cases of B_{12} deficiency, replacement responsive, with psychiatric features appearing in the absence of subacute combined degeneration of the cord and with unremarkable bone marrow and blood studies (save an abnormally low serum B_{12} level). Though the concept of psychiatric presentations antedating all other features of B_{12} deficiency states is intriguing, it is not satisfactorily proven. The suggested relationship may reflect no more than random association. Given the insidious onset of B_{12} deficiency, it seems more likely that psychiatric features might often be responsible for bringing the patient to medical attention, although other clinical features of the deficiency state may be readily discernible upon examination. The most useful screening method for possible B_{12} deficiency is careful review of routine hematological parameters including red cell indices and peripheral blood smear. These should serve as a starting point for possible utilization of B_{12} levels.

With B_{12} treatment, the reticulocyte count begins to rise by the fourth day, reaches a maximum on the eighth to ninth day, and is normal by the fourteenth day. Subjective improvement usually commences within 2 to 3 days (De Gruchy, 1970). The resolution of psychiatric presentations in B_{12} deficiency with treatment has been observed to approach 80 percent (Holmes, 1956). However, it has been noted that correction of the B_{12} deficiency does not always influence the mental state (Shulman, 1967), and long-term controlled studies are still needed in this matter. Spontaneous remission and the possibility that B_{12} deficiency does not have the same causal relationship to all psychiatric syndromes have been discussed by Shulman (1967) who reported a few cases in which routine psychotropics corrected the psychiatric disturbance prior to B_{12} injections.

Folic Acid Deficiency. Deficiency of folic acid can result from intestinal malabsorption, increased demand, the action of folic acid antagonists, or inadequate intake. Folic acid is a water-soluble, B-complex vitamin required for the synthesis of purine, thymines, and methionine, the amino acid required for a multitude of transmethylation reactions. The adult daily requirement is 50 to 75 mcg; normal human reserves are adequate for a short time (Herbert, 1962).

There has emerged growing interest in the psychiatric aspects of folic acid deficiency. The current status of work in the area is best reflected by the statement of Carney and Sheffield (1978), "The neurology and psychiatry of folic acid deficiency need to be defined and, with respect to B_{12} deficiency, brought up to date," (p. 143). Adding to the lack of clarity, there is disagreement between American and British hematologists as to the possibility that folic acid deficiency alone results in neurologic pathology. The majority of citations in the following discussion are the works of British investigators taking the affirmative position in this unresolved debate.

Herbert's folate fast (1962) demonstrated multiple sequelae attendant to restricting daily intake of folate to less than 5 μg for 5 months. The initial hematologic abnormality was hypersegmentation of the neutrophilic polymorphonuclear leukocytes in the peripheral blood at 7 weeks. Macroovalocytosis appeared peripherally at 18 weeks. The marrow became megaloblastic at 19 weeks. At 14 weeks, Herbert reported the onset of forgetfulness and insomnia, both progressing and joined by increasing irritability at 19 weeks. Both anemia and mental changes remitted within 48 hours of restoring folic acid to the diet. Herbert noted a transient euphoria and sternal bone pain as well with the restoration of folic acid.

Folic acid deficiency (due to inborn errors of metabolism) has been reported as a cause of mental retardation (Arakawa, 1970). Folic acid responsive homocystinuria and schizophrenic-like behavior has been described in a mildly retarded adolescent girl (Freeman et al., 1975). Treatment of folic acid deficiency in organic (dementiform) presentations has yielded unexpected, sustained behavioral improvement or even total correction (Strachan and Henderson, 1967; Read et al., 1965). Manzoor and Runcie (1976), describing 10 cases of folic acid responsive neuropathy, noted all their subjects experienced an improvement in mood with folic acid treatment (10 mg TID). Two psychotic presentations resolved; four of five patients with pretreatment confusion showed cognitive improvement. The psychic improvement "was discernible within 2 weeks of starting treatment and preceded the improvement in reflex abnormalities by many weeks, and even months," (p. 1177). Others have reported improvement in the mental state of chronically folic acid-deficient patients when given folic acid (Carney and Sheffield, 1978). Regrettably, few of these reports reflect well-designed studies originally intended to address psychiatric alterations.

As with B_{12}, it has been suggested that folic acid-related psychiatric abnormality may develop in the absence of overt megaloblastic anemia (Strachan and Henderson, 1967). Nor does a normal hemoglobin exclude a folic acid-dependent neuropathy with behavioral features according to Manzoor and Runcie (1976). Evidence supporting a fundamental role for folic acid in maintaining the integrity of the nervous system has been offered (Wells, 1965; Wells and Casey, 1967). In contrast to vitamin B_{12}, folic acid is selectively concentrated in the cerebrospinal fluid as compared with plasma (Wells, 1965).

Biochemical surveys of psychiatric populations have found serum folate levels to be associated with both depressive disorders and organic states and low B_{12} levels with organic presentations (Carney, 1967). These surveys found high incidences of low folate and B_{12} levels, but these may not have reflected true deficiency due to the effects of drugs and other factors (Carney and Sheffield, 1978). Also, serum folate levels may not accurately reflect whole body folate deficiency; however, hypersegmentation of granulocytes is usually a reasonable reflection of tissue depletion of folic acid.

The aforementioned surveys and case reports suggest that organic and depressive psychiatric presentations could be early indicators of folic acid deficiency, perhaps antedating or appearing concurrently with neurological features. Clinically, the patient may manifest glossitis, diarrhea, hyperpigmentation, anorexia, and general features of anemia. Macrocytosis is a sensitive indicator of occult folate deficiency, but this effect may be masked by concurrent iron deficiency. As with B_{12}, hypersegmented granulocytes in the peripheral smear may assist in the decision to determine serum levels. The hypersegmentation and oval macrocytes are indistinguishable from those of vitamin B_{12} deficiency.

Folic acid deficiency is the usual cause of megaloblastic anemia associated with pregnancy, sprue, malnutrition, chronic hemolytic anemia, and the use of anticonvulsants. Reynolds et al. (1966) found megaloblastic hemopoiesis in 38 percent, and subnormal serum folates in more than 75 percent, of a series of 54 outpatient epileptics. Reynolds (1967) has suggested these metabolic disturbances may play a part in the production of the schizophreniform psychoses of epilepsy. Carney and Sheffield (1970) note that neuroleptics, tricyclic antidepressants, minor tranquilizers, and monoamine oxidase inhibitive (MAOI) drugs are likely to have antifolate activity. Oral contraceptives, cytotoxics (such as methotrexate), alcohol, and renal dialysis are all known to contribute to or engender folic acid deficiency states. The major cause of folic acid deficiency in alcoholics is dietary deprivation, but alcohol does interfere with folic acid metabolism, and there is evidence of decreased jejunal absorption of folic acid in alcoholics (Eichner, 1973). Macrocytosis may prove to be a reliable indication of alcoholic abuse (Carney and Sheffield, 1978).

The clinician's index of suspicion regarding folic acid deficiency should rise when any of the preceding variables is known to be involved. It should be noted that the therapeutic use of folic acid can precipitate subacute combined degeneration of the cord in subjects with occult B_{12} deficiency. This points to the merits of determining serum B_{12} and folate levels together.

Symptomatic Anemias. Anemias associated with disorders including infection, renal failure, malignancy, liver disease, endocrine dysfunction, collagen diseases, and scurvy are usually normocytic and normochromic in type. These so-called "symptomatic" anemias respond only to the correction or alleviation of the causative disorder. Associated psychiatric presentations are best viewed in the context of the specific causative disorder in combination with the general clinical aspects of anemia noted earlier.

Increased Red Cell Destruction

Psychiatric presentations are seldom early or initial indicators of hemolytic anemias. The life span of the red cell in these disorders is shortened due either to an intracorpuscular defect or an extracorpuscular abnormality involving an abnormal hemolytic mechanism (De Gruchy, 1970). The hereditary hemoglobinopathies, such as sickle cell disease, exemplify the former in which the fault lies in the cells themselves. In these disorders, psychiatric disturbances emerge as the consequence of obstruction of cerebral vessels. The presentations vary with the site and extent of the obstruction. Seizures, headaches, paralysis, disorders of consciousness, and death may also evolve from such vascular phenomena.

In hemolytic anemias involving an extrinsic abnormality, psychiatric presentations are encountered attendant to vascular occlusion, or secondary to processes such as disseminated intravascular coagulation (DIC), thrombotic thrombocytic purpura (TTP), or infections. For example, Blocker et al. (1968), examining psychiatric manifestations of cerebral malaria, noted anoxia (due either to thrombosis or reduced oxygen-carrying capacity of the infected erythrocytes) produced psychotic states as well as neurologic signs. Psychiatric presentations may also accompany the hemolysis induced by drugs and chemicals. Though psychiatric features may be encountered in the acquired hemolytic anemias, they will almost invariably be found in conjunction with multiple signs of a systemic process rather than in isolation.

MYELOPROLIFERATIVE DISORDER

Polycythemia Vera

Polycythemia vera is an uncommon condition marked by an excess production of the formed elements of the blood by a hyperplastic bone marrow (De Gruchy, 1970). The cause is unknown, and the disease is classified as a myeloproliferative disorder. It is usually insidious in onset, most often presenting in the sixth decade. (Relative polycythemia and stress polycythemia often first appear in the fourth decade.) Incidence is slightly higher in males and in Jews.

Psychic changes usually prevail in the initial stage of the disease (Ekiert et al., 1967). In a series of 231 cases of polycythemia vera, Lawrence (1955) noted that many of the patients had initially been thought to be suffering from neurasthenia and the true diagnosis was not made for as much as several years. Early clinical symptoms are usually attributable to hypervolemia and hyperviscosity (Weinstein, 1973) and generally involve the central nervous system. De Gruchy (1970) has observed that cerebral symptoms (e.g., psychiatric and neurologic) constitute the most common presentation, likely resulting from vascular distention, stasis, and perhaps tissue hypoxia. Headache, syncope, vertigo, tinnitus, visual changes, and paresthesias are noted. The constellation has been likened to mountain sickness (Wintrobe et al., 1974). Psychiatric features include anxiety, irritability, apathy, sleep dysfunction, depression, hallucinations, confusion, and loss of memory. Myoclonia, chorea, seizures, narcolepsy, and catalepsy have also been observed. Lethargy and fatigue are nonspecific symptoms of polycythemia vera, known to persist after normalization of laboratory values. Weinstein (1973) attributed these to associated depression. Though noting the absence of definitive studies of the psychiatric aspects of polycythemia vera, he contended that psychiatric syndromes, including severe organic mental disorders, are rare in true polycythemia. However, Ekiert et al. (1967) found decreased intellectual function (but no psychosis) in a series of 20 patients with polycythemia vera. De Gruchy (1970) suggested that depression and other psychiatric disturbances "occur occasionally" in the disorder (p. 489).

EEG findings in polycythemia have not been shown to differ markedly from an age matched control group (Ekiert et al., 1967). In later stages of the disorder, symptoms such as diaphoresis, anorexia, weight loss, and diarrhea are usually indicative of panmyelosis or significant myeloid metaplasia.

The clinician's recognition of the disorder in the face of a psychiatric presentation may be aided by the ruddy complexion, complaints of pruritus (especially after bathing), urticaria, vague digestive complaints ("almost universally present," Weinstein, 1973: p. 95), plethora of hands, feet, ears, and mucous membranes, engorgement of the retinal veins, and splenomegaly. True polycythemia must be distinguished from the spurious forms and secondary forms of erythrocytosis, especially as regards treatment.

DISORDERS OF THE WHITE CELL, LYMPHOID TISSUE AND THE DYSPROTEINEMIAS

Infectious Mononucleosis

Infectious mononucleosis is a relatively common acute infectious disease whose onset is usually insidious and characterized by an absolute lymphocytosis with the appearance of abnormal lymphocytes in the peripheral blood.

Acute psychosis or delirium may constitute the presenting or predominant symptomatology of this disorder and obscure recognition of "the true identity of the disorder," (Schnell et al., 1966: p. 51). Actual involvement of the CNS is rare, occurring in less than 2 percent of cases and overshadowing the usual presenting symptoms. When present, meningitis, encephalitis, and polyneuritis usually appear 1 to 3 weeks after disease onset. Neck stiffness, palsies, and cerebellar features may be found. The cerebrospinal fluid (CSF) shows an increment of cells (lymphocytes) and protein. Schnell et al. (1966) described nine cases with primary CNS involvement. Eight showed psychiatric changes consisting of delirium, loss of memory, and "irrational behavior," (p. 52). In none of these cases did the neurologic or psychiatric manifestations herald the onset of the illness, though one patient developed an acute psychosis after a brief prodromal illness. Electroencephalographic changes were noted in seven of the nine cases.

The most common symptoms of infectious mononucleosis are malaise, lassitude, headache, and generalized muscle aching or soreness. These may precede sore throat and lymphadenopathy; they may constitute the total symptomatology in mild cases (De Gruchy, 1970). Anorexia and nausea may also contribute to the clinical picture. Accordingly, the presentation may be confused with neurasthenia or an affective disorder. Fever, superficial lymph node enlargement (particularly posterior cervical group), enathem, and splenomegaly assist in accurate diagnosis. There is no specific treatment; prognosis of cases with psychiatric features is excellent (Schnell et al., 1966).

A depressive syndrome or anxiety state is often noted to emerge during convalescence from infectious mononucleosis. Peszke and Mason (1969) found patients with heterophile antibody titres greater than 1/96 more likely to seek psychiatric aid. Cadre et al. (1976) supported the view that infectious mononucleosis frequently leads to depression, but found only women to be so affected.

Leukemias and Dysproteinemias

Psychiatric presentations seldom are initial or early indicators of leukemic processes. Stasis of leukocytes in the vessels of the CNS, most commonly seen in acute myelogenous leukemia and less commonly in acute lymphocytic leukemia, can however give rise to neurologic and presumptively psychiatric constellations. Direct leukemoid invasion of menninges may also engender a psychiatric presentation. Such an occurrence is most often encountered in a known leukemic who has been in remission. In addition, leukoencephalopathies and CNS infections may result as sequelae to chemotherapy and present with psychiatric features.

Mitchell (1967) reviewed etiologic factors producing psychiatric constellations in patients with neoplastic diseases. He noted general effects of neoplasia, including the propensity to cachexia, infection, and compromised metabolic and organ function. Other factors cited were the malignancy's effects on the CNS (metastatic and nonmetastatic), and the hormonal activity of certain tumors. Finally, Mitchell detailed psychiatric considerations of tumors due to their effects on blood. These include the neurasthenic pictures of anemia and erythrocytemia, the increased hemorrhagic and thrombotic tendencies due to coagulation disturbances, and sequelae of the dysproteinemias (particularly thromboses of small vessels of the brain).

Although neurologic complications of dysproteinemias, particularly Waldenström's macroglobulinemia, have received careful attention (Solomon, 1965; Logothetis et al., 1960), psychiatric presentations of these disturbances are not well delineated. In fact, Solomon (1965) reported no mental aberrations in 27 patients with macroglobulinemia, refuting Fessel's earlier observations (1962). Logothetis et al. (1960), reviewing 182 cases, found 25 percent with progressive neurological manifestations, including chronic encephalopathy, strokes, and subarachnoid hemorrage. Nine patients were also noted to show psychiatric features, ranging from personality change to organic mental syndromes. The emergence of psychiatric features was associated with shortened survival time. Pathological findings included lymphocyte and plasma cell accumulation in the subarachnoid, and Virchow-Robin spaces correlated consistently with the presence of mental symptoms. In a multiple myeloma patient with "periodic dementia," Nelson et al. (1966: p. 489) demonstrated cerebral cortical lesions at autopsy. The lesions were marked by nerve cell loss, microglial proliferation, and astronuclear swelling and vesiculation.

Increased serum viscosity in the dysproteinemias is thought to promote: (1) aggregation of cellular blood elements in small vessels, and (2) decreased cerebral blood flow, producing hypoxic changes. "Headache and mental dullness may occur with frankly psychotic behavior in some cases," (Wintrobe et al., 1974: p. 255). No specific psychiatric intervention has been reported.

Tumors of Lymphoid Tissue

Reviewing a series of 229 patients with malignant lymphoma, Hutchinson et al. (1958) found 17 with psychiatric alterations varying from depression to profound dementia. Although delineating a case in which affective disturbance was the presenting sign of Hodgkin's disease, these authors note that most often psychiatric aberrations coincided with a deterioration in the patient's condition. They conclude that these features, as other neurological aspects, suggest a rapidly advancing disease course. Postmortem examination failed to demonstrate intracranial deposits of malignant tissue of any of six autopsied patients among the group with psychiatric features.

Direct involvement of the CNS consists usually of meningeal invasion, though the cerebral cortex may be compressed by tumor from without (De Gruchy, 1970). An encephalopathic syndrome (with confusion, memory deficits, and mood disturbance) has been observed in patients with lymphomas (Mitchell, 1967) and may constitute the initial indicator of the malignancy. Its mechanism is as yet obscure. Lymphomas have also been associated with the production of a parathormone-like polypeptide, giving rise to hypercalcemia. In turn, such hypercalcemia is often associated with psychiatric symptoms, particularly organic mental disorders or affective disturbances (Mitchell, 1967).

DISORDERS OF HEMOSTASIS

Disorders of hemostasis may result from defects in the vascular, platelet, or coagulation components of the hemostatic process. Psychiatric presentations attendant to these disorders have rarely been the subject of systematic inquiry. With a few exceptions, psychiatric changes are unlikely to serve as early indicators of such disturbances. More often they reflect sequelae and serious complications including intracranial bleeding.

Acquired Vascular Defects of Hemostasis

Among these disorders, dysproteinemias, autoerythrocyte sensitization, uremia, Cushing's disease, amyloidosis, scurvy, and several others may entail psychiatric constellations. Most often, psychiatric features are likely to emerge well after the primary disorder has been recognized. However, this may not be the case with the dysproteinemias (as noted earlier) and amyloidosis. Weakness, fatigue, weight loss, paresthesias, light-headedness, or syncope are the most common presenting symptoms of primary amyloidosis, affording the clinician a 1- to 2-year period for diagnosis (Kyle and Bayrd, 1975). Cutaneous abnormalities and enlargement of the liver, spleen, and tongue are principal initial findings. Purpura involving the face and neck is frequent and periorbital purpura may be striking after proctoscopy. Orthostatic hypotension may be prominent and should alert the clinician to the diagnosis (Kyle and Bayrd, 1975). Kyle and Bayrd (1975) found peripheral neuropathy in 17 percent of their subjects, usually involving weakness of the legs, often impotence, and infrequently incontinence.

Scurvy

Scurvy is an often overlooked cause of a hemorrhagic diathesis and afflicts alcoholics, food faddists, and the malnourished. It is caused by inadequate intake of vitamin C (ascorbic acid) and marked by perifollicular hemorrhage, bleeding gums, anemia (normocytic or slightly macrocytic), ecchymoses, and a disturbance of folate metabolism with low serum folate levels (Cox et al., 1967). The latter phenomenon may be crucial to the genesis of psychiatric presentations. Features including depression, irritability, and weakness may occur concomitantly with other clinical features of the disease (Freedman and Kaplan, 1972). With adequate ascorbic acid administration, the anemia is usually promptly corrected, though folic acid is required in some cases (De Gruchy, 1970). Rapid relief of symptoms accompanies adequate replacement.

Autoerythrocyte Sensitization

Autoerythrocyte sensitization (AES) is an unusual syndrome characterized by crops of painful ecchymoses and multiple systemic complaints. The disorder, first described by Gardner and Diamond (1955), appears confined to adult women whose symptoms include severe headache, transient paresthesias, transient paresis, bouts of syncope, nausea and vomiting, abdominal pain, dyspnea, and myalgias. The pathogenesis is poorly understood. Gardner and Diamond (1955) postulated that the patients had become sensitized to their own erythrocytes, usually after trauma. Although the lesions may, at times, be factitious, self-infliction has apparently been adequately excluded in a number of reports (Gottlieb, 1972). A high incidence of emotional disturbance has been uniformly observed in these patients together with hysterical and masochistic character traits. Ratnoff and Agle (1968) suggested the term *psychogenic purpura* to be more appropriate than AES, proposing the development of new lesions to be critically related to emotional issues. New bruises have appeared at sites suggested during hypnosis (Agle et al., 1967). There is no specific treatment for AES syndrome.

Thrombocytopenia

Thrombocytopenia is caused by decreased production, increased destruction, or sequestration of platelets. Production of platelets depends upon the availability of vitamin B_{12} and folate. Deficiencies in these nutrients may engender thrombocytopenia as well as psychiatric presentations (as noted earlier). Intracranial bleeding is a particular danger in thrombocytopenic patients. Such bleeding is a major cause of death in patients with platelet counts less than 20,000/mm^3 (Zieve and Levin, 1976). It may also give rise to various organic mental syndromes, dependent upon the area of involvement.

Of the varied etiologies of increased destruction of platelets, thrombotic thrombocytopenic purpura (TTP) is distinguished by the likelihood of a psychiatric presentation as an early or initial indicator of the disorder. TTP is a syndrome characterized by thrombocytopenia, hemolytic anemia, and fluctuating neurologic deficits with psychiatric concomitants. Renal dysfunction and fever are also usually part of the clinical picture. The thrombocytopenia and hemolytic anemia are probably caused by mechanical damage to blood elements traversing an abnormal microcirculation (Zieve and Levin, 1976). The occlusion of small vessels by hyaline thrombi is presumed to account for most signs and symptoms (Zieve and Levin, 1976).

Neurologic manifestations are thought to constitute the initial symptom in more than 50 percent of these patients (Wintrobe et al., 1974). Silverstein (1968) found that varying degrees of organic mental syndromes were the most frequent initial "neurologic" manifestation, occurring in 75 of 168 of his cases. Mental changes ranged from confusion to delirium and stupor. Improvement was more likely in patients initially showing focal manifestations (as aphasia or hemiparesis) rather than organic mental signs. EEG findings usually showed diffuse abnormalities. In the great majority of reported cases, the patient has died.

Drug-associated thrombocytopenia may entail immune phenomena or damage to platelets by mechanisms poorly understood. Alcohol is among the latter group, apparently reducing platelet survival and suppressing production (Eichner, 1973). The relative contribution of such thrombocytopenia to psychiatric presentations encountered in alcoholism is questionable.

Coagulation Disorders

Psychiatric presentations in coagulation disorders have not received attention as early or initial features of the respective diseases. Inquiry has instead largely been directed to the emotional sequelae of these chronic diseases and adaptational responses (Jonas, 1977; Spencer, 1971). Bleeding into the CNS is the most common cause of death in hemophiliacs (Zieve and Levin, 1976). Such bleeding may also evoke organic mental syndromes.

Disseminated intravascular coagulation (DIC), or consumption coagulopathy, may occur as a complication of a number of disorders and clinical situations. Its manifestations include bleeding of varying degree and organ damage due to ischemia. The latter is attributed to the effect of diffuse intravascular thrombosis, particularly upon kidney and brain (De Gruchy, 1970). Accordingly, DIC may engender psychiatric disturbances together with bleeding. Laboratory diagnosis and treatment of DIC has been reviewed by Zieve and Levin (1976).

DISORDER OF PIGMENT METABOLISM

Acute Intermittent Porphyria

The porphyrias are a group of metabolic disorders characterized by the excretion of biochemical precursors of heme into the urine and feces. The various forms of porphyria are divided into two groups based on the main site of abnormal porphyrin formation, either liver or bone marrow. Of the hepatic porphyrias, acute intermittent porphyria (AIP), hereditary coproporphyria, and porphyria variegata may incorporate psychiatric presentations. Variegate porphyria is usually marked by chronic skin lesions upon sunlight exposure. Apart from this, these three forms are not clearly distinguishable on clinical grounds (including psychiatric), though their patterns of excretion of porphyrin metabolites are distinctive (Marver and Schmid, 1972). Discussion will, however, be restricted to AIP, which has been studied in greater detail than the other two forms.

AIP is inherited as a Mendelian dominant with limited penetrance. The disease exists in latent or asymptomatic forms. Women are more frequently affected than men; onset of symptoms is usually in the third to fifth decade. Diagnosis is made by detecting the porphyrin metabolites in the urine. Attacks are known to be precipitated by agents including barbiturates, oral contraceptives, chloroquine, sulphonamides, aldomet and griseofulvin (Granville-Grossman, 1971). Acute attacks are episodic, may last days to months, and the presenting clinical triad includes abdominal pain (95 percent of cases), and neurologic and psychiatric features. The abdominal pain is colicky, severe, and usually accompanied by emesis. Ileus may result. Several days after the onset of abdominal pain, nervous system manifestations often appear and may include peripheral neuropathy, and cranial and bulbar palsies. Motor disturbance may vary from weakness to quadriplegia. In most cases, paralysis is of the lower motor neuron type with absent deep tendon reflexes. Sensory disturbances, particularly in the legs, include paresthesias and hypalgesia. Diplopia, nystagmus, ptosis, dysphonia, dysphagia, and even respiratory paralysis may result from cranial and bulbar involvement.

Seizures, hypertension, tachycardia, leukocytosis, hypouricemia, inappropriate ADH secretion, abnormal glucose tolerance test, and increased glutamic oxalacetic transaminase (SGOT) are frequent accompaniments of AIP (Scully et al., 1975).

Psychiatric presentations are often prominent and sometimes are the initial presenting symptoms in AIP (Granville-Grossman, 1971). Reviewing 69 cases, Markovitz (1954) found 15 percent with psychiatric changes as their first symptom. The incidence of psychiatric alterations has been observed to range from 40 to 75 percent (Goldberg and Rimington, 1962; Stein and Tschudy, 1970; Markovitz, 1954). A full spectrum of psychiatric presentations has been reported; organic mental syndromes and affective disturbances (unipolar) predominate in most accounts. The picture has been suggested to resemble a toxic delirium (Wintrobe et al., 1974). Hysterical symptoms have also been noted. The atypical nature of both the abdominal and neurological symptomatology in AIP may predispose to labeling a patient's responses as hysterical and may contribute to an erroneous diagnosis. Ridley (1969) found patients with neuropathy in AIP to have psychiatric disturbances as well in 25 of 29 instances. Kaelbling et al. (1961) screened 2500 psychiatric patients for urinary porphobilinogen; of 35 positive urines, 12 patients had clinical features of AIP, and 7 of these were diagnosed as organic mental disorder. Psychiatric manifestations, particularly depression, may also be seen between attacks (Scully et al., 1975). In the acute attacks, certain psychiatric features may emerge attendant to electrolyte disturbance, not the primary disorder (De Gruchy, 1970). EEG is usually abnormal in an acute attack (Wintrobe et al., 1974).

Differential diagnosis includes poliomyelitis, Guillain-Barré syndrome, hemoglobinuria, lead and arsenic poisoning, and occult neoplasm.

Phenothiazines have been shown to ameliorate both psychiatric presentations and pain in AIP (Monaco et al., 1957). Lithium carbonate has been utilized to treat AIP-evoked depressive constellations (Stein and Tschudy, 1970). Additional management measures are largely supportive and symptomatic. Electrolyte balance must be maintained in the face of a proclivity to hyponatremia (due to inappropriate ADH secretion). ALA synthetase may be "repressed" by a glucose loading (De Gruchy, 1970). Respiratory assistance may be needed in severe cases. Degree of recovery is quite variable (Goldberg, 1959) and may take as long as 5 years. The infusion of hematin has recently been shown to correct both biochemical and clinical manifestations of AIP (Watson et al., 1977; Peterson et al., 1976).

FACTITIOUS BLOOD DISEASE

Though very rarely encountered and infrequently documented, factitious blood disease presents marked difficulties in appropriate diagnosis and clinical management. Abram and Hollender (1974) reviewed 36 cases involving surreptitious use of anticoagulants ("Dicumarol eaters": p. 692), noting most patients to be young women who were either members of the medical profession or had been previously treated with an anticoagulant. They further reviewed factitious bleeding ("hemorrhagic histrionica") and factitious anemia resulting from self-bloodletting. Abram and Hollender emphasized the depressive, masochistic features of these patients, the bizarreness of their tactics, the recalcitrance of patient and family alike to psychiatric intervention, the underlying psychic need to assume the patient role, and the usual poor prognosis. Agle et al. (1970) offered a more encouraging account of psychiatric intervention with anticoagulant malingers diagnosed by demonstrating the offending drug in the patient's plasma. Lindebaum (1974) has described two cases of "hemoglobin munchausen" involving classical, although factitious, symptoms of sickle cell disease.

CONCLUSION

Cognitive dysfunction and affective disturbance, including neurasthenic features, predominate among the psychiatric presentations that may herald or accompany hematological disorders. The preceding discussion indicates that clinical recognition and treatment of the hematological disorder may be delayed by the emergence of psychiatric constellations. To expedite diagnostic clarity and preclude possible sequelae of untreated hematological disorder, the clinician encountering a psychiatric presentation may be assisted by examining the following points.

First, the patient's age, sex, personal, and family psychiatric history should be reviewed with respect to their consistency with known onset patterns and genetic features of psychiatric illness. Discussing pernicious anemia in 1929, McAlpine said, "More frequent examination of the gastric contents and of the blood, especially for megalocytosis, is called for in primary neuroses and psychoses occurring after the age of 35 . . . ." This contention accurately addressed the likelihood that late onset psychiatric presentations may reflect underlying medical illness. This prospect is heightened if the family history is negative for psychiatric disorder.

Second, McAlpine also called attention to the merits of hematological screening measures in the face of psychiatric symptoms. Any neurasthenic or affective constellation emerging from a careful review of systems warrants, at a minimum, a complete blood count (e.g., hemoglobin, red cell indices, white cell count, differential, platelet count) and an examination of the peripheral blood smear with attention to morphology. Ascribing neurasthenic complaints or depressive signs to a psychiatric basis without such screening must be viewed as hazardous practice. Careful history-taking may also elicit variables known to be associated with or predispose to specific hematological disorders. Identifying past medical problems, dietary and drug practices, toxic and infectious exposures, and current and prior medications may heighten the clinician's index of suspicion regarding an underlying hematological disorder, which may be insidious in its evolution.

Third, the clinical examination should include special attention to alterations in vital signs, inspection for known signs of hematological disorder, and a detailed neurological and mental status examination. As cognitive dysfunction is often the nature of the psychiatric presentation in hematological disease, the clinician should check carefully for defects in memory, information processing, arousal, perception, and attention. Corroborative history may be helpful in appreciating the often insidious onset and progression of cognitive deficits and behavioral change. When the clinician finds organic deficits, a full workup for the etiology of the organic mental disorder should follow. Regarding hematological disease, this should include a complete blood count (e.g., hemoglobin, red cell indices, white cell count and differential, platelet count, and review of the peripheral smear), serum folate and B_{12} levels, erythrocyte sedimentation rate, and a coagulation screen. Psychometric testing, EEG, and additional hematological studies may be indicated upon critical review of the preliminary laboratory results.

As in other disease entities, premorbid physical and emotional health plus adaptive capacities are critical to the resultant psychiatric presentations of hematological disorders. In many cases, the psychiatric presentations, including organicity, are fully reversible, and the likelihood of this outcome is enhanced by prompt clinical recognition and intervention. In some of the hematological disorders reviewed here, the emergence of psychiatric features has been shown to be associated with shortened survival time, a rapidly advancing disease course, or deterioration in the patient's condition due to critical CNS involvement. Most often, psychiatric intervention may be obviated by correction of the hematological disorder, if that proves possible.

REFERENCES

Abram, H. S., and Hollender, M. H. Factitious blood disease. *S. Med. J.* 67:691–696 (1974).

Agle, D. P., Ratnoff, O. D., and Spring, G. K. The anticoagulant malingerer: Psychiatric studies of three patients. *Ann. Intern. Med.* 73:67–72 (1970).

Agle, D. P., Ratnoff, O. D. and Wasman, M. Studies in autoerythrocyte sensitization: The induction of purpuric lesions by hypnotic suggestion. *Psychosom. Med.* 29:491–503 (1967).

Arakawa, T. Congenital defects in folate utilization. *Am. J. Med.* 48:594–598 (1970).

Blocker, W. W., Kastl, A. J., and Daroff, R. D. The psychiatric manifestations of cerebral malaria. *Am. J. Psychiat.* 125:192–196 (1968).

Cadre, M., Nye, F. J., and Storey, P. Anxiety and depression after infectious mononucleosis. *Brit. J. Psychiat.* 128:559–561 (1976).

Carmel, R., and Johnson, C. S. Race patterns in pernicious anemia. *N. Eng. J. Med.* 298:647–650 (1978).

Carney, M.W.P. Serum vitamin B_{12} values in 374 psychiatric patients. *Behav. Neuropsychiat.* 1:19–22 (1969).

Carney, M.W.P. Serum folate values in 423 psychiatric patients. *Brit. Med. J.* 4:512–516 (1967).

Carney, M.W.P., and Sheffield, B. F. Serum folic acid and B_{12} in 272 psychiatric inpatients. *Psychol. Med.* 8:139–144 (1978).

Carney, M.W.P., and Sheffield, B. F. Associations of subnormal serum folate and vitamin B_{12} values and effects of replacement therapy. *J. Nerv. Ment. Dis.* 150:404–412 (1970).

Cox, E. V., Meynell, M. J., Northam, B. E., and Cooke, W. T. The anemia of scurvy. *Am. J. Med.* 42:220–227 (1967).

De Gruchy, G. C. *Clinical Haematology in Medical Practice,* 3rd ed. Blackwell Scientific Publications, Oxford, England (1970).

Eichner, E. R. The hematological disorders of alcoholism. *Am. J. Med.* 54:621–630 (1973).

Ekiert, H., Gogol, Z., Jarzeboska, E., Lezko, B., and Stunkiewicz, D. Psychic disturbances and EEG patterns in polycythemia vera. *Pol. Med. J.* 6:1041–1047 (1967).

Fessel, W. J. Clinical analysis of 142 cases with high molecular weight serum proteins. *Acta Med. Scand.* Supp. 391, 173:1–32 (1962).

Freedman, A. M., and Kaplan, H. I. *Comprehensive Textbook of Psychiatry.* Williams & Wilkins Company, Baltimore, Maryland (1972), pp. 733.

Freeman, J. M., Finklestein, J. D., and Mudd, S. H. Folate responsive homocystinuria and "schizophrenia". *N. Eng. J. Med.* 292:491–496 (1975).

Gardner, F. H., and Diamond, L. K. Autoerythrocyte sensitization. A form of purpura producing painful bruising following autosensitization of red blood cells in certain women. *Blood.* 10:675–690 (1955).

Goldberg, A. Acute intermittent porphyria. *Quart. J. Med.* 28:183–209 (1959).

Goldberg, A., and Rimington, C. *Diseases of Porphyrin Metabolism.* Charles C. Thomas, Springfield, Illinois (1962), pp. 64–109.

Gottlieb, A. J. Autoerythrocyte and DNA Sensitivity, in *Hematology.* W. J. Williams, E. Beutler, A. J. Erslev, and R. W. Rundles, eds. McGraw-Hill Book Co., New York (1972), pp. 1182–1183.

Granville-Grossman, K. *Recent Advances in Clinical Psychiatry.* J & A Churchill, London, England (1971), pp. 234–239.

Herbert. V. Experimental nutritional folate deficiency in man. *Trans. Assn. Am. Phys.* 74:307–320 (1962).

Herbert, V., Gottlieb, C. W., and Altschule, M. D. Apparent low serum vitamin B_{12} levels associated with chlorpromazine. *Lancet.* 2:1052–1053 (1965).

Hillman, R. S. Acute blood loss anemia, in *Hematology.* W. J. Williams, E. Beutler, A. J. Erslev, and R. W. Rundles, eds. McGraw-Hill Book Co., New York (1972), pp. 521–526.

Holmes, J. M. Cerebral manifestations of vitamin B_{12} deficiency. *Brit. J. Med.* 2:1394–1398 (1956).

Hutchinson, E. C., Leonard, B. J., Maudsley, C., and Yates, P. O. Neurological complications of the reticuloses. *Brain.* 81:75–92 (1958).

Jefferson, J. W. The case of the numb testicles. *Dis. Nerv. Syst.* 38:749–751 (1977).

Jonas, D. L. Psychiatric aspects of hemophilia. *Mt. Sinai J. Med.* 44:457–463 (1977).

Kaelbling, R., Craig, J. B., and Pasamanick, B. Urinary porphobilinogen. Results of screening 2500 psychiatric patients. *Arch. Gen. Psychiat.* 5:494–508 (1961).

Kyle, R. A., and Bayrd, E. D. Amyloidosis: Review of 236 cases. *Med.* 54:271–299 (1975).

Langdon, F. W. Nervous and mental manifestations of pre-pernicious anemia. *Am. Med. Assn.* 45:1635–37 (1905).

Lawrence, J. H. Polycythemia. *Physiology, Diagnosis, and Treatment Based on 303 Cases.* Modern Medical Monographs, Grune and Stratton, New York and London, England (1955), pp. 2–69.

Lindebaum, J. Hemoglobin munchausen. *J.A.M.A.* 228:498 (1974).

Logothetis, J., Silverstein, P., and Coe, J. Neurological aspects of Waldenström's macroglobulinemia. *Arch. Neurol.* 3:564–573 (1960).

Manzoor, M., and Runcie, J. Folate-responsive neuropathy: Report of 10 cases. *Brit. Med. J.* 1:1176–1178 (1976).

Markovitz, M. Acute intermittent porphyria: A report of 5 cases and a review of the literature. *Ann. Intern. Med.* 41:1170–1188 (1954).

Marver, H. S., and Schmid, R. The porphyrias, in *The Metabolic Basis of Inherited Disease.* J. B. Stanbury, J. B. Wyngaarden, and D. S. Fredrickson, eds. McGraw-Hill Book Co., New York (1972), pp. 1087–1140.

McAlpine, D. A review of the nervous and mental aspects of pernicious anemia. *Lancet.* 217:643–647 (1929).
Mitchell, W. E. Etiological factors producing neuropsychiatric syndromes in patients with malignant diseases. *Int. J. Neuropsychiat.* 3:464–468 (1967).
Monaco, R. N., Leeper, R. D., Robbins, J. J., and Calvy, G. L. Intermittent acute porphyria treated with chlorpromazine, *N. Eng. J. Med.* 256:309–311 (1957).
Nelson, J. S., Woolsey, R. M., and Brown, G. O. Cortical degeneration associated with myeloma and dementia. *J. Neuropathol. Exp. Neurol.* 25:489–97 (1966).
Peszke, M. A., and Mason, W. M. Infectious mononucleosis and its relationship to psychological malaise. *Conn. Med.* 33:260–262 (1969).
Peterson, A., Bossenmaier, R., Cardinal, R., and Watson, C. J. Hematin treatment of acute porphyria. *J.A.M.A.* 235:520–522 (1976).
Ratnoff, O. D., and Agle, D. P. Psychogenic purpura: A re-evaluation of the syndrome of autoerythrocyte sensitization. *Med.* 47:475–500 (1968).
Read, A. E., Gough, K. R., Pardoe, J. L., and Nicholas, A. Nutritional studies on the entrants to an old people's home, with particular reference to folic acid deficiency. *Brit. Med. J.* 2:843–848 (1965).
Reynolds, E. H. Schizophrenia-like psychoses of epilepsy and disturbances of folate and vitamin B_{12} metabolism induced by anti-convulsant drugs. *Brit. J. Psychiat.* 113:911–919 (1967).
Reynolds, E. H., Chanarin. J., Milner, G., and Matthews, D. M. Anti-convulsant therapy, folic acid, and vitamin B_{12} metabolism and mental symptoms. *Epilepsia.* 7:261–270 (1966).
Ridley, A. The neuropathy of acute intermittent porphyria. *Quart. J. Med.* 38:307–333 (1969).
Roos, D., and Willanger, R. Various degrees of dementia in a selected group of gastrectomized patients with low serum B_{12}. *Acta Neurol. Scandinav.* 55:363–376 (1977).
Samson, D. C., Swisher, S. N., Christian, R. M., and Engel, G. L. Some observations on the mechanism of delirium in pernicious anemia. *J. Clin. Invest.* 30:669–670 (1951).
Schnell, R. G., Dyck, P. J., Boure, E.W.J., Klass, D. W., and Taswell, H. F. Infectious mononucleosis: neurologic and EEG findings. *Med.* 45:51–63 (1966).
Scully, R. E., Goldabini, J. J., and McNeely, B. V. Case records of the Massachusetts General Hospital, Case 41-1975. *N. Eng. J. Med.* 293:817–823 (1975).
Shulman, R. Vitamin B_{12} deficiency and psychiatric illness. *Brit. J. Psychiat.* 113:252–256 (1967).
Silverstein, A. TTP, the initial neurological manifestations. *Arch. Neurol.* 18:358–362 (1968).
Solomon, A. Neurological manifestations of macroglobulinemia, in *The Remote Effects of Cancer on the Nervous System.* W. R. Brain and F. Norris, eds. Grune and Stratton, New York and London, England (1965), pp. 112–124.
Spencer, R. F. Psychiatric impairment versus adjustment in hemophilia: Review and five case studies. *Psychiat. Med.* 2:1–12 (1971).
Stein, J. A., and Tschudy, D. P. Acute intermittent porphyria: A clinical and biochemical study of 46 patients. *Med.* 49:1–16 (1970).
Strachan, R. W., and Henderson, J. G. Dementia and folate deficiency. *Quart. J. Med.* 142:189–204 (1967).
Strachan, R. W., and Henderson, J. G. Psychiatric syndromes due to avitaminosis B_{12} with normal blood and marrow. *Quart. J. Med.* 34:303–317 (1965).
Sullivan, L. W. Differential diagnosis and the management of the patient with megaloblastic anemia. *Am. J. Med.* 48:609–617 (1970).
Watson, C. J., Pierach, C. A., Bossenmaier, J., and Cardinal, R. Postulated deficiency of hepatic heme and repair by hematin infusions in the "inducible" hepatic porphyrias. *Proc. Nat. Acad. Sci.* 74:2118–2120 (1977).
Weinstein, J. M. Clinical manifestations, in *Polycythemia: Theory and Management.* H. Klein, ed. Charles C. Thomas, Springfield, Illinois (1973), pp. 90–111.
Wells, C.E.C. The clinical neurology of macrocytic anemia. *Proc. Roy. Soc. Med.* 58:721–724 (1965).

Wells, D. G., and Casey, H. J. Lactobacillus casei CSF folate activity. *Brit. Med. J.* 3:834–836 (1967).

Wintrobe, M. M., Lee, G. R., Boggs, D. R., Bithell, T. C., Athens, J. W., and Foerster, J. *Clinical Hematology,* 7th ed. Lea & Febiger, Philadelphia, Pennsylvania (1974), pp. 988–1002, 943–945, 1025.

Zieve, P. D., and Levin, J. Disorders of hemostasis: Volume X in the series, *Major Problems in Internal Medicine*. Lloyd H. Smith, Jr., ed. W. B. Saunders Company, Philadelphia, Pennsylvania (1976), pp. 24–39, 51–64, 71–79.

Psychiatric Presentations of Medical Illness

CHAPTER 15

Seizure Disorders

BRIAN KIRKPATRICK, M.D.
RICHARD C.W. HALL, M.D.

GENERAL CONSIDERATIONS

Approximately 1 in 200 patients has a seizure disorder. The etiology of these disorders ranges from drug abuse, abscess, metabolic imbalance, and tumor to posttraumatic scarring, which may not become apparent for years. Correct diagnosis of the patient with a psychiatric presentation of epilepsy is particularly important, for such patients are usually under the age of 30, and may suffer from a surgically remediable lesion, such as abscess or benign tumor, or have a disease amenable to medical intervention.

The physician's preconception of psychiatric patients may interfere with correct diagnosis. Perhaps "the number of patients with schizophrenia diagnosed and treated as psychomotor epilepsy by neurologists is . . . equaled only by the number of patients with psychomotor epilepsy diagnosed and treated as schizophrenia by psychiatrists" (Treffert, 1964).

A disorder of the temporal lobe is usually found in the patient with a psychiatric presentation of epilepsy, but occipital, frontal, and parietal foci may cause many of the same symptoms, often by secondary involvement of the temporal lobe (Schneider et al., 1961; Ajmone Marsan and Goldhammer, 1973; Ludwig et al, 1975; Ludwig and Ajmone Marsan, 1975; Sherwin, 1976).

DIFFERENTIATING TRUE SEIZURES FROM PSEUDOSEIZURES

Distinguishing true ictal psychiatric symptons from pseudoseizures may be difficult, even in patients with well-documented seizure disorders. Amnesia and postictal confusion, which are helpful differentiating signs, are not always present following seizures and may occur in hysterical patients. When present, severe tongue-biting, incontinence of urine or feces, Babinski's sign, intraictally fixed and dilated pupils, and loss of corneal reflex are more reliable for differentiating true seizures from pseudoseizures.

Certain guidelines and procedures pertaining to the use of the electroencephalogram (EEG) will increase the clinician's ability to diagnose epilepsy properly:

1. The use of sphenoidal (nasopharyngeal) leads may define deep foci, which would otherwise produce a confusing surface picture.
2. Sleep studies increase the likelihood of finding foci of all types.
3. EEG's should be interpreted by an experienced electroencephalographer.
4. When possible, the EEG should be obtained at the time of symptom occurrence.
5. Sleep-deprived EEG's will increase the yield of positive reports by a factor of 2 or 3.

Seizure disorders with a psychiatric presentation usually do not remain monosymptomatic. Therefore, where diagnosis is uncertain, psychiatric observation may provide useful diagnostic information by documenting infrequent or fleeting signs and symptoms, such as automatisms, focal seizures, reflex changes, intermittent confusion, incontinence, or pupillary dilatation.

PSYCHIATRIC PRESENTATIONS OF EPILEPSY

The psychiatric presentations of seizure disorders will be categorized as follows: hallucinations, affective symptoms, behavioral disorders, disorders of higher function, disorders of motor function, special experiences, sexual disorders, and pediatric presentations (See Tables 1 and 2.)

Hallucinations

Most clinicians associate hallucinations with functional psychosis or toxic encephalopathy, but seizure disorders may also produce visual, olfactory, auditory, kinesthetic, and gustatory hallucinations. These are usually secondary to involvement of the temporal lobe, occurring in about 18 percent of such patients (Currie et al., 1971). Hallucinations may also occur in patients with parietal, frontal, and occipital lobe foci (Ajmone Marsan and Goldhammer, 1973; Ludwig and Ajmone Marsan, 1975). Hallucinations of occipital and temporal origin can usually be distinguished on clinical grounds. Frontal and parietal foci usually

TABLE 1. PSYCHIATRIC PRESENTATION OF SEIZURE DISORDERS

HALLUCINATIONS

Olfactory
Gustatory (and postictal loss of taste)
Auditory – formed and unformed
Visual – formed and unformed
palinopsia
darkness
metamorphopsia

AFFECTIVE SYMPTOMS

Depression
Fear
Anxiety
Unpleasant experiences (usually indescribable)
Lowering of interictal rage threshold
Euphoria, other pleasurable states

BEHAVIOR DISORDERS

Aggression and violence (controversial)
Confused struggling
Epilepsia cursiva
Binge eating

DISORDERS OF MOTOR FUNCTION

Automatism: reactive
stereotyped
Paroxysmal kinesgenic choreoathetosis
(classification as seizure disorder is controversial)

SPECIAL SUBJECTIVE EXPERIENCES

Somatosensory: vertigo
paresthesias
sensations of heat and cold
visceral and cephalic sensations
(usually discomfort)
Disorders of time perception: déjà vu
jamais vu
other disorders
Repetitive or intrusive thoughts
Depersonalization/derealization
Distortions of bodily proportions
Autoscopy
Nightmares
Focal pleasure
Focal pain
Sensations of eye movement
Indescribable experiences

TABLE 1. PSYCHIATRIC PRESENTATION OF SEIZURE DISORDERS (Cont.)

DISORDERS OF HIGHER FUNCTION

- Memory: transient global amnesia (doubtful)
  - postictal amnesia
- Confusional psychotic states (TLE and absence)
- Speech disorders: aphasia
  - dysphasia
  - speech iteration
  - undescribed
- "Typical personality" (controversial)

SEXUAL DISORDERS

- Hyposexuality
- Hypersexuality
- Fetishism (doubtful)
- Somatosensory symptoms of genitals or breasts

PEDIATRIC PRESENTATIONS (includes many of the above)

- Postictal blindness
- Postictal deafness
- Atonic seizures
- Focal paralysis
- School phobia ("abdominal epilepsy")

TABLE 2. OCCURENCE OF SIGNS AND SYMPTOMS OF TEMPORAL LOBE EPILEPSY

HALLUCINATIONS – Total Frequency Unknown

Visual – 18%
Auditory – 16%
Olfactory – 12%
Gustatory – 3%

AFFECTIVE SYMPTOMS – 19%

Unpleasant (often indescribable) – 14%
Panic attacks – 1%

BEHAVIORAL DISORDERS – Total Frequency Unknown

Rage attacks – 2%
Violent outbursts – 1%

DISORDERS OF HIGHER FUNCTION – Total Frequency Unknown

Speech disorders – 22%
  a. not classifiable – 3%
  b. dysphasia – 16%
  c. speech iteration – 3%
Disorders of thinking – 27%

DISORDERS OF MOTOR FUNCTION – Total Frequency Unknown

Other than grand mal – 14%
  a. adversive – 0.5%
  b. masticatory – 10%
Grand mal – 57%

SPECIAL SUBJECTIVE EXPERIENCES

Somatosensory symptoms
  a. vertigo – 19%
  b. others – 14%
Déjà vu – 14%
Visceral symptoms – 40%

cause hallucinations by excitation of the temporal lobe, and consequently mimic temporal foci.

Hallucinations caused by excitation of the temporal lobe are often quite complicated and detailed, with scenes, characters, and actions, which may be related or unrelated to the patient's past. Such hallucinations are usually differentiated from those of functional origin by the lack of accompanying affect (Goldensohn, quoted in Dreifuss, 1975).

Occipital hallucinations are usually simpler and less structured than those of temporal origin, appearing as colored lines, stars, or circles, which may move across the visual field. Characteristically, they appear in the field or homonymous fields contralateral to the affected lobe (Gassel, 1974; Holtzmann and Goldensohn, 1977). The persistence of an object or scene in a visual field, despite the actual disappearance of the image from the patient's retina, also suggests an occipital foci (Bender et al., 1968). The precise localization of a lesion within the occipital cortex can often be determined by clinical findings alone. For instance, continuously moving lights correlate strongly with calcarine lesions (Russell and Whitty, 1955).

Other symptoms such as metamorphopsia (i.e., the distortion of a perceived object's dimensions), and paroxysmal darkening of the visual fields, are of no help in localizing a lesion since they may occur secondary to such conditions as transient ischemic attack, and metabolic disturbances. Lesions that appear on the EEG as bilateral synchronous occipital foci usually produce no visual symptoms.

The physician should not immediately assume that auditory hallucinations are secondary to a functional psychosis, since some epileptics experience hallucinations that vary from crude sounds to those of actual voices or music. Organic auditory hallucinations can be differentiated from those of a functional nature in that: (1) unformed hallucinations are five times more common than the formed variety in patients with epilepsy; (2) the voice is often perceived as inside the patient's head by the epileptic, while psychotics often perceive the sound as coming from without; (3) the tongue of the epileptic may feel stiff, with the patient being unable to speak during the hallucination; and (4) the content of the hallucination caused by epilepsy is not bizarre, threatening, or condemning as is common if the hallucination is the result of a functional psychosis (Karagulla and Robertson, 1955; Currie et al., 1971).

Olfactory hallucinations are often considered classic of temporal lobe lesions, yet they occur in only 4 to 12 percent of such patients (Currie et al., 1971; Strobos, 1974). Six percent of patients with occipital lobe foci also experience such symptoms (Ludwig and Ajmone Marsan, 1975). Patients with disorders such as dental abscess, nasal polyps, and empyema also experience olfactory abnormalities that may be mistaken for hallucinations. Epileptic olfactory hallucinations are distinguished by two clinical features: (1) the odors perceived are distinctly pungent and unpleasant (burning rubber, burning hair, dead fish), and (2) their occurrence is intermittent and often associated with ictal fear, or to a lesser extent, depression. These symptoms may occur simultaneously with the olfactory change, precede, or follow it (Macrae, 1954; Weil, 1955, 1956).

Slowly growing temporal lobe tumors are frequently found in patients experiencing olfactory hallucinations; consequently, these tumors should be suspected when such symptoms occur (Strobos, 1974).

Gustatory hallucinations occur in 3 percent of patients with temporal lobe epilepsy, and are frequently associated with olfactory hallucinations. Such symptoms are fleeting, in contrast to those produced by metabolic disorders or drugs, which tend to persist over time and to occur without an olfactory component. A sudden loss of taste persisting for 24 hours or longer occurs postictally in approximately 1 percent of patients with temporal lobe epilepsy (Currie et al., 1971).

Affective Symptoms

Episodic emotional disturbances directly related to seizures occur in one fifth of patients with temporal foci (Currie et al., 1971). They are poorly understood and difficult to differentiate, since the subjective state experienced by the patient is often indescribable. Furthermore, no one-to-one correspondence exists between the location of a foci and any particular affective state (Dongier, 1959). In about half of such "emotional seizures," fear predominates, while in the other half, depression is primary (Weil, 1959).

Isolated ictal fear or anxiety represents the presenting complaint of 1 percent of patients with temporal lobe and 4 percent of patients with occipital lobe foci (Currie et al., 1971; Ludwig and Ajmone Marsan, 1975). Occasionally, patients with an absence disorder experience intraictal anxiety.

Intermittent depression as a solitary epileptic complaint is indicative of a focal disorder of the temporal lobe. Expressions of fear or anxiety during seizures occur more frequently than is reported, since patients are usually unable to remember these episodes (Gloor, 1975; Bouchard, 1977). Unlike the phobic patient, the epileptic who does remember an episode of ictal fear will usually discuss it dispassionately (Dreifuss, 1975).

Behavioral Disorders

The relationship between epilepsy and violence remains a controversial issue, and the diagnosis of intraictal violence demands rigorous proof (Ervin et al., 1969; Mark et al., 1969; Williams, 1969; Bach-y-Rita et al., 1971; Rodin, 1973; Coleman, 1974; Breggin, 1975; Gloor, 1975; Kligman and Goldberg, 1975; Keiji, 1975; Lion, 1975; Mark et al., 1975; Williams, D., 1975; Nassi and Abramowitz, 1976). Epilepsy is rarely a direct cause of purposeful violence (Goldstein, 1974). The majority of cases involving epileptic violence represent nonpurposeful, nondirected aggression occurring during the postictal period confusion. Attempts to restrain the postical patient may induce fear and struggling, subsequently reported as directed aggression. The diagnosis of "epileptic furor" should be considered only if all of the following criteria are present: (1) aggression is sudden, and without premeditation, (2) no precautions are taken to protect against self-injury or being apprehended, and (3) an altered state of consciousness is present. More widely accepted than the existence of purposeful intraictal violence is the concept that chronic disruption of the limbic system produces a lowering of the interictal rage threshold and frustration tolerance, which predisposes epileptics to angry outbursts (Gloor, 1975; Livingston, 1976).

Episodes of sudden flight without provocation occur as another behavioral manifestation of epilepsy. Such "epilepsia cursiva" may occur as a seizure component, or during the postictal confusional state. This phenomenon occurs in 1 percent of temporal lobe epileptics and should be suspected if: (1) episodes of flight are associated with alteration of consciousness or amnesia; (2) the stimulus from which the patient appears to flee is not consistent; (3) episodes are of short duration; and (4) the patient is unaware of the reason for flight (Strauss, 1960).

Binge eating may represent a behavioral symptom of epilepsy (Green and Rau, 1974, Davis et al., 1974; Weiss and Levitz, 1976). Patients who meet the following criteria may respond to medical therapy: (1) a history of impulsive, unpredictable, episodic, rapid ingestion of large quantities of food over short periods of time; (2) eating until physical discomfort occurs; (3) an associated feeling of guilt, remorse, perplexity, or self-contempt; and (4) for the year prior to treatment, binges have occurred at least once weekly with no binge-free periods of more than 3 weeks duration (Wermuth et al., 1977).

Disorders of Higher Function

Seizure disorders may produce generalized impairment of higher cognitive function, as well as symptoms suggesting focal lesions. Many clinicians believe that temporal lobe epilepsy is associated with a particular personality constellation manifested by circumstantiality, an increased interest in philosophical issues, lability, diminished frustration tolerance, and sudden outbursts of anger (Waxman and Geschwind, 1975). Patients exhibiting such manifestations describe themselves as humorless, dependent, and obsessional. Patients with right temporal foci are more apt to be emotionally labile, while those with left-sided foci are more likely to experience paranoid or grandiose delusions (Bear and Fedio, 1977). However, the relationship between temporal lobe epilepsy and personality type is by no means certain and remains a controversial issue (Stevens, 1975).

Psychotic episodes may occur as a result of epilepsy during the preictal or postictal confusional period, or between seizures. In the latter instance, the condition presents as a chronic interictal psychosis. Intraictal psychosis has also been reported (Wells, 1975).

Interictal psychoses, which occur most frequently in association with lesions of the temporal lobe, may be misdiagnosed as schizophrenia, since these patients present with an alert state of consciousness, changes in abstract thought, and paranoid delusions (Bruens, 1974). These patients, compared to temporal lobe epileptics who are not psychotic, have a higher incidence of bilateral or dominant hemisphere (left-sided) foci (Currie et al., 1971; Flor-Henry, 1974). The inappropriate affect and history of social isolation characteristic of schizophrenia are usually absent. Application of strict diagnostic criteria usually excludes the diagnosis of schizophrenia (Dongier, 1959; Kennard, 1960; Flor-Henry, 1969, 1972, 1974; Bruens, 1974). A right-sided foci is most likely to produce prominent affective symptoms, often misdiagnosed as a major depressive disorder. Thought disorders are more prominent with left-sided lesions (Flor-Henry, 1974).

The intraictal behavioral disturbances that occur with nonmotor status epilepticus may also be misdiagnosed as schizophrenia or hysteria (Wells, 1975).

Absence disorders are a rare manifestation of nonmotor status epilepticus before age 10. They are unusual during adolescence, but may be the only manifestation of such a disorder in the adult, particulary the geriatric patient (Andermann and Robb, 1972). However, they are usually associated in the older patient with a history of myoclonus, an aura, minor motor attacks, or grand mal seizures. The extent of amnesia occurring during absence episodes correlates poorly with the degree of ictal confusion, and is therefore not reliable for differentiating absence status from dissociative phenomena, hysteria, or malingering.

Clinical signs other than confusion may facilitate the diagnosis of absence status epilepticus. Such signs and symptoms include rhythmic blinking of the eyes, small amplitude jerking of the face and arms, hippus, or quivering of the lips. An apprehensive expression may be present as well as fluctuations of the patient's level of consciousness. The psychiatric presentation is typified by: (1) an abrupt onset of psychosis in a patient with no previous psychiatric disorder, (2) an unexplained intermittent delirium, (3) a history of similar episodes characterized by abrupt exacerbations and remissions, and (4) a history of fainting or falling spells (Wells, 1975).

Temporal lobe status epilepticus is often associated with reactive automatisms (i.e., the patient produces simple responses to stimuli). For instance, a patient may drink a glass of water that is handed to him (Escueta, 1974, 1977). Such reactive automatisms are usually associated with oneiroid states, whereas sterotyped (nonreactive) automatisms usually occur with seizures producing a more marked impairment of consciousness. The physician should not be misled into making a diagnosis of hysteria in patients with reactive automatisms simply because they are well-coordinated and occur in association with reported amnesia (Escueta, 1974).

Oneiroid psychoses are ictal confusional states that may occur secondary to either absence disorders or temporal lobe epilepsy; the two etiologies may be difficult to differentiate clinically in the adult (Friedlander and Feinstein, 1956; Bornstein et al., 1956; Lugaresi et al., 1971). During psychotic episodes, these patients exhibit signs of organicity, slowed or impoverished speech, and an inability to abstract. They may be able to continue to perform simple tasks and may appear irritable to the casual observer. An aura often precedes the attack, and the patient may be somewhat aware of the cognitive difficulties he experiences. The attacks can end spontaneously with the patient achieving sleep, or the attacks can generalize, producing a grand mal seizure. Episodes of nonmotor status epilepticus, producing an oneiroid psychosis, may last for as long as 72 hours (Goldensohn and Gold, 1960).

Speech disturbances are often overlooked as a sign of epilepsy, yet they occur in 20 percent of all temporal lobe disorders (Serafetinides and Falconer, 1963; Currie et al., 1971). Dysphasia accounts for two thirds of the speech disorders seen and is usually associated with a lesion of the dominant hemisphere. These dysphasic episodes are usually remembered by the patient. Conversely, speech automatisms (speech iteration) occur with lesions of either hemisphere and are usually associated with amnesia (Driver et al., 1964). Alexia may also occur intraictally (Holtzmann and Goldensohn, 1977). Both aphasia and dysphasia are more common in children and adolescents than in adults (Gascon et al., 1973; Shoumaker et al., 1974; McKinney and McGreal, 1974; dePasquet et al., 1976; Deuel and Lenn, 1977).

Temporal lobe epilepsy may produce a syndrome of transient global amnesia. This syndrome, which occurs most frequently in patients between the ages of 40 and 70, consists of total amnesia accompanied by isolated episodes of anxiety and confusion which persist for several hours. On mental status examination, the patient is able to perform immediate memory retention tasks, but has poor short-term memory (3-minute recall), and subsequent amnesia for testing. This syndrome is rare and usually occurs in a patient with no other signs, symptoms, or history of epilepsy (Jaffe and Bender, 1966; Joynt et al., 1973; Vroom, 1973).

Disorders of Motor Function

Paroxysmal kinesthetic choreoathetosis (paroxysmal choreoathetosis, extrapyramidal epilepsy) is an uncommon and frequently misdiagnosed disorder having many characteristics of pseudoseizure. There is no amnesia, ictal or postictal change of consciousness, tonic or clonic movement, or EEG change. These episodes are characteristically precipitated by environmental stress and are preceded by an aura. Some patients may be able to consciously abort an impending attack. The clinical picture is one of twisting, writhing, and thrashing movements that begin distally and proceed to involve the trunk and head. An attack averages from 15 to 30 seconds and is heralded by a period of sudden immobility, followed by erratic body movement. Onset peaks between the ages of 6 and 15, with symptoms becoming most severe during early adulthood. Genetic studies suggest transmission by an autosomal recessive or poorly penetrant autosomal dominant gene. Dispute exists concerning the etiologic classification of the disorder, since it responds to L-dopa, as well as to phenytoin and carbamazepine (Stevens, 1966; Walter, 1977).

Temporal lobe automatisms may also present as motor disorders. Masticatory automatisms occur in 10 percent of patients with temporal lesions; 0.5 to 6 percent of temporal lobe patients experience such adverse movement disorders (Currie et al., 1971). Automatisms are not specific to lesions of the temporal lobe. They also occur in 30 percent of patients with occipital foci, in some patients with frontal lesions (Rasmussen, 1963; Ludwig and Ajmone Marsan, 1975), and in patients with absence disorders (Penry et al., 1975).

Special Experiences

It is often difficult for patients to describe their ictal somatosensory symptoms. Forty percent of patients with temporal lobe disorders report unusual cranial or abdominal sensations. Vertigo occurs in 19 percent. Fourteen percent report other unusual somatosensory symptoms (Williams, D.J., 1967; Kornhuber, 1976). These symptoms are also common in patients with occipital foci (Ludwig and Ajmone Marsan, 1975). Lesions in either area also produce complaints of epigastric discomfort, numbness, and tingling of the extremities and sensations of warmth or cold, which may suggest a diagnosis of hyperventilation syndrome. These sensory distortions may be either focal or generalized.

Distortion of time perception is a common ictal phenomena. Déjà vu occurs in 14 percent of patients with temporal, and 5 percent of those with occipital, epilepsy (Currie et al., 1971; Ludwig and Ajmone Marsan, 1975). The patient may report, "I felt that time stopped," or "I felt that everything was happening in rhythm." Jamais vu, the sensation that familiar surroundings or events have never been encountered, also occurs, but is less common (Niedermeyer, 1974: p. 113).

Other epileptic symptoms may suggest a psychiatric disorder. Depersonalization and derealization were found in 35 percent of the patients with temporal lobe epilepsy who were admitted to psychiatric wards. These phenomena may also be seen with occipital epilepsy (Kenna and Sedman, 1965). Autoscopy, the sensation of viewing oneself from outside the body, is another complaint of temporal lobe patients (Daly, 1975). Schizophrenia may be suggested by reports of intrusive or repetitive thoughts, which frequently occur secondary to foci in the temporal or frontal lobes. Epileptic intrusion and thought repetition are different from similar schizophrenic symptoms, in that the former are poorly remembered and have little associated affect (Rasmussen, 1963).

Symptoms suggestive of neurosis or hysteria also occur and include: nightmares, unusual "anatomically incorrect" pain, sudden and intensely pleasurable focal sensations, subjective sensations of eye movement without such movements actually occurring, distortion of bodily size or proportion, and sudden intermittent postictal blindness (Boller et al., 1975; Fine, 1967; Wilkenson, 1973; Warneke, 1976; Holtzmann and Goldensohn, 1977; Walsh and Hoyt, 1969).

Sexual Disorders

Changes in sexual interest, drive, and performance are commonly reported by patients with diencephalic and temporal lobe epilepsy. Epilepsy should be included in the differential diagnosis of any patient who has been previously well-adjusted sexually, and suddenly develops an unusual or pressured sexual drive. Global hyposexuality, with loss of interest in sex and diminished erotic arousability to visual stimuli, are the most frequent epilepsy-related sexual changes. Cases of hypersexuality and seizure-related fetishism have been reported (Gastaut and Collomb, 1954; Mitchell et al., 1954; Hierons and Saunders, 1966; Blumer and Walker, 1967; Blumer, 1970; Walker and Blumer, 1975). Interictal copulatory movements are usually a form of automatism (Currie et al., 1971). Ictal sensations (paresthesias, etc.) focused on the genitals or breasts may occur as variations of somatosensory distortion.

Pediatric Presentations

No psychiatric presentation of seizure disorder is specific to children, but some symptoms occur with increased frequency in this age group. These include: postictal blindness, dysphasia, aphasia, and epilepsia cursiva (flight). Focal paralysis, the "classic" Freudian hysterical symptom, occurs more frequently in children than in adults as an ictal phenomenon (Waltregny et al., 1970; Beaussart and Beaussart-Boulengé, 1970). It should also be remembered that paroxysmal choreoathetosis most frequently presents between the ages of 6 and 15 (Waller, 1977).

It is important for the physician to remember that epilepsy may mimic school phobia. A child with frequent morning episodes of abdominal pain does not necessarily dislike school, but may have "abdominal epilepsy" (Walsh, 1974). Similarly, absence seizures, which can occur several times hourly, may interfere with a child's learning and be reported as a behavioral disorder by teachers.

REFERENCES

Ajmone Marsan, C., and Goldhammer, L. Clinical ictal patterns and electrographic data in cases of partial seizures of fronto-centro-parietal origin, in *Epilepsy: Its Phenomena in Man,* M. A. B. Brazier, ed. Academic Press, New York (1973), pp. 236–260.

Andermann, F., and Robb, J. P. Absence status: A reappraisal following review of thirty-eight patients. *Epilepsia.* 13:177–187 (1972).

Bach-y-Rita, G., Lion, J. R., Climent, C. E., and Ervin, F. R. Episodic dyscontrol: A study of 130 violent patients. *Am. J. Psychiat.* 127: 1473–1478 (1971).

Bear, D. M., and Fedio, P. Quantitative analysis of interictal behavior in temporal lobe epilepsy. *Arch. Neurol.* 34:454–467 (1977).

Beaussart, M., and Beaussart-Boulengé, L. Partial atonic seizures. *Electroenceph. Clin. Neurophysiol.* 29:536 (1970).

Bender, M. B., Feldman, M., and Sobin, A. J. Palinopsia. *Brain.* 91:321–338 (1968).

Blumer, D. Hypersexual episodes in temporal lobe epilepsy. *Am. J. Psychiat.* 126:1099–1106 (1970).

Blumer, D., and Walker, A. E. Sexual behavior in temporal lobe epilepsy: A study of the effects of temporal lobectomy on sexual behavior. *Arch. Neurol.* 16:37–43 (1967).

Boller, F., Wright, D. G., Cavalieri, R., and Mitsumoto, H. Paroxysmal "nightmares": Sequel of a stroke responsive to diphenylhydantoin. *Neurol.* 25:1026–1028 (1975).

Bornstein, M., Coddon, D., and Song, S. Prolonged alterations in behavior associated with a continous electroencephalographic (spike and dome) abnormality. *Neurol.* 6:444–448 (1956).

Bouchard, G. Behavioral and psychiatric problems in epilepsy, in *Neurosurgical Treatment in Psychiatry, Pain, and Epilepsy,* W. H: Sweet, S. Obrador, and J. G. Martin-Rodriguez, eds. University Park Press, Baltimore, Maryland (1977), pp. 539–552.

Breggin, P. R. Psychosurgery for the control of violence: A critical review, in *Neural Bases of Violence and Aggression.* W. S. Fields and W. H. Sweet, eds., W. H. Green, St. Louis, Missouri (1975), pp. 350–378.

Bruens, J. H. Psychoses in epilepsy, in *Handbook of Clinical Neurology,* Vol. 15, P. J. Vinken and G. W. Bruyn, eds. North-Holland, Amsterdam, Holland (1974), pp. 593–610.

Coleman, L. S. Perspectives on the medical research of violence. *Am. J. Orthopsychiat.* 44:675–687 (1974).

Currie, S., Heathfield, K.W.G., Henson, R. A., and Scott, D. F. Clinical course and prognosis of temporal lobe epilepsy: A survey of 666 patients. *Brain.* 94:173–190 (1971).

Currier, R. D., Little, S. C., Suess, J. F., and Andy, O. J. Sexual seizures. *Arch. Neurol.* 25:260–264 (1971).

Daly, D. D. Ictal clinical manifestations of complex partial seizures, in *Advances in Neurology,* Vol. 11. J. K. Penry and D. D. Daly, eds. Raven Press, New York (1975), pp. 57–84.

Davis, K. L., Qualls, B., Hollister, L. E., and Stunkard, A. J. EEGs of "binge" eaters (ltr. to ed.). *Am. J. Psychiat.* 131:1409 (1974).

dePasquet, E. G., Gaudin, E. S., Bianchi, A., and Mendilaharsu, S. A. Prolonged and monosymptomatic dysphasic status epilepticus. *Neurol.* 26:244–247 (1976).

Deuel, R. K., and Lenn, N. J. Treatment of acquired epileptic aphasia. *J. Pediat.* 90:959–961 (1977).

Dongier, S. Statistical study of clinical and electroencephalographic manifestations of 536 psychotic episodes occurring in 516 epileptics between clinical seizures. *Epilepsia.* 1:117–142 (1959).

Dreifuss, F. E. The differential diagnosis of partial seizures with complex symptomatology, in *Advances in Neurology,* Vol. 11 J. K. Penry and D. D. Daly, eds. Raven Press, New York (1975), pp. 187–200.

Driver, M. V., Falconer, M. A., and Serafetinides, E. A. Ictal speech automatism reproduced by activation procedures: A case report with comments on pathogenesis. *Neurol.* 14:455–463 (1964).

Ervin, F. R., Delgado, J., Mark, V. H., and Sweet, W. H. Rage: A paraepileptic phenomenon? *Epilepsia.* 10:417 (1969).

Escueta, A. V., Boxley, J., Stubbs, N., Waddell, G., and Wilson, W. A. Prolonged twilight state and automatisms: A case report. *Neurol.* 24:331–339 (1974).

Escueta, A. V., Kunze, U., Waddell, G., Boxley, J., and Nadel, A. Lapse of consciousness and automatisms in temporal lobe epilepsy: A videotape analysis. *Neurol.* 27:144–155 (1977).

Ferguson, S. M., Rayport, M., Gardner, R., Kass, W., Weiner, H., and Reiser, M. F. Similarities in mental content of psychotic states, spontaneous seizures, dreams, and responses to electrical brain stimulation in patients with temporal lobe epilepsy. *Psychosom. Med.* 31:479–498 (1969).

Fine, W. Posthemiplegic epilepsy in the elderly. *Brit. Med. J.* 23:199–201 (1967).

Flor-Henry, P. Psychosis and temporal lobe epilepsy: A controlled investigation. *Epilepsia.* 10:363–395 (1969).

Flor-Henry, P. Ictal and interictal psychiatric manifestations in epilepsy: Specific or non-specific? A critical review of some of the evidence. *Epilepsia.* 13:773–783 (1972).

Flor-Henry, P. Psychosis, neurosis, and epilepsy: Developmental and gender-related effects and their aetiological contribution. *Brit. J. Psychiat.* 124:144–150 (1974).

Friedlander, W. J., and Feinstein, G. H. Petit mal status (epilepsia minoris continua). *Neurol.* 6:357–362 (1956).

Gascon, G., Victor, D., Lombroso, C. T., and Goodglass, H. Language disorder, convulsive disorder, and electroencephalographic abnormalities: Acquired syndrome in children. *Arch. Neurol. 28:*156–162 (1973).

Gassel, M. M. Occipital lobe tumors, in *Handbook of Clinical Neurology*, Vol. 17, P. J. Vinken and G. S. Bruyn, eds. North-Holland, Amsterdam, Holland, (1974), pp. 310–349.
Gastaut, H., and Collomb, H. Etude du comportement sexual chez les epileptiques psychomoteurs. *Ann. Medico-psychologiques*. 112:657 (1954).
Gloor, P. Electrophysiological studies of the amygdala, in *Neural Bases of Violence and Aggression*. W. S. Fields and W. H. Sweet, eds. W. H. Green, St. Louis, Missouri (1975), pp. 5–40.
Goldensohn, E. S., and Gold, A. P. Prolonged behavioral disturbances as ictal phenomena. *Neurol*. 10:1–9 (1960).
Goldstein, M. Brain research and violent behavior. *Arch. Neurol*. 30:1–35, (1974).
Green, R. S., and Rau, J. H. Treatment of compulsive eating disturbances with anticonvulsant medication. *Am. J. Psychiat*. 131:428–432 (1974).
Hierons, R., and Saunders, M. Impotence in patients with temporal lobe lesions. *Lancet*. 2:761–764 (1966).
Holtzmann, R.N.N., and Goldensohn, E. S. Sensations of ocular movement in seizures originating in occipital lobe. *Neurol*. 27:554–556 (1977).
Jaffe, R., and Bender, M. B. EEG studies in the syndrome of isolated episodes of confusion with amnesia: "Transient global amnesia." *J. Neurol. Neurosurg. Psychiat*. 29:472–474 (1966).
Joynt, R. J., Satran, R., and Charlton, M. Transient global amnesia and psychomotor epilepsy. *Epilepsia* 14:99 (1973).
Karagulla, S., and Robertson, E. E. Psychical phenomena in temporal lobe epilepsy and the psychoses. *Brit. Med. J*. 11:748–752 (1955).
Keiji, S. Posterior hypothalamic lesions in the treatment of violent behavior, in *Neural Bases of Violence and Aggression*. W. S. Fields and W. H. Sweet, eds. W. H. Green, St. Louis, Missouri (1975), pp. 401–428.
Kellaway, P., Crawley, J. W., and Kagawa, N. Paroxysmal pain and autonomic disturbances of cerebral origin: A specific electro-clinical syndrome. *Epilepsia*. 1:466–483 (1960).
Kenna, J. C., and Sedman, C. Depersonalization in temporal lobe epilepsy and the organic psychoses. *Brit. J. Psychiat*. 111:293–299 (1965).
Kennard, M. A. Paroxysmal behavior and its EEG correlates. *Epilepsia*. 1:484–492 (1960).
Kligman, D., and Goldberg, D. A. Temporal lobe epilepsy and aggression: Problems in clinical research. *J. Nerv. Ment. Dis*. 160:324–341 (1975).
Kornhuber, H. H. Differential diagnosis of dizziness. *Arch. Otorhinlaryngol*. 212:339–349 (1976).
Kosnik, E., Paulson, G. W., and Laguna, J. F. Postictal blindness. *Neurol*. 26:248–250 (1976).
Lance, J. W. Simple formed hallucinations confined to the area of a specific visual field defect. *Brain*. 99:719–734 (1976).
Lion, J. R. Conceptual issues in the use of drugs for the treatment of aggression in man. *J. Nerv. Ment. Dis*. 160:76–82 (1975).
Livingston, K. E. Limbic system dysfunction induced by "kindling": its significance for psychiatry, *Neurosurgical Treatment in Psychiatry, Pain, and Epilepsy*. W. H. Sweet, S. Obrador, and J. G. Martin-Rodgriguez, eds. University Park Press, Baltimore, Maryland (1977) pp. 63–76.
Ludwig, B. I., Ajmone Marsan, C., and Van Buren, J. Cerebral seizures of probable orbitofrontal origin. *Epilepsia*. 16:141–158 (1975).
Ludwig, B. I., and Ajmone Marsan C. Clinical ictal patterns in epileptic patients with occiptal electroencephalographic foci. *Neurol*. 25:463–471 (1975).
Lugaresi, E., Pazzaglia, P., and Tassinari, C. A. Differentiation of "absence status" and "temporal lobe status." *Epilepsia*. 12:77–87 (1971).
Macrae, D. Isolated fear: a temporal lobe aura. *Neurol*. 4:497–505 (1954).
Mark, V. H., Ervin, F. R., Sweet, W. H., and Delgado, J. Remote telemeter stimulation and recording from inplanted temporal lobe electrodes. *Confinia Neurologica* 31:86–93 (1969).
Mark, V. H., Sweet, W. H., and Ervin, F. Deep temporal lobe stimulation and destructive lesions in episodically violent temporal lobe epileptics, in *Neural. Bases of Violence and Aggression*, W. S. Fields and W. H. Sweet, eds. W. H. Green, St. Louis, Missouri (1975), pp. 379–391.

McKinney, W., and McGreal, D. A. An aphasic syndrome in children. *Canad. Med. Assn. J.* 110:637 (1974).
Mitchell, W., Falconer, M. A., and Hill, D. Epilepsy with fetishism relieved by temporal lobectomy. *Lancet.* 2:626–630 (1954).
Nassi, A. J., and Abramowitz, S. I. From phrenology to psychosurgery and back again: Biological studies of criminality. *Am. J. Orthopsychiat.* 46:591–607 (1976).
Niedermeyer, E. *Compendium of the Epilepsies.* Charles C. Thomas, Springfield, Illinois (1974).
Parsonage, M. J. Treatment with carbainazepine: Adults, in *Advances in Neurology,* Vol. 11. J. K. Penry and D. D. Daly, eds. Raven Press, New York (1975), pp. 221–236.
Penry, J. K., Porter, R. J., and Dreifuss, R. E. Simultaneous recording of absence seizures with videotape and electroencephalography: A study of 374 seizures in 48 patients. *Brain* 98:427–440 (1975).
Rasmussen, T. Surgical therapy of frontal lobe epilepsy. *Epilepsia.* 4:181–198 (1963).
Rodin, E. A. Psychomotor epilepsy and aggressive behavior. *Arch. Gen. Psychiat.* 28:210–213 (1973).
Russell, W. R., and Whitty, C.W.M. Studies in traumatic epilepsy. 3. Visual fits. *J. Neurol. Neurosurg. Psychiat.* 18:79–96 (1955).
Schneider, R. C., Crosby, E. C., Bagchi, B. K., and Calhoun, H. D. Temporal or occipital lobe hallucinations triggered from frontal lobe lesions. *Neurol.* 11:172–179 (1961).
Serafetinides, E. A., and Falconer, M. A. Speech disturbances in temporal lobe seizures: A study in 100 epileptic patients submitted to anterior temporal lobectomy. *Brain.* 86:333–346 (1963).
Sherwin, I. Temporal lobe epilepsy: neurological and behavioral aspects. *Ann. Rev. Med.* 27:37–47 (1976).
Shoumaker, R., Bennett, D., Bray, P., and Curless, R. Clinical and EEG manifestations of an unusual aphasic syndrome in children. *Neurol.* 24:10–16 (1974).
Stevens, H. Paroxysmal choreo-athetosis: A form of reflex epilepsy. *Arch. Neurol.* 14:415–420 (1966).
Stevens, J. R. Interictal clinical manifestations of complex partial seizures, in *Advances in Neurology,* Vol. 11, J. K. Penry and D. D. Daly, eds. Raven Press, New York (1975) pp. 85–112.
Strauss, H. Paroxysmal compulsive running and the concept of epilepsia cursiva. *Neurol.* 10:341–344 (1960).
Strobos, R. J. Temporal lobe tumors, in *Handbook of Clinical Neurology,* Vol. 17, P. J. Vinken and E. W. Bruyn, eds. North-Holland, Amsterdam, Holland (1974), pp. 281–295.
Taylor, D. C. Mental state and temporal lobe epilepsy. *Epilepsia.* 13:727–765 (1972).
Treffert, D. A. The psychiatric patient with an EEG temporal lobe focus. *Am. J. Psychiat.* 120:765–771 (1964).
Vroom, F. Q. Electroencephalographic findings in transient global amnesia. *Electroenceph. Clin. Neurophysiol.* 34:734–735 (1973).
Walker, A. E., and Blumer, D. Long term effects of temporal lobe lesions on sexual behavior and aggressivity, in *Neural Bases of Violence and Aggression,* W. S. Fields and W. H. Sweet, eds. W. H. Green, St. Louis, Missouri (1975), pp. 392–400.
Waller, D. A. Paroxysmal kinesigenic choreoathetosis or hysteria? *Am. J. Psychiat.* 134:1439–1440 (1977).
Walsh, F. B., and Hoyt, W. F. Clinical neuro-ophthalmology. Williams & Wilkins, Baltimore, Maryland (1969).
Walsh, G. O. Unusual presentations of epilepsies. *Pediat.* 53:548–551 (1974).
Waltregny, A., Roger, J., Régis, H., and Gastaut, H. Polygraphic and movie recording of a partial clinical atonic seizure. *Electroenceph. Clin. Neurophysiol.,* 29:530 (1970)
Warneke, L. B. A case of temporal lobe epilepsy with an orgasmic component. *Canad. Psychiat. Assn. J.* 21:319–324 (1976).
Waxman, S. G., and Geschwind, N. The interictal behavior syndrome of temporal lobe epilepsy. *Arch. Gen Psychiat.* 32:1580–1586 (1975).

Weil, A. A. Depressive reactions associated with temporal lobe uncinate seizures. . *J. Nerv. Ment. Dis.* 121:505–510 (1955).

Weil, A. A. Ictal depression and anxiety in temporal lobe disorders. *Am. J. Psychiat.* 113:149–157 (1956).

Weil, A. A. Ictal emotions occuring in temporal lobe dysfunction. *Arch. Neurol.* 1:101–111 (87-97) (1959).

Weiss, T., and Levitz, L. Diphenylhydantoin treatment of bulimia (ltr. to ed.) *Am. J. Psychiat.* 133:1093 (1976).

Wells, C. E. Transient ictal psychosis. *Arch. Gen. Psychiat.* 32:1201–1203 (1975).

Wermuth, B. E., Davis, K. L., Hollister, L. E., and Stunkard, A. J. Phenytoin treatment of the binge-eating syndrome. *Am. J. Psychiat.* 134:1249–1253 (1977).

Wilkenson, H. A. Epileptic pain: An uncommon manifestation with localizing value. *Neurol.* 23:518–520 (1973).

Williams, D. Neural factors related to habitual aggression. *Brain.* 92:503–520 (1969).

Williams, D. Studies of persons confined for crimes of violence, in *Neural Bases of Violence and Aggression,* W. S. Fields and W. H. Sweet, eds. W. H. Green, St. Louis, Missouri (1975), pp. 285–293.

Williams, D. J. Central vertigo. *Proc. Roy. Soc. Med.* 60:961–964 (1967).

Psychiatric Presentations of Medical Illness

CHAPTER 16

Disorders of Fluid and Electrolyte Balance

William L. Webb, Jr., M.D.
Mohan Gehi, M.D.

Disorders of fluid and electrolyte balance may occur as a complication of an underlying illness, or as a consequence of therapeutic endeavor. It is imperative that these disorders are recognized early to prevent or decrease morbidity and mortality, and that they are treated accordingly. These disorders may present with a multitude of signs and symptoms and thus create a diagnostic dilemma for the physician.

Disorders of fluid and electrolyte balance can produce a wide variety of neuropsychiatric signs and symptoms. We will attempt to describe in this chapter the role of electrolytes; common clinical causes of fluid and electrolyte imbalance, neuropsychiatric manifestations associated with electrolyte imbalance; pathology and pathogenesis, if known; and the principles of treatment.

CALCIUM

Calcium, the most prevalent cation of the body, is maintained in the plasma under the strict control of complex homeostatic mechanisms. It exists in plasma in three states: ionized, attached to protein, and complexed to lactates and citrates. The active form is the ionized fraction, and any change in that fraction activates feedback mechanisms that restore normal levels.

Regulation of Calcium Metabolism

The principal factors in calcium homeostasis are parathormone, vitamin D metabolites, circulating levels of inorganic phosphorus, and calcitonin. Parathormone is a peptide secreted by the parathyroid glands whenever there is a reduction in ionized calcium in plasma. Its principal effects on the kidney are to enhance tubular reabsorption of calcium and to promote the excretion of phosphorus, bicarbonate, sodium, potassium, and amino acids. Parathormone mobilizes calcium from bone by stimulating osteocytes to osteolysis. The exchange of calcium between bone and plasma is a major factor in homeostasis. Intestinal absorption of calcium and glomerular filtration occupy an important, but lesser, status in homeostasis (Bledsoe, 1976).

Vitamin D is ordinarily produced in the skin under the influence of ultraviolet light. Cholecalciferol is converted to the biologically active 1,25-Dihydroxycholecalciferol (1,25-DHCC) through a two-step process: first, to 25-Hydroxycholecalciferol (25-HCC) in the liver, and then to 1,25-DHCC in the kidney. The biologically active 1,25-DHCC promotes the intestinal absorption of calcium and supports the activity of parathormone on bone. The major effect of vitamin D metabolites is to increase the proximal tubular reabsorption of calcium and phosphorus. The lack of sunlight experienced by inhabitants of northern climates is thought to exert an effect on serum calcium. This is particularly true in the elderly population of Britain, where the diet is deficient in calcium (Crammer, 1977). Katz and Foulkes (1970) investigated dissociative reactions among Alaskan Eskimos and their relation to hypocalcemia. Although no statistical correlation between abnormal mental states and serum calcium levels could be proven, a relationship was strongly suggested.

Calcium and inorganic phosphorus plasma concentrations are closely related. Calcium phosphate is a major component of bone. The relationship is such that a rise in plasma concentration of one ion produces a decline in the other. The major effect of parathormone is to promote a phosphorus diuresis.

The "C" cells of the thyroid secrete a small chain peptide, calcitonin, in response to hypercalcemia. Calcitonin exerts an effect antagonistic to parathormone on bone and promotes the renal tubular secretion of phosphorus.

Other hormones exert an effect on calcium homeostasis. Estrogens modulate the release of calcium from bone. The importance of this mechanism is demonstrated in the osteoporosis of menopause. Corticosteroids and thyroid hormone also decrease intestinal absorption of calcium and increase its renal excretion.

The sensitive and complex regulation of calcium in the plasma is obviously necessary to support its multitude of vital functions. Calcium is directly involved in bone formation, lactation, coagulation, and muscle contraction. Most pertinent to psychiatry is the stabilization of cell membranes and the regulation of membrane permeability. The stabilizing effect is derived from the capacity of calcium to bind with negatively charged axonal membrane sites. The binding reduces permeability to other cations. Since increased permeability is associated with depolarization, calcium has an important effect on impulse initiation and propagation (Winokur and Beckman, 1977).

Calcium is known to have an important role in the release of neurotransmitters, such as norepinephrine and acetylcholine. Removal of calcium from perfusion fluid in vitro will markedly decrease the release of neurotransmitter substances. Lowering calcium ion concentration increases the excitability of neural tissue. Clinically, this is manifested by reflex hyperactivity or tetany. The introduction of calcium into the cerebrospinal fluid of animals causes sedation and antagonizes the action of morphine. The latter suggests some effect on endorphins or morphine receptors.

Hypercalcemia

Causes and Neuropsychiatric Manifestations

Elevated serum calcium (hypercalcemia) may be asymptomatic or present with vague nonspecific symptoms. There is evidence that the cerebrospinal fluid concentrations may remain constant, despite significant elevations of serum calcium. This finding suggests that the central nervous system manifestations of hypercalcemia may be related to a breakdown of the blood-brain barrier (Crammer, 1977).

The prominence and character of mental symptoms produced by hypercalcemia are related to its serum levels. Peterson (1968) demonstrated that when calcium levels exceed 14 to 16 mg%, patients develop signs of organic brain syndrome. However, in a number of surveys on medical outpatients, numerous cases were found where patients had significantly elevated calcium levels, but remained asymptomatic. EEG abnormalities are regularly found in patients with serum calciums above 13 mg%. Etheridge, on the other hand, found, in 15 cases of hypercalcemia without other medical complications, only 2 cases evidencing minor EEG changes (Etheridge and Grabos, 1971). Swash and Rowan (1972) reported 14 EEG recordings on a single patient during periods of hypercalcemia and hypocalcemia. Characteristic patterns could be recognized by independent observers. Bursts of high-voltage slow activity were characteristic of all degrees of hypercalcemia, but present only in severe hypocalcemia.

Symptoms of hypercalcemia are manifested primarily in the nervous system and gastrointestinal tract. Mental symptoms include lack of energy, fatigue, irritability, headache, somnolence, and memory deficit. Severe hypercalcemia may produce stupor or coma and constitutes a medical emergency. It should be noted that any of these symptoms can simulate an affective disorder or senility. Because they are common in the elderly, affective disorder and senility are more likely to be suspected than hypercalcemia. Gastrointestinal symptoms include anorexia, nausea, vomiting, constipation and, occasionally, abdominal pain. The differential diagnosis of hypercalcemia includes primary hyperparathyroidism, ectopic parathormone producing malignancy, milk alkali syndrome, bony metastasis of malignant tumors, sarcoidosis, adrenal insufficiency, acute immobilization, and the late stages of chronic secondary hyperparathyroidism.

Primary hyperparathyroidism most commonly presents with mental symptoms associated with renal colic, epigastric pain, weight loss, weakness, and fatigue. Mental symptoms including lassitude, depression, loss of interest, and anhedonia appear in from 30 to 50 percent of cases (Gatewood et al., 1975). Polyuria, polydipsia, and bone pain usually appear as late complications of the illness. The preponderance of reported cases have occurred in women between the ages of 20 and 60. Some have speculated that the mental symptoms of hyperparathyroidism may be a reflection of the central nervous system activity of parathormone. Although the symptoms respond immediately to the reduction of serum calcium, whether or not parathormone per se produces central nervous system effects is still unknown.

Hypercalcemia associated with malignant bone disease, with or without ectopic production of parathormone, usually occurs late in the illness, when the diagnosis is obvious. At other times, its differentiation from hyperparathyroidism is very difficult (Bledsoe, 1976).

Overly vigorous therapy with vitamin D for arthritis, or milk and alkali for peptic ulcer, may produce hypercalcemia. Both of these syndromes are rare, but a careful history should be taken, both from the patient and others, to elucidate the possibility of medication misuse.

Hypercalcemia occurs in both adrenal cortical insufficiency and thyrotoxicosis. Since mental symptoms are associated with both, the role of hypercalcemia is unclear. Some authors suggest that the lassitude, somnolence, and depression of Addison's disease are produced by hypercalcemia. However, the hyponatremia characteristic of this disorder is also known to produce them (Crammer, 1977).

Patients with a high turnover of bone from either growth or underlying disease (hyperthyroidism, Paget's disease, or hyperparathyroidism) may develop hypercalcemia if immobilized. This may be missed or confused with other diagnoses as the following case illustrates:

> The patient, a 71-year-old spinster, living alone, had been treated for the past year with a combination of Elavil and Valium by a local mental health center. Her initial complaints were of periods of listlessness, depression, and withdrawal. Over time, she simply remained in bed. Except for chronic emphysema, she was in good health. She was always of an independent disposition and had few friends. Her only contacts, outside of the TV and the daily paper, were with her niece and two sisters. She had been mildly responsive to Elavil and supportive psychotherapy, but for the past 6 months, showed a downhill course with more complaints of listlessness and decreased physical activity. She began to complain at length of severe

low back and hip pain with radiation down the left leg. She became completely bedridden and was described by her sister as "out of her head at times." X-rays revealed "punched-out areas" throughout her pelvis and vertebrae with a compression fracture at L4 and L5. Her serum calcium was 12.5 mg%. A diagnosis of Paget's disease resulted in treatment with calcitonin and a back brace. Following return of calcium to normal levels, she showed marked improvement in her mental and physical state. The most dramatic change was abatement of her depression and stabilization of her mood.

Various conditions, including vitamin-D-deficient rickets, renal disease with defective calcium absorption, inborn errors of vitamin D metabolism, and idiopathic hypercalcemia (Fanconi's syndrome) can produce secondary hyperplasia of the parathyroids and hypercalcemia. Correction of the disease process producing hypercalcemia results in a slow recovery of calcium homeostasis, with the patient at times requiring more than a year to achieve normal calcium levels.

Idiopathic hypercalcemia, a rare condition inherited as an autosomal recessive trait, is associated with mental retardation. The metabolic defect is an excessive response to vitamin D. The clinical picture includes irritability, intellectual deficit, a peculiar elfin facial appearance, short stature, hypotonia, hypertension, and renal calculi (Cytryn and Lourie, 1975).

Treatment

The treatment of hypercalcemia in these various states is directed to the underlying management of the disorder; for example, primary hyperparathyroidism is most frequently a manifestation of an adenoma (usually benign) of the parathyroid and the treatment is surgical removal. Attempts to correct calcium loss usually rectify secondary hyperparathyroidism.

Hypocalcemia

Causes and Neuropsychiatric Manifestations

Reduced ionized calcium produces symptoms of increased neuromuscular irritability. This can be illustrated in a normal subject who deeply and rapidly overbreathes for a short time, producing the typical hyperventilation syndrome of perioral numbness, increased nervousness, irritability, and the appearance of early signs of tetany (Chvostek's or Trousseau's signs). The overbreathing produces a respiratory alkalosis that reduces the ionized fraction of calcium in plasma.

The magnitude of mental symptoms produced by hypocalcemia runs the gamut from anxiety and increased emotional lability to stuporous or catatonic states. Laryngospasm may be a feature, particularly in children. Predisposed individuals may develop epileptic seizures.

Although the most common cause of low serum calcium is low albumin, this seldom affects the ionized calcium fraction, and therefore, produces no symptoms of tetany. Hypoparathyroidism and deficiency of the active metabolite of vitamin D are the conditions most commonly responsible for symptomatic hypocalcemia. A calcium level below 7 mg% usually produces mental changes and EEG abnormalities.

Hypoparathyroidism is most often produced by inadvertant surgical removal of the parathyroids during thyroidectomy. Primary hypoparathyroidism is a rare entity. Only 200 cases are reported in the literature. Its onset is usually in childhood. Only 7 percent of patients show signs of tetany; one-third present with an organic brain syndrome. Treatment, which usually alleviates all mental abnormalities, is accomplished by the administration of calcium and vitamin D.

Secondary hypoparathyroidism is produced by severe hypomagnesemia, which interferes with parathormone synthesis.

The condition of pseudohypoparathyroidism occurs when bone and kidney are unresponsive to parathormone. Pseudohypoparathyroidism is an autosomal recessive disorder that may result in convulsions, tetany, and skeletal abnormalities. Mental retardation may develop secondary to the many seizures. Hypocalcemia can also occur in advanced carcinoma of the breast.

The rapid improvement of neuromuscular irritability following calcium replacement prompted some authors to suspect that calcium may play a role in the production of anxiety neurosis. Pitts and McClure (1967) hypothesized that in certain predisposed individuals, stress produced a buildup of lactate, a calcium complexing metabolite, which subsequently reduced calcium and precipitated attacks of anxiety. Unfortunately, the Pitts hypothesis has not been clinically verified, so the role of hypocalcemia in the production of anxiety states still remains unclear.

PHOSPHORUS

Phosphorus, the major intracellular anion, has received much less attention than calcium. This is hardly commensurate with the many vital biological functions performed by phosphorus. Adenosine diphosphate (ADP), adenosine triphosphate (ATP), and phosphorus are vital to all synthetic and catabolic processes. Phosphorus regulates many enzyme systems, and by regulating the level of ATP and 2,3-Diphosphoglycerate (2,3-DPG) in erythrocytes, plays a principal role in oxygen delivery. Adequate phosphorus levels are also essential for leukocyte phagocytosis, platelet function, the structural integrity of muscle, and proper central nervous system function (Knochel, 1977).

Hypophosphatemia

Causes and Neuropsychiatric Manifestations

Recent automated laboratory measurements of phosphorus have shown hypophosphatemia to occur in a number of conditions and to be associated with serious morbidity. However, the abundance of phosphorus in natural foods is such that phosporus deficiency in normal man is rare. The clinical syndrome of hypophosphatemia was not realized until Lotz induced phosphorus deficiency in normals and hyperparathyroids by a phosphorus-deficient diet and the ingestion of phosphate-binding antacids. The subjects became weak, tremulous, irritable, and complained of bone pain (Lotz et al., 1968).

It is now appreciated that moderate hypophosphatemia occurs in a number of medical conditions that affect the homeostasis of phosphorus. These include the intravenous administration of glucose and fructose, vitamin D deficiency, gram negative septicemia, and following administration of glucagon, epinephrine, diuretics, corticosteroids, and androgens. Since parathormone inhibits the tubular reabsorption of phosphorus, moderate hypophosphatemia frequently occurs in cases of hyperparathyroidism (Betro and Pain, 1972; Ansar, 1970).

Profound hypophosphatemia occurs primarily in three conditions: alcoholic withdrawal, diabetic ketoacidosis, and during hyperalimentation (Silvis and Paragas, 1972; Vianna, 1971). Hypomagnesemia and the respiratory alkalosis of alcoholic withdrawal potentiate the central nervous system effects of hypophosphatemia. The myopathy of chronic alcoholism may result from phosphorus depletion.

Franks et al. (1948) believed that diabetic coma was shortened by administration of phosphorus supplements. Severe disturbances of central nervous system function and EEG abnormalities associated with hyperalimentation were eliminated when phosphorus supplements were included.

The central nervous system effects of hyperphosphatemia have not been clearly elucidated, since hyperphosphatemia occurs in the face of other significant changes (hypocalcemia or hyperkalemia). Profound hypophosphatemia, on the other hand, produces very definite medical symptoms, which include irritability, apprehension, muscular weakness, numbness, paresthesias, dysarthria, confusion, obtundation, convulsive seizures, and coma. Hypophosphatemia may contribute to the symptoms of delirium tremens in alcohol withdrawal, but does not produce the distinctive visual hallucinations that occur with that disorder.

The mechanisms by which phosphorus affects central nervous system function include impairment of glucose metabolism and anoxia due to diminution of 2,3 DPG in the red cell.

The pathophysiology and central nervous system effect of hypophosphatemia have only recently been appreciated. Since phosphorus is such a vital element in a multitude of energy transformations and enzyme reactions, it is likely that changes in phosphorus levels may have more of a role in the production of emotional and behavioral disorders than has been currently proven.

SODIUM

Sodium is the principal cation in extracellular fluid. It accounts for the major part of extracellular osmotic activity; therefore, any change in serum sodium concentration is associated with a shift of fluid into or out of the cell.

The activity of nerve cells is directly influenced by their metabolic environment, with the nervous system being particularly susceptible to changes in electrolyte concentration. The neuronal membrane separates the intracellular and the extracellular fluids, which have widely different ionic compositions. (In normal neuronal function, a resting membrane potential is maintained, that is controlled by the difference in the concentration of sodium and potassium across the neuronal membrane.) An increase or decrease of serum sodium or potassium concentration may manifest clinically in a wide range of symptoms and signs, e.g., changes in sensorium, muscular weakness, or seizures.

Regulation of Sodium Metabolism

Sodium concentration is closely regulated despite fluctuations in intake. The renal mechanism for regulation includes the renin-angiotension-aldosterone system; hemodynamic alterations in response to variations of sodium intake; and a "third factor" that may be mediated (Walker and Whelton, 1976). Low sodium concentration in the extracellular fluid results in a decreased plasma volume and glomerular filtration rate. Renin release and aldosterone levels increase producing an increased reabsorption of sodium. A high sodium concentration in the extracellular fluid causes the opposite effect. Renin release and aldosterone secretion are reduced while a "third factor" causes a decreased amount of tubular sodium to be reabsorbed.

During recovery from depression, there may be a decrease in exchangeable body sodium. Gibbons (1960) measured exchangeable body sodium in a group of patients with endogenous depression. Following treatment with electroconvulsive therapy, there was a statistically significant decrease of exchangeable body sodium. Ueno was able to show a statistically significant decrease of sodium concentration in cerebrospinal fluid in depressed patients (Ueno et al., 1961).

However, in an earlier study by Altschule (1953), no such decrease in sodium was noted.

In a study conducted by Shaw et al. (1969), the brains of depressed patients who commited suicide were found to have a decreased concentration of sodium and potassium as well as an increased water content when compared to the brains of controls. However, there were factors that were not controlled, such as mode of death, drugs used prior to death, and postmortem changes that occurred prior to autopsy.

In manic patients, Ueno et al. (1961) found normal concentrations of sodium, potassium, calcium, and chloride in both serum and cerebrospinal fluid (CSF). There was a small decrease in CSF potassium upon recovery from mania. Coppen et al. (1966) found a striking increase of intracellular sodium in manic depressive patients during their manic phase. However, Baer and associates (1970) failed to confirm Coppen's findings.

Sodium Metabolism in Lithium Therapy

Animals treated with low dose lithium show significant changes in cerebral sodium metabolism. Patients placed on a constant sodium diet and treated with lithium exhibit a significant increase in sodium excretion during the first day of lithium therapy. Sodium retention occurs by the third treatment day and is followed by a return to normal levels by the sixth or seventh day (Baer et al., 1971). The mechanism responsible for this lithium-induced change is independent of the glomerular filtration rate. A possible mechanism by which lithium may influence sodium and potassium is by displacing these cations from the intracellular and extracellular compartments (Baer, 1973). It is possible that lithium can substitute for sodium in the central nervous system membrane transport system. This could lead to altered electrical transmission and has been shown to change the evoked cortical potential (Gartside et al., 1966). Electrolyte abnormalities, including hyponatremia and decreased brain sodium concentration, are all known to produce EEG changes similar to those observed with lithium (Johnson et al., 1970). Sodium is required for the uptake and storage of norepinephrine (Bogdanski et al., 1968). These studies support the hypothesis that altered electrolyte metabolism may be involved in some fundamental way in the production of affective disorders (Baer, 1973).

Hypernatremia

Hypernatremia is defined as a serum sodium concentration above 150 mEq per liter. It usually results from a loss of water, producing a relative excess of sodium in the body fluids.

Causes

Hypernatremia may occur in patients of any age who have an impaired sensorium, since such patients can neither appreciate nor respond to their own thirst mechanism. It may also occur in mental patients who refuse to drink water.

Severe water loss from the gastrointestinal tract, e.g., diarrhea and vomiting, may also produce it. A complete loss of gastrointestinal secretions for 24 hours would deprive the body of about 8 liters of water or nearly one fifth of the total body water.

Diabetes insipidus, an antidiuretic hormone insufficiency usually results in hypernatremia. The symptoms of diabetes insipidus may be secondary to a tumor, basilar meningitis, sarcoidosis, histiocytosis, or brain injury. Ectopic pinealoma, when located in the hypothalamus, may be associated with hyponatremia, usually secondary to the loss of thirst (Ross and Christie, 1969; Leaf 1967).

Cushing's syndrome is produced by prolonged excessive production of cortisol. It may be caused by tumor, but more commonly results from adrenal hyperplasia. There may be an excess of glucocorticoids or, more commonly, an excess of all adrenal steroids.

In Cushing's syndrome, there is retention of sodium and, to a lesser extent, chloride ions. Patients may manifest the characteristic "moon face," buffalo hump, centripetal fat distribution, muscular weakness and wasting, acne, and hirsutism. Often present are mental changes that vary from symptoms of depression to mania. Some patients become delusional.

In *primary aldosteronism,* there is prolonged excessive secretion of aldosterone from an adrenocortical adenoma. The characteristic features are hypokalemia, hypernatremia, alkalosis, muscle wasting, polyuria, polydipsia, and hypertension.

In patients with *cerebral or essential hypernatremia* (DeRubertis et al. 1975; Pleasure and Goldberg, 1966), forced hydration leads to increased excretion of excess water, with maintenance of increased plasma sodium levels.

Additional causes of hypernatremia include: acute renal failure (Ross and Christie, 1969), postoperative water restriction, hyperalimentation (Engel and Jaeger, 1954), accidental salt poisoning, and salt water ingestion.

Neuropsychiatric Manifestions

Neuropsychiatric signs and symptoms are present in at least one fourth of all patients with a plasma sodium of 160 mEq per liter or greater. Personality changes appear first. Characteristically, the patient is restless, hyperactive, and irritable. Irritability is the most frequent presentation in children (Bruck et al., 1968).

Acute organic brain syndrome is characterized by depression of the sensorium, which may vary from lethargy to frank coma. There may be disorientation, impaired memory and ability to concentrate, diminished attention span, and inability to abstract. Hallucinations may appear with visual forms being more common (Logothetis, 1966). Neurological symptoms include hyperactive deep tendon reflexes, nonspecific tremors, muscular twitching, myoclonus, and focal or generalized seizures.

The electroencephalogram (EEG) may be normal or show slowing of background frequencies. Some patients evidence focal epileptic activity (Bruck et al., 1968). EEG changes usually revert to normal within 1 to 6 weeks following treatment (Logothetis, 1966).

Patients with hypernatremia evidence a significant morbidity and mortality. Luttrell and Finberg (1959), followed 32 hypernatremic patients for 8 years, and found 1 to be monoplegic, 2 to develop seizure disorders, and 8 to evidence persistent electroencephalographic abnormalities. It is possible that patients who recovered completely had cerebral edema only, whereas, those with permanent lesions suffered cerebral infarction or hemorrhage.

Pathogenesis of Neuropsychiatric Signs and Symptoms

Hypernatremia produces a hyperosmolar state with a resultant loss of brain fluid, neural shrinkage, and tissue damage, secondary to tearing of cerebral blood vessels (Luttrell and Finberg, 1959). There may be subdural, subarachnoid, or intracerebral hemorrhage. Multiple petechial hemorrhages occur throughout the cortex and in the subcortical white matter. Thrombotic occlusion of capillaries, veins, and sinuses produces infarction.

Animal experiments demonstrate that blood vessel damage and resultant hemorrhage occur rapidly following the intraperitoneal injection of hypertonic solutions. In cats killed 4 hours following injection, cerebral lesions were present.

Treatment

Treatment is accomplished by giving fluids, either by mouth or intravenously. If hypernatremia is corrected too rapidly, cerebral edema and convulsions may result.

Hyponatremia

Causes

Hyponatremia is a common accompaniment of such systemic diseases as congestive heart failure and cirrhosis. It may also result from dietary restriction;

prolonged hyperthermia; excessive diaphoresis; salt-losing nephritis; the administration of excessive amounts of intravenous fluids, particularly in the elderly and as a consequence of diuretic treatment. Patients with edema usually develop some degree of hyponatremia unless fluid intake is restricted. "Essential" hyponatremia has also been reported.

Schwartz Bartter syndrome is produced by the chronic inappropriate secretion of antidiuretic hormone, secondary to central nervous system neoplasms, other central nervous system disorders, oat-cell carcinoma of the lung, or intermittent porphyria. In this syndrome, the osmolality of urine is always higher than that of plasma, suggesting excessive antidiuretic hormone secretion particularly when the glomerular filtration rate (GFR) is normal.

Hyponatremia is a characteristic of Addison's disease, since aldosterone deficiency decreases tubular reabsorption of sodium and chloride and increases the retention of potassium. Symptoms and signs include muscular weakness and easy fatigability, organic brain syndrome, pigmentation of skin and buccal mucosa, anorexia, nausea, vomiting, weight loss, decreased body hair, hypoglycemia, and a decreased ability to withstand metabolic stress.

Hyponatremia, produced by increased water intake secondary to compulsive drinking, was first described by Rountree (1923). In this condition, although the renal capacity is normal, the patient is unable to excrete water at a rate equal to his intake. The symptoms of water intoxication differ significantly from those caused by pure hyponatremia, suggesting that other factors are involved in their production. Resnick and Patterson (1969) described a case of compulsive water drinking associated with the delusion that the Virgin Mary had commanded the patient to drink holy water. He drank enough water to produce convulsions, and ultimately, coma. A lead article in *Lancet* (1953) stated that water cannot harm thirsty patients. However, there are several reports of patients with normal renal function who developed hyponatremia secondary to excessive water intake. Of the 21 reported cases of water intoxication due to polydipsia, 15 have been associated with psychiatric illness (Noonan and Ananth, 1977). Hobson and English (1963) speculated that a hypothalamic disorder in some schizophrenic patients may produce the inappropriate secretion of antidiuretic hormone. The possibility that purely psychogenic polydipsia may result in water intoxication remains controversial.

Beresford (1970) reported two cases of compulsive water drinking in which the patients developed an acute hyponatremic encephalopathy after receiving a therapeutic dose of hydrocholorothiazide.

Neuropsychiatric Manifestations

Depression may be suspected, since the presentation is often one of apathy, weakness, lethargy, anorexia, and taste impairment. McCance (1936) found that when sodium was experimentally lowered from an average of 147 to 131 mEq per liter in healthy volunteers, these subjects experienced impaired taste, anorexia, constant thirst, muscular cramps, a clouded sensorium general exhaustion, and dyspnea on exertion. Other neurological manifestations were not observed until plasma sodium fell below 125 mEq per liter. The severity of symptoms produced by hyponatremia is determined by both the absolute serum level and the rapidity of decline.

Hyponatremic encephalopathy is an organic brain syndrome produced by hyponatremia. The organic brain syndrome that results may be acute or chronic, depending on whether it is reversible or irreversible. The acute phase is marked by impaired orientation and concentration, and a decreased attention span. Physical signs and symptoms include: muscular weakness, incoordination, headache, nausea, vomiting, and seizures, which may be of the myoclonic, focal, or generalized type. Cerebrospinal fluid pressure is increased in some cases. Papilledema may be present. Chronic patients complain of headache, lethargy, somnolence, impaired attention, concentration, and recent memory. In addition, focal weakness, hemiparesis, ataxia, and Babinski sign may occur (Weiner and Epstein, 1972; Rankind, 1974).

Following is a case history of hyponatremia:

> A 53-year-old female was admitted to the coronary care unit through the emergency room. The patient presented with signs of pulmonary edema, secondary to congestive heart failure. She was a known case of hypertensive heart disease. Her blood pressure had been difficult to control, necessitating treatment with diuretics, digoxin, and an antihypertensive. She had run out of medications a week prior to admission. On the fifth day of hospitalization, she was noted by the nurses to "look depressed"; she initiated no conversation, answered questions with yes/no answers, had a poor appetite and manifested emotional lability with inappropriate outbursts of weeping. A psychiatric consultation was requested to evaluate for depression. In addition to the above findings, on evaluation by the psychiatrist, she was found to have impairment in concentration and a poor memory for recent events. She was noted to have a serum sodium of 125 mEq per liter. The psychiatric manifestations were thought to be secondary to hyponatremia. On the eighth day of hospitalization, the patient's sodium level was back in the normal range. She was not depressed. Her mood, memory, attention span, and concentration were all normal.

Pathophysiology

Cerebral edema with brain stem herniation is a major cause of death in patients with severe hyponatremia (Arieff and Guisado, 1976). Patients dying several days after correction of their hyponatremia die of other causes (i.e., have no evidence of cerebral edema) (Lipsmeyer and Ackerman, 1966). The seizures that occur with hyponatremia are probably related to cerebral edema and/or to low intracellular concentrations of sodium and potassium.

In severe hyponatremia, electroencephalography shows a loss of alpha waves and irregular discharge of high amplitude slow wave activity, which are characteristic (Epstein et al., 1961; Pampiglione, 1973). These changes generally return to normal following correction of the hyponatremia.

Treatment

Treatment is directed to correction of the underlying etiologic deficit. If sodium stores are intact, restriction of water intake alone is sufficient. It is not known how fast one can safely raise serum sodium levels. When neurological symptoms are present, hypertonic solutions should be infused slowly, since the rapid infusion of large quantities of hypertonic solution can precipitate congestive heart failure or subdural and intracerebral hemorrhage.

POTASSIUM

Potassium is the major cation of intracellular fluid, where it plays a major role in maintaining the membrane potential. The concentration of potassium in extracellular fluid is stabilized between 3.5 and 5 mEq per liter, while the intracellular concentration is in the range of 150 mEq per liter. Potassium is a co-factor for many enzymatic reactions and maintains the excitability of neural and muscle tissue. One cannot equate the serum potassium concentration to total body stores, since 98 percent of the latter is located intracellularly (Lindeman, 1976). Isotope dilution studies and muscle biopsy have been utilized to demonstrate that intracellular stores can be decreased in a variety of clinical conditions, e.g., diabetic ketoacidosis (Aikawa et al., 1953), chronic congestive heart failure, and cirrhosis (Birkenfeld et al., 1958); while serum potassium levels remain within normal limits. However, serum potassium concentration is the only practical clinical measure of potassium stores, and needs to be considered along with the clinical status of the patient if one is to satisfactorily estimate potassium balance (Lindeman, 1976).

Regulation of Potassium Metabolism

A number of factors interact to regulate total body potassium and its concentration in extracellular fluid; among these are dietary intake of other nutrients, the acid base balance, and losses from the intestine, skin, and kidneys.

Shaw and Coppen (1966) showed that the intracellular potassium concentrations of depressed patients was low when compared to values obtained from normal controls. Cox et al. (1971) demonstrated that in depression and dementia there is a loss of intracellular potassium and a retention of intracellular sodium, while the plasma levels of these electrolytes remain normal. In a study of the brains of suicide victims (Shaw et al., 1969), potassium concentration was found to be below normal when compared to a control group.

Hypokalemia

Causes

Hypokalemia is produced by the total dietary depletion of this ion for 2 to 3 weeks. Such depletion occurs clinically in patients with anorexia nervosa, pituitary cachexia, and in those on prolonged parenteral therapy without potassium supplement. Alkalosis may produce a lowering of serum levels, suggesting deficiency by causing a shift of potassium to the intracellular space. Excessive gastrointestinal losses may occur following severe vomiting, diarrhea, or malabsorption. Other causes include: Cushing's syndrome (Christie and Laragh, 1961), chronic renal disease, congenital renal defects, and thyrotoxicosis (Sanghvi et al., 1959).

Diuretics are probably the most frequent cause of hypokalemia in hospital and outpatient populations. Excessive, concealed self-administration of oral diuretics, especially in women, must be considered in the differential (Katz et al., 1972). The potassium-losing actions of the various thiazides and loop diuretics (furosemide, ethacrynic acid) are dependent on the increase in sodium load delivered to the distal sodium-potassium exchange site. There appears to be no advantage of one diuretic over another in preventing potassium loss while accomplishing a desired natriuresis (Lindeman, 1976).

Laxative abuse may cause hypokalemia (Schwartz and Relman, 1953). In a study of two patients who were apparently abusing laxatives, neither of whom had any overt neuromuscular symptoms or signs, the discovery of severe hypokalemia was made by T-wave changes observed on a routine electrocardiogram. Licorice extract, used as an additive to alcoholic drinks, for the treatment of ulcer disease, and as a flavoring agent for drugs, can produce hypokalemia and pseudoaldosteronism (Gross et al., 1966). Hypokalemia is also produced by corticosteroids, acetylsalicylic acid (Robin et al., 1959) penicillin, and carbenicillin (Linderman, 1976).

Lastly, it may result from idiopathic hypokalemic alkalosis, a familial illness, with no apparent identified cause (France et al., 1973).

Neuropsychiatric Manifestations

In 1882, Shakhnovitch (1884) reported the case of a patient with a 25-year history of intermittent paraplegia (periodic hypokalemia). The patient was considered to be suffering from a new form of neurosis, for which Shakhnovitch coined the term "paraplegia spinalis intermittens nervosa." Psychiatric misdiagnosis is common, since the neuropsychiatric manifestations take many different forms. Conversion reactions are frequently suspected. Mitchell and Feldman (1968) reported the case of a 30-year-old female with three hospital admissions for weakness of her extremities and inability to walk. The patient would progressively regain her strength and leave the hospital a few days later. On the first two admissions, she was diagnosed as having a conversion reaction. Her symptoms were thought to be psychogenic, brought on by marital difficulties. It was only on the third admission that this patient was found to have a serum potassium level of 1.8 mEq per liter. Subsequently, a diagnosis of renal tubular acidosis was made.

Patients may present with symptoms of anxiety, characterized by nervousness, irritability, headaches, paresthesias, and other vague aches and complaints. Depression, manifested by dysphoric mood, loss of appetite, weakness, excessive fatigue, feeling of a lack of well being, and withdrawal from one's usual activities may occur. The presence of these "unexplained" symptoms may further contribute to the patient's "depression."

Following is a case history of hypokalemia:

> A 36-year-old school teacher was admitted to the hospital with severe asthma. She had made a few visits to the emergency room in the past for acute asthma attacks. Each time she was treated with bronchodilators and discharged. During this admission, her asthma attack was more severe and did not respond to bronchodilators. She was, therefore, hospitalized and treated with steroids, fluids, and bronchodilators. On the seventh day of hospitalization, her medical condition had significantly improved. She was breathing without any difficulty and had a respiratory rate of 24 per minute. At this time, she was receiving 20 mg of prednisone a day. Psychiatric consultation was requested following a threat of suicide. She was tearful, had not eaten for 1 day, had difficulty sleeping, and was in a depressed mood. The medical intern, who was very familiar with this patient, was surprised at this dramatic change in her mental status. A serum potassium level of 2.9 mEq per liter was obtained. Over the next 3 days, her depression improved as her potassium level returned to normal.

Another frequent presentation of hypokalemia is that of acute organic brain syndrome, manifested by impairment of sensorium, ranging from lethargy through somnolence to frank coma, associated with diminished concentration and attention span, impairment of memory and ability to abstract, hallucinations, confabulation, emotional lability, and poor judgement.

Kitzes et al. (1976) have described cases of acute organic brain syndrome in the elderly, secondary to diuretic-induced hypokalemia. These patients have an age-related decrease of total body potassium stores and are thus vulnerable to this disorder. At times, acute organic brain syndrome produced by hypokalemia may be superimposed on an existing chronic brain syndrome, especially in the elderly. Therefore, sudden worsening in the mental status of a patient with already compromised mental functioning should alert the treating physician to initiate a complete metabolic workup.

Treatment

In most patients, hypokalemia is one facet of a complex metabolic disorder, which responds to appropriate treatment of the underlying abnormality. Intravenous administration of potassium may result in sinus bradycardia, or even cardiac arrest in systole if the plasma levels are increased too rapidly. The administration of more than 40 mEq per hour, or concentrations in excess of 40 mEq per liter, is generally excessive and should only be administered when electrocardiographic monitoring is available. In such situations, serum potassium levels must be monitored frequently.

Hyperkalemia

Causes

Hyperkalemia is defined as an increase in serum potassium greater than 5 mEq per liter. Common clinical causes include: acute renal failure (Thomson, 1973); rapid administration of potassium supplements; tissue breakdown, following burns, infarction or inflammation; adrenal insufficiency (Pollen and Williams, 1960); a shift of potassium from intracellular to extracellular fluid as in acidosis; and the use of potassium-sparing diuretics such as spironolactone.

"Pseudohyperkalemia" represents an increase in potassium in vitro caused by release of intracellular potassium from white cells, platelets, and hemolyzed red blood cells. A tight constricting tourniquet, or an exercising forearm, can cause a localized increase in serum potassium distal to the tourniquet (Farber et al., 1951).

Neuropsychiatric Manifestations

The neuropsychiatric manifestations of hyperkalemia include confusion, clouding of consciousness, weakness, dysphasia, dysarthria, and paralysis (Bull et al., 1953). Some patients become syncopal secondary to bradycardia or asystole. Associated abdominal distension and diarrhea may prompt further electrolyte and water loss, thereby worsening the patient's confusion and organic brain syndrome.

Treatment

Treatment is directed toward correction of the specific cause of potassium excess; decreasing the potassium intake; or facilitating the removal of potassium with cation exchange resins, intravenous glucose containing insulin, or peritonealdialysis or hemodialysis.

MAGNESIUM

Magnesium is a major intracellular cation with a normal serum concentration of between 1.5 to 2 mEq per liter. One third of the total body magnesium is bound to protein. Residual magnesium is stored in the skeletal muscle and parenchymatous tissue with a high concentration being found in liver, bone, kidney, and brain.

Magnesium is essential for the activity of many enzymatic systems (Fishman, 1965). Along with ATP, it is currently thought to be the main electrolyte required for uptake of catecholamines into neural vesicles (Euler and Lishajko, 1963). Magnesium is also concerned with the release of acetylcholine at the motor end plate. High concentrations may thus produce motor paralysis.

Regulation of Magnesium Metabolism

Our knowledge of magnesium metabolism is limited. Decreased magnesium concentrations in the extracellular fluid promote increased reabsorption of magnesium from the tubules, while an increased concentration promotes decreased tubular reabsorption (Guyton, 1971).

Magnesium and calcium act as co-regulating ions. For example, the action of calcium in promoting release of acetylcholine from synaptic vesicles in cholinergic nerve endings is inhibited by magnesium, while the central nervous system depression and neuromuscular block produced by high plasma levels of magnesium can be overcome by the intravenous injection of calcium.

Hypomagnesemia

Causes

Inadequate dietary intake of magnesium is rare since magnesium is present in abundant quantities in most foods. Clinically significant hypomagnesemia most often results from vomiting, diarrhea, malabsorption, chronic alcoholism, hypercalcemia, prolonged loss of body fluids, or administration of intravenous fluids free of magnesium, pancreatitis, diuretic therapy, diabetic acidosis, hyperaldosteronism, or porphyria. In burn patients, the daily irrigation of large surface areas in fluids containing negligible amounts of magnesium may result in a significant magnesium deficit and produce toxicity (Broughton et. al., 1968).

Neuropsychiatric Manifestations

Personality changes manifested by increasing irritability, nervousness, and restlessness are usually the first symptoms noted, later followed by depression (Hall and Joffe, 1973). A case of iatrogenic hypomagnesemia, uncomplicated by other factors, presented as an organic brain syndrome (Hall and Joffe, 1973). The hypomagnesemia occurred secondary to intravenous fluid replacement and suction loss. Physical signs included: cramping, nystagmus, tremor, myoclonic jerks, and Chvostek's sign. Psychiatric signs were the first to appear and persisted for 48 hours after serum levels had returned to normal and other signs and symptoms had cleared.

The mental symptoms that occur in burn patients in some instances are due to or aggravated by magnesium deficiency (Broughton et al., 1968). Replacement magnesium therapy usually promptly relieves both the mental symptoms and neuromuscular excitability exhibited by these patients. Hallucinations are common in rapidly developing and severe cases. Neurological symptoms and signs include: tremors, generalized hyperreflexia, athetoid and choreiform movements, Chvostek's and Trousseau's signs, and seizures.

Treatment

Hypomagnesemia should be treated by administering magnesium sulfate or chloride intravenously or intramuscularly.

Hypermagnesemia

Hypermagnesemia may occur following the excessive administration of magnesium containing antacids and in patients with renal failure. It may produce lethargy leading to coma (Gilroy and Meyer, 1975), respiratory failure, or death. Treatment consists of the intravenous administration of fluids containing 10 percent calcium gluconate. In severe cases, renal dialysis may be necessary.

CONCLUSION

Electrolyte abnormalities occur frequently in patients seen in hospital and clinic settings. Knowledge of the neuropsychiatric symptoms produced by electrolyte imbalance can alert the physician to their presence. Failure to diagnose these conditions early may convert an acute organic brain syndrome (reversible) to a chronic (irreversible) form.

REFERENCES

Aikawa, J. K., Felts, J. H., Jr., and Harrel, G. J. Isotope studies of potassium metabolism in diabetes. *J. Clin. Invest.* 32:15–21 (1953).

Altschule, M. D. Bodily physiology in mental and emotional disorders. Grune and Stratton, New York (1953), pp. 156–168.

Ansar, A. Antacid induced phosphorus depletion and repletion. *Minn. Med.* 53:837–838 (1970).

Arieff, A. I., and Guisado, R. Effects on the central nervous system of hypernatremic and hyponatremic states. *Kidney Int.* 18:104–116 (1976).

Baer, L. Electrolyte metabolism in psychiatric disorders, in *Biological Psychiatry*. J. Mendels, ed. Wiley-Interscience, New York (1973), pp. 199–234.

Baer, L., Platman, S. R., and Fieve, R. R. The role of electrolytes in affective disorders: Sodium potassium and lithium ions. *Arch. Gen. Psychiat.* 22:108–113 (1970).

Baer, L., Platman, S. R., Kassin, S., and Fieve, R. R. Mechanisms of renal lithium handling and their relationship to mineralcorticoids: A dissociation between sodium and lithium ions. *J. Psychiat. Res.* 8:91–105 (1971).

Beresford, H. R. Polydipsia, hydrochlorothiazide, and water intoxication. *J.A.M.A.* 214:879–883 (1970).

Betro, M. G., and Pain, R. W. Hypophosphatemia and hyperphosphatemia in a hospital population. *Brit. Med. J.* 1:274–276 (1972).

Birkenfeld, L. W., Leibman, J., O'Meara, M. P., and Edelman, I. S. Total exchangeable sodium, total exchangeable potassium, and total body water in edematous patients with cirrhosis of the liver and congestive heart failure. *J. Clin. Invest.* 37:687–698 (1958).

Bledsoe, T. Calcium and bone, in *The Principles and Practice of Medicine*. A. M. Harvey, R. J. Johns, A. H. Owens, and R. S. Ross, eds. Appleton-Century-Crofts, New York (1976), pp. 1047–1072.

Bogdanski, D. F., Tissani, A., and Brodie, B. B. The effect of inorganic ions on the uptake, storage, and metabolism of biogenic amines in nerve endings. *Psychopharmacology:* A review of progress 1957–1967. D. H. Efron, ed. U. S. Government Printing Office, Washington, D. C. (1968), pp. 17–26.

Broughton, A., Anderson, I.R.M., and Bowden, C. H. Magnesium deficiency syndrome in burns. *Lancet* 2:1156–1158 (1968).

Bruck, E., Abul, G., and Aceto, T. Pathogenesis and pathophysiology of hypertonic dehydration with diarrhea. *Am. J. Dis. Child.* 115:122–144 (1968).

Bull, G. M., Carter, A. B., and Lowe, K. G. Hyperpotassaemic paralysis. *Lancet* 2:60–63 (1953).

Christie, N. P., and Laragh, J. H. Pathogenesis of hypokalemic alkalosis in Cushing's syndrome. *N. Eng. J. Med.* 265:1083–1088 (1961).

Coppen, A., Shaw, D. M., Malleson, A., and Costain, R. Mineral metabolism in mania. *Brit. Med. J.* 1:71–75 (1966).

Cox, J. R., Rosemary, E. P., and Speight, C. J. Changes in sodium, potassium, and fluid spaces in depression and dementia. *Geront. Clin.* 13:232–245 (1971).

Crammer, J. D. Calcium metabolism and mental disorders. *Psychol. Med.* 7:557–560 (1977).

Cytryn, L., and Lourie, R. Mental retardation, in *Comprehensive Textbook of Psychiatry*. A. M. Freedman, H. I. Kaplan, and B. J. Sadock, eds. Williams & Wilkins, Baltimore, Maryland (1975), pp. 1158–1197.

DeRubertis, F. R., Michelis, M. F., and Davis, B. B. "Essential" hypernatremia. *Arch. Int. Med.* 134:889–895 (1975).

Engel, F. L., and Jaeger, C. Dehydration with hypernatremia, hyperchloremia, and azotemia, complicating nasogastric tube feeding. *Am. J. Med.* 17:196–204 (1954).

Epstein, F. H., Leviten, H., Glasser, G., and Lavietes, P. Cerebral hyponatremia. *N. Eng. J. Med.* 265:513–518 (1961).

Etheridge, J. E., and Grabos, T. D. Hypercalcemia without EEG abnormalities. *Dis. Nerv. Syst.* 32:479–482 (1971).

Euler, U.S.V., and Lishajko, F. Catecholamine release and uptake in isolated adrenergic nerve granules. *Acta Physiol. Scand.* 57:468–480 (1963).

Farber, S. J., Peligrino, E. D., Conant, N. J., and Earle, D. P. Observations on the plasma potassium level of man. *Am. J. Med. Sci.* 221:678–687 (1951).

Fishman, R. A. Neurological aspects of magnesium metabolism. *Arch. Neurol.* 12:562–569 (1965).

France, R., Stone, W. J., Michelakis, A. M., Island, D. P., and Merrel, J. M. Renal potassium wasting of unknown cause in a clinical setting of chronic potassium depletion. *S. Med. J.* 66:115–128 (1973).

Franks, M., Berris, R. F., Kaplan, N. O., and Myers, G. B. Metabolic studies in diabetic acidosis. II. The effect of the administration of sodium phosphate. *Arch. Int. Med.* 81:42–55 (1948).

Gartside, I. S., Lipold, O.C.J., and Meldurm, B. S. The evoked cortical somatosensory response in normal man and its modification by oral lithium carbonate. *Electroenceph. Clin. Neurophysiol.* 20:282–390 (1966).

Gatewood, J. E., Organ, C. H., and Mead, B. T. Mental changes associated with hyperparathyroidism. *Am. J. Psychiat.* 132:129–132 (1975).

Gibbons, J. L. Total body sodium and potassium in depressive illness. *Clin. Sci.* 19:133–138 (1960).

Gilroy, J., and Meyer, J. S. *Medical Neurology*. MacMillan, New York (1975), pp. 225–229.

Gross, E. G., Dexter, J. D., and Roth, R. G. Hypokalemic myopathy with myoglobinuria associated with licorice ingestion. *N. Eng. J. Med.* 274:602–606 (1966).

Guyton, A. C. Basic human physiology: Normal function and mechanism of disease. W. B. Saunders Company, Philadelphia, Pennsylvania (1971), pp. 288–304.

Hall, R.C.W., and Joffe, J. R. Hypomagnesemia: physical and psychiatric symptoms. *J.A.M.A.* 224:1749–1751 (1973).

Hobson, J. A., and English, J. T. Self-induced intoxication from compulsive water drinking. *Ann. Int. Med.* 58:324–332 (1963).

Johnson, G., Maccario, M., Gershon, S., and Korein, J. The effect of lithium on electroencephalogram, behavior, and serum electrolytes. *J. Nerv. Ment. Dis.* 151:273–289 (1970).

Katz. F. H., Eckert, R. C., and Gebott, M. D. Hypokalemia caused by surreptitious self administration of diuretics. *Ann. Int. Med.* 76:85–90 (1972).

Katz, S., and Foulkes, E. F. Mineral metabolism and behavior: Abnormalities of calcium homeostasis. *Am. J. Phys. Anthropol.* 32:299–304 (1970).

Kitzes, R., Cohen, L., and Rosenfield, J. Neuropsychiatric manifestations of potassium depletion. *Harefuah.* 90:78–79 (1976).

Knochel, J. P. The pathophysiology and clinical characteristics of severe hypophosphatemia. *Arch. Int. Med.* 137:203–220 (1977).

Lancet. Water intoxication. (Lead article.) 1:425–426 (1953).

Leaf, A. The clinical physiological significance of the serum sodium concentration. *N. Eng. J. Med.* 276:24–30 (1967).

Linderman, R. D. Hypokalemia causes, consequences, and correction. *Am. J. Med. Sci.* 271:5–17 (1976).

Lipsmeyer, E., and Ackerman, G. L. Irreversible brain damage after water intoxication. *J.A.M.A.* 196:286–288 (1966).

Logothetis, J. Neurological effects of water and sodium disturbances. I. General mechanisms of hypernatremic syndromes. *Postgrad. Med. J.* 40:408–417 (1966).

Lotz, M., Zisman, E., and Bartter, F. C. Evidence for phosphorus depletion syndrome in man. *N. Eng. J. Med.* 278:409–415 (1968).

Luttrell, C. N., and Finberg, L. Hemorrhagic encephalopahty induced by hypernatremia, clinical laboratory, and pathological observations. *Arch. Neurol. Psychiat.* 81:424–432 (1959).

McCance, R. A. Experimental sodium chloride deficiency in man. *Proc. Roy. Soc. Lond.* (Biol.) 119:245–268 (1936).

Mitchell, W., and Feldman, F. Neuropsychiatric aspects of hypokalemia. *Canad. Med. Assn. J.* 98:49–51 (1968).

Noonan, J.P.A., and Ananth, J. Compulsive water drinking and water intoxication. *Comp. Psychiat.* 18:183–187 (1977).

Pampiglione, G. The effects of metabolic disorders on brain activity. *J.R. Coll. Phys. London.* 7:347–364 (1973).

Peterson, P. Psychiatric disorders in primary hyperparathyroidism. *J. Clin. Endocrinol* 38:1491–1495 (1968).

Pitts, F. N., and McClure, J. N. Lactate metabolism in anxiety neurosis. *N. Eng. J. Med.* 277:1329–1336 (1967).

Pleasure, D., and Goldberg, M. Neurogenic hypernatremia. *Arch Neurol.* 15:78–87 (1966).

Pollen, R. H., and Williams, R. H. Hyperkalemic neuromyopathy in Addison's disease. *N. Eng. J. Med.* 263:273–278 (1960).

Rankind, M. Psychosis, polydipsia, and water intoxication: Report of a fatal case. *Arch. Gen. Psychiat.* 30:112–114 (1974).

Resnick, M. E., and Patterson, C. Coma and convulsions due to compulsive water drinking. *Neurol.* 19:1125–1126 (1969).

Robin, E. D., Davis, R. P., and Rees, S. B. Salicylate intoxication with special reference to the development of hypokalemia. *Am. J. Med.* 26:869–882 (1959).

Ross, E. J., and Christie, S.B.M. Hypernatremia. *Med. (Baltimore)* 48:441–473 (1969).

Rountree, L. G. Water intoxication. *Arch. Int. Med.* 32:157–174 (1923).

Sanghvi, L. M., Gupta, K. D., Banerjee, K., and Bose, K. Paraplegia, hypokalemia, and neuropathy with muscle lesions of potassium deficiency associated with thyrotoxicosis. *Am. J. Med.* 27:817–823 (1959).

Schwartz, W. B., and Relman, A. S. Metabolic and renal studies in chronic potassium depletion resulting from overuse of laxatives. *J. Clin. Invest.* 32:258–271 (1953).

Shakhnovitch: *Russk Vrach* 32:537–538 (1882). Abstracted in *London Med. Rec.* 12:130 (1884).

Shaw, D. M., and Coppen, A. Potassium and water distribution in depression. *Brit. J. Psychiat.* 112:260–276 (1966).

Shaw, D. M., Frizel, D., Camps, F. E., and White, S. Brain electrolytes in depressive and alcoholic suicides. *Brit. J. Psychiat.* 115:69–79 (1969).

Silvis, S., and Paragas, P. Paresthesias, weakness, seizures, and hypophosphatemia in patients receiving hyperalimentation. *Gastroenterol.* 62:4:514–519 (1972).

Swash, M., and Rowan, A. T. Electroencephalographic criteria of hypocalcemia and hypercalcemia. *Arch. Neurol.* 26:218–227 (1972).

Thomson, G. E. Acute renal failure. *Med. Clin. N. Am.* 57:1579–1589 (1973).

Ueno, Y., Aoki, N., Yabuki, T., and Kuraishi, F. Electrolyte metabolism in blood and cerebrospinal fluid in psychosis. *Folia Psychiat. Neurol. Jap.* 15:304–326 (1961).

Vianna, J. H. Severe hypophosphatemia due to hypokalemia. *J.A.M.A.* 215:1497–1500 (1971).

Walker, W. G., and Whelton, A. Sodium metabolism, in *The Principles and Practice of Medicine.* A.M. Harvey, R. J. Johns, A. H. Owens, and R. S. Ross eds. Appleton-Century-Crofts, New York (1976), pp. 85–94.

Weiner, M. W., and Epstein, F. H. *Signs and Symptoms of Electrolyte Disorders in Clinical Disorders of Fluid and Electrolyte Metabolism.* M. H. Maxwell, and C. R. Kleeman, eds. McGraw-Hill Book Co., New York (1972), pp. 629–661.

Winokur, A., and Beckman, A. L. *Principles of neurophysiology in* The Biological Bases of Psychiatric Disorders. A. Frazer and A. Winokur, eds. Spectrum Publications, New York (1977), pp. 37–83.

Psychiatric Presentations of Medical Illness

CHAPTER 17

Mental Disturbances Related To Metals

NEIL EDWARDS, M.D.

INTRODUCTION

Of the 90 naturally occurring elements, 69 are metals. Some exist in great quantities, such as aluminum and iron; some are quite rare, such as silver, gold, and the radioactive elements; the others occupy positions intermediate in their abundance. Metals are ubiquitous in our environment. Added to this are man's natural curiosity and drive to better his condition, leading to even greater contact with these elements because of their beauty and utility. With this extensive contact, certain consequences are inevitable. Many of these metals, being part of the environment, have become essential to most organisms including man, e.g., sodium, magnesium, potassium, calcium, vanadium, chromium, manganese, iron, cobalt, copper, zinc, and molybdenum (Tarjan and Morava, 1976). These authors note that nickel and tin have been found to be essential to various farm animals, but not as yet to man. Thirty-nine metals have been found to be important in various enzyme systems, but have not as yet been proven essential to man (Davies, 1972). Hence, there are 12 essential metals, and, if we don't break the usual rules of evolution, several others are likely to be demonstrated in man in the future. With essentiality, the first natural consequence of the ubiquitous presence of metals, come two natural subconsequences: (1) that deficiency syndromes will occur whether from insufficient intake, excessive loss, or acquired improper metabolism (acquired deficiency); and (2) inborn errors of metabolism resulting in both deficiency and excess syndromes will occur. The second major consequence of the omnipresence of metals is that toxic disorders due to simple excessive intake, or acquired lack of excretion of both essential and non-essential metals, will occur.

All of the aforementioned types of disorders of metals do occur in man, and many have psychiatric symptoms as part of the clinical picture.

DISORDERS OF THE ESSENTIAL METALS

As Scheinberg and Sternlieb (1976) have noted, active processes of absorption, distribution, and excretion have evolved for the homeostatic regulation of the essential elements. Hence, the human organism is not only subject to exogenous toxic overload of these elements but also to mutagenic derangement of their regulating mechanisms. Examples of the latter are Wilson's disease (hepatolenticular degeneration), Menkes' Kinky-Hair disease, ideopathic hemochromatosis, acrodermatitis enteropathica, the various genetic hemoglobinopathies, and ideopathic hypomagnesemia. The essential metals, as mentioned above, are also subject to simple exogenous deficiency. Thus, the disorder of any essential metal can be broken down into: (1) hereditary disorders of regulation, which can result in either toxicity or deficiency; (2) acquired toxicity; and (3) acquired deficiency. The discussions of disorders relevant to each metal will generally follow this outline.

Copper

Hereditary Disorders

Copper is required in the function of several enzymes (Davies, 1972). It would therefore be expected that hereditary lack of one or more of these enzymes might lead to a toxic overload of this metal. This is indeed the case in Wilson's disease or hepatolenticular degeneration (HLD) where ceruloplasmin is lacking and where there is probably also an impairment of lysosomal excretion of copper into the bile (Scheinberg and Sternlieb, 1976). One would expect that copper deficiency, by causing decreased activity of several enzymes, might result in a syndrome with many systems affected. Menkes' Kinky-Hair disease is such a syndrome and is apparently due to an hereditary deficiency in the copper transport system in the gut (Danks et al., 1972).

Hepatolenticular Degeneration. HLD is inherited as an autosomal recessive, has affected every race studied, and has a prevalence of one in 200,000 (Scheinberg and Sternlieb, 1976). Its onset is usually in the first three decades of life. As mentioned before, there are apparently two pathogenic defects in this disorder, viz. the liver's inability (relative or absolute) to synthesize ceruloplasmin (the plasma copper transport protein) and an impairment of liver lysozymal excretion of copper into the bile. As a result, free copper is deposited in various organs, notably the liver and brain, to which organs the prominent symptoms and signs are referable. Free copper is also deposited in the periphery of the cornea in Descemet's membrane, resulting in the pathognomonic Kayser-Fleischer ring.

It is difficult to ascertain what percentage of patients with HLD present with psychiatric symptomatology. Scheinberg (1975) has stated, "Essentially every patient with Wilson's disease manifests a psychiatric disorder at some time during his disease, and a psychiatrist is the first physician consulted by about 25 percent of patients". Walker (1969) studied 12 patients with HLD and found that they all had psychiatric symptomatology before any other signs or symptoms developed. All had seen psychiatrists, had received psychiatric diagnoses, and had psychiatric intervention recommended. In his classical description of this disorder, Wilson (1911–1912) noted prominent psychiatric symptomatology in 8 of his 12 patients. Walshe (1975) has cautioned us that we must have a higher index of suspician for HLD when evaluating elementary-school-age children for personality changes, poor school performance, and writing or speech problems, since many children with HLD give this kind of "premorbid" data. Two different sets of psychiatric symptomatology are being addressed, and it is important that the distinction be made. Walshe is speaking of "softer" psychiatric symptomatology, which precedes the onset of hepatic and/or neurologic disease by as much as several years. Scheinberg and Wilson are addressing the "harder" psychiatric symptomatology, seen during, or immediately prior to, overt organic illness. Walker speaks to both types.

The types of psychiatric problems that precede organic illness by some time and that have been dubbed "soft," tend to lie in the areas of personality change, behavior disorder, school phobia, and mental retardation. The "hard" psychiatric symptoms seen during, or immediately prior to, overt organic disease, present as schizophreniform psychoses, organic brain syndromes, major affective disorders, and hysterical states. The psychiatric manifestations of Wilson's disease are protean, and Scheinberg (1975) has stated that HLD can mimic almost any psychiatric illness. Since other signs and symptoms may not be present early in the disease, a careful history, physical examination, and laboratory screening may save a life. A careful family history may reveal that a relative has died at an early age of liver disease, neurological disease, or while in a mental hospital. Tremor, not obvious at rest, may be elicited by fine motor movements. An enlarged liver may be palpated below the costal margin. The Kayser-Fleischer ring (golden-brown or greenish-brown) may not be present at this stage but should be looked for with the slit lamp. Liver function studies may be abnormal. Serum ceruloplasmin and copper are low while urinary copper and amino acids are high. This constellation of laboratory findings is diagnostic.

The diagnosis after, or immediately prior to, the appearance of organic illness is, of course, more readily made, although there are still some important pitfalls. These patients often display a theatric quality leading to confusion with hysterical states. Often, friends or the patient himself may report withdrawal from interests and a feeling of sadness. If this is combined with a loss of appetite and weight loss from an as yet unapparent liver disease, a misdiagnosis of major affective disorder may be made. Sometimes the clinical picture is dominated by a Parkinsonian presentation with fixed facial expression and loss of associational movements of the arms in walking. This can be confused with the blunted affect and stereotypy of movement of schizophrenia, expecially in the young patient. It is important, then, to study such cases thoroughly with respect to family history, physical examination, and laboratory findings.

Physical examination may demonstrate a tremor, not obvious at rest, but elicited by fine motor movements. Rigidity, sometimes constant, sometimes intermittent, of the voluntary musculature may be present. Dysarthria, ataxia, and a complaint of clumsiness are frequent findings. Careful mental status examination will often reveal deficits in cognitive skills, e.g., poor mathematical calculation, poor recent memory, difficulty in concentration, poor judgement and insight, and affective lability. Jaundice may be present as well as splenomegaly, ascites, hepatomegaly, hematemesis from esophageal varices, and spider angiomata.

When the disease becomes advanced, the diagnosis is apparent. Most patients by this time will display cirrhosis of the liver, signs of basal ganglion disease, an organic brain syndrome, and Kayser-Fleischer rings. The patient's appearance is characteristic and not easily mistaken for psychiatric illness: The facial muscles are fixed in a wide, vacuous smile, the neck and trunk are rigid, the upper extremities are fixed in flexion at the elbow, and wrist and metacarpal joints and the legs are fixed in extension.

The prognosis for HLD if untreated is invariably death in as little as a few months or as long as 30 to 40 years; usually in 5 to 10 years. Life can be prolonged and symptomatology largely ameliorated by the combined therapy of potassium sulfide to prevent absorption of copper in the gut and penicillamine to chelate copper and remove it from the tissues.

Menkes' Kinky-Hair Disease. This entity was first described by Menkes et al., (1962). These authors described five male babies all in the same family who had peculiar white stubby hair, early and severe mental retardation, growth retardation, and severe neurological impairment. These infants present, usually in the first month of life, with poor head control, weak Moro reflexes, difficulty following light, and often seizures. They fail to meet developmental milestones and progress through spastic paresis to terminal opisthotonus. Death without treatment is inevitable and occurs as early as 7 months and sometimes as late as 3½ years. Danks et al. (1972) studied seven children affected with this disease and found them all to have the clinical signs and symptoms mentioned above, plus hypothermia. The authors demonstrated very low serum copper and copper-oxidase levels in all the patients as well as greatly increased loss of copper in the stool and normal red blood cell copper levels.

Treatment with high doses of oral copper resulted in a slight, transient improvement in one of the patients studied by Danks et al. (1972), but intravenous cupric chloride resulted in circulatory collapse and discontinuation of the therapy. Intravenous copper does result in marked rise in serum copper and ceruloplasmin (Dekaban et al., 1975). These authors had some modest success in treating Menkes' Kinky-Hair disease with subcutaneous copper sulfate (temporary arrest in the mental deterioration, slight motor improvement and darkening and strengthening of the hair). The future of such patients, however, is not encouraging.

Acquired Copper Toxicity. Copper toxicity from external sources certainly occurs in man, is mainly secondary to prolonged use of copper sulfate-containing fungicides, algecides, or molluskicides, and causes symptoms and signs mainly referable to hematologic, gastrointestinal, and cardiovascular systems (Scheinberg and Sternleib, 1976).

Acquired Copper Deficiency. Graham and Cordano (1976) have stated that with the rare exception of the very small premature infant fed an unmodified cow's milk diet, exogenous copper deficiency is usually due to a combination of a copper-deficient diet and loss of large amounts of copper through diarrhea in infants. However, Solomons et al. (1976) studied 13 patients on total parenteral alimentation for various gastrointestinal disorders and found that all had a precipitous decline in their serum copper. Hence, at least in this restricted population and perhaps in other populations beyond infancy where dietary copper is severely limited, exogenous copper deficiency is a possibility. In fact, Dudrick (1978) adds copper and zinc routinely to hyperalimentation fluid when hyperalimentation is to be prolonged.

Copper deficiency has been shown to cause nervous disorders in the neonates of various species (lambs, goats, pigs, guinea pigs, and rats). Called neonatal ataxia, it is associated with central nervous system hypomeylination and lowered central nervous system concentrations of norepinephrine and dopamine (O'Dell, 1976). Neonatal ataxia has been prevented in farm animals by prenatal copper supplementation. In an affected animal, copper supplementation corrects the dopamine deficit but alleviates neither the hypomyelination nor the ataxia. These observations raise interesting questions: (1) Does copper deficiency play a role in some cases of human cerebral palsy? (2) Is copper, via its apparent effect on dopamine and norepinephrine, important in the pathogenesis of some cases of schizophrenia and major affective disorders? At present, there do not appear to be any studies in the literature bearing on the first of these questions. However, increased serum copper levels have been reported in schizophrenics (Pfeiffer and Iliev, 1972; Rahman et al., 1976) and in autistic children (Kirscher, 1978). On the other hand, Greiner et al. (1975) measured concentrations of copper, as well as those of various other metals, in white and gray matter in schizophrenics, brain-damaged patients, and normals, and found no differences. Copper does cross the blood-brain barrier. Hence, one would expect elevated serum levels to reflect themselves in brain tissue. Furthermore, if copper were exerting an influence on the brain dopamine in some schizophrenics, it is difficult to envisage how this would occur without the presence of elevated brain copper levels. Elucidation of these conflicting data awaits further definitive research.

Magnesium

This metal poses a unique problem. Although the data are conflicting, it would appear that hypomagnesemia, through mechanisms at present poorly understood, results in hypocalcemia (Shils, 1976; Nordio et al., 1971; Lombeck et al.,1975a; Medalle et al., 1976). Hypomagnesemia also appears to render organisms of various species refractory to parathyroid hormone (Shils, 1976). Further, hypercalcemia due to hyperparathyroidism results in hypomagnesemia (Gatewood et al., 1975). It is not clear from the literature if elevated serum magnesium results in a change in serum calcium, or if hypocalcemia results in hypomagnesemia. What is clear is that in any given case of hypomagnesemia, hypocalcemia or hypercalcemia may also be present. Hypomagnesemia and hypocalcemia share certain symptoms, notably: irritability, psychosis, organic brain syndrome, depression, anxiety, restlessness, and tetany. Hypomagnesemia and hypercalcemia also share certain symptoms, e.g., depression, psychosis, and organic brain syndrome. Therefore, it is often unclear in a given case (clinically and from the literature) whether magnesium or calcium is the culprit in the presenting picture, and it is incumbent upon the clinician to obtain laboratory measurements of both metals.

With this caveat in mind, we can now go on to discuss the various syndromes related to magnesium.

Hereditary Disorders

Primary Hypomagnesemia. According to Lombeck et al. (1975a), 12 cases of this disorder have been reported in the literature. Primary hypomagnesemia is an autosomal recessive disorder. The homeostatic defect appears to be intestinal malabsorption of magnesium. It is characterized by hypomagnesemia, hypocalcemia, tetany, carpopedal spasms, and tetanic seizures beginning in the first few months of life. One of the cases reported by Lombeck et al. (1975a) had a square face, moderate ocular protrusion, and white stripes in the distal aspects of the fingernails. One case reported by Nordio et al. (1971) displayed irritability and psychomotor retardation beginning at 4 weeks of life. This child had an IQ of 68 at age 32 months. One of the cases reported by Lombeck et al. (1975) died at 5 months in tetanic convulsions that started in the third week of life. Treatment with calcium produces no change in these patients, but treatment with oral magnesium sulfate in large doses results in normalization of the clinical and laboratory findings. The requirement in these infants is 30 to 70 mg/kg/day of magnesium (over 10 times the adult daily requirement) Lombeck et al., (1975a).

Acquired Magnesium Toxicity. Exogenous magnesium toxicity usually occurs as a complication of the medical use of magnesium sulfate intravenously as an antihypertensive or anticonvulsant, or orally as a cathartic and, since magnesium is rapidly excreted by the kidneys, usually in the presence of compromised renal function (Harrison, 1970; Fishman, 1965). Magnesium is a powerful nervous system depressant, causing lowered blood pressure at blood levels above 4 mEq per liter; decreased responsiveness above 5 mEq per liter; depressed deep tendon reflexes, weakness, and ataxia at levels between 7 and 10 mEq per liter; respiratory depression at levels of 10 mEq per liter and above; coma at 12 mEq per liter; and death at higher levels (Fishman, 1965). In view of this, it is surprising that there have not been a great many articles published on the psychiatric symptoms of early magnesium toxicity, expecially in renal dialysis patients. In fact, however, this author could find none despite considerable personal experience with patients with slightly elevated magnesium levels who have displayed lassitude, depression, and organic brain syndromes, both psychotic and nonpsychotic. Calcium quite effectively antagonizes the neurological and neuromuscular actions of magnesium, and therefore can be used as a specific antidote in magnesium toxicity. Intravenous calcium gluconate (10 ml of a 10 percent solution) repeated as needed to control symptoms, is recommended by Harrison (1970).

Acquired Magnesium Deficiency. Magnesium deficiency occurs through a number of different mechanisms, viz. lack of replacement in intravenous fluids, excessive losses via vomiting and diarrhea in various gastrointestinal disorders, excessive loss through the kidneys as in the excessive use of diuretics and in hyperaldosteronism, hyperparathyroidism, and inadequate intake. Inadequate intake, as the sole cause of hypomagnesemia, except in the chronic alcoholic who is not eating, is probably quite rare because of the abundant quantities present in many foods.

As mentioned above, hypomagnesemia can produce anxiety, immobility, restlessness, depression, psychosis, and organic brain syndrome. Such symptoms can occur singly or in various combinations and often occur in concert with various neurological symptoms and signs. The latter may also occur singly or in various combinations and include: pronounced startle response, muscular twitches, myoclonic jerks, course tremor, irritability of muscles to percussion, hyperreflexia, positive Chvostek sign, seizures (tetanic, grand mal, or multifocal), tetany, carpopedal spasm, athetoid and choreiform movements, positive Babinski sign, clonus, ataxia, nystagmus, fasciculations, vertigo, paresthesias, auditory hyperacusis, gait disturbances, and muscular weakness (Flink et al., 1954; Fishman, 1965; Hall and Joffe, 1973). Any combination of these psychiatric and neurological signs and symptoms can be present in any given patient, but the usual picture is that of an anxious, irritable, uncooperative patient with some degree of organic brain syndrome (which often contains psychotic elements) plus signs of neurological and neuromuscular irritability, such as a pronounced startle response, muscular twitching, course tremor, carpopedal spasm, and seizures. The electroencephalogram (EEG) may show a "tetanic pattern," which consists of trains of 13 to 20 cps spikes very similar to those seen in the tonic phase of a grand mal seizure or generalized slowing reminiscent of metabolic derangement. Diagnosis can be confirmed by serum magnesium levels less than 1.9 mEq per liter.

Treatment of hypomagnesemia consists of intravenous, intramuscular, or oral administration of magnesium sulfate, the route chosen depending upon: (1) the extent of the patients' obtundation, and (2) the likelihood that enough magnesium will be absorbed by the gastrointestinal tract to correct the deficit. There is no particular advantage of one parenteral route over the other, except that the intravenous route is preferable if: (1) a loading dose is required as in the presence of seizures, or (2) intravenous fluids are required for other reasons. Different parenteral dosage schedules have been proposed by various authors, but those suggested by Flink (1969) for magnesium deficiency (regardless of etiology) seem to be preferable since they are based upon probable total body deficit. For intramuscular administration, he suggests 2 grams of magnesium (via a 50 percent magnesium sulfate solution) every 2 hours for three doses, and then every 4 hours for four doses on the first day. On the second day, the schedule is 1 gram every 4 hours for six doses; and on the third through fifth days, 1 gram every 6 hours. By the intravenous route, he recommends 6 grams of magnesium in 1000 ml of glucose solution over 3 hours, then two 1-liter glucose solutions containing 5 grams each throughout the remainder of the first day. On days two through five, 6 grams of magnesium should be distributed throughout the total fluids of each day. For oral administration, Fishman's (1965) schedule seems quite adequate. He suggests that 4 to 10 grams of magnesium as a 4 percent magnesium sulfate solution be administered daily, preferably in orange juice. Patients experiencing heavy losses where the underlying disorder is not readily correctable (e.g., regional enteritis and gastric and jejunal bypass surgery) may require prolonged replacement. The aforementioned replacement schedules should be safe, vis-á-vis, magnesium toxicity if renal function is good. Therefore, it is important that renal function be checked before replacement starts and, if compromised, the dosage schedule should be modified and frequent serum magnesium levels should be obtained.

It is important to keep in mind that calcium may also be low in most hypomagnesemic states or high when the underlying disorder is hyperparathyroidism. When magnesium deficit is causing hypocalcemia, the latter will be corrected by magnesium replacement. However, when hyperparathyroidism is the basic problem, magnesium replacement will probably do no harm but is superfluous to the definitive treatment, usually parathyroid adenectomy, which will bring both levels back to normal.

Hypomagnesemia and Alcoholic Encephalopathies. Stendig-Lindberg (1974) has noted that magnesium deficiency is frequently found in chronic alcoholics, especially when delerium tremens is present. In this same article, she also reviews the work of several other groups who have found similar results. The mechanism of the deficit in these patients is complex and probably includes inadequate dietary intake, gastrointestinal losses from malabsorption and vomiting, and increased urinary losses presumably due to decreased tubular reabsorption (Fishman, 1965). Flink et al. (1954) suggested that the hypomagnesemia in such patients may be etiologically related to their delerium tremens, and treated 30 patients with magnesium sulfate with good success. However, these authors note that the differences in results between patients treated with magnesium sulfate and patients treated with the standard techniques available at that time were " . . . slight and not firmly established." (Flink et al., 1954). Further, Fishman (1965) contends that magnesium deficiency is not important etiologically in these patients, despite the similarities of their disorder to experimental magnesium deficiency in animals since many delerium tremens patients do not improve with magnesium replacement. Faillace (1978) reports that he has treated large numbers of such patients without specific magnesium replacement with no untoward results.

It would appear, then, that the etiologic importance of magnesium deficiency in these patients is, at best, controversial, although it is difficult to resist the speculation that it is at least contributory. Of more interest, however, are the empirical observations of Stendig-Lingberg (1974): (1) of ten patients with delerium tremens or predelirium who had normal serum magnesium, none developed alchoholic encephalopathies (Korsakoff's syndrome, Wernicke's syndrome, dementia alcoholitica, and intellectual reduction of a degree that makes social readjustment impossible) as a sequel, and of 11 patients with delerium tremens who had low serum magnesium, six developed chronic alcoholic encephalopathies as a result; and (2) four patients with recent onset of alcoholic encephalopathy treated with magnesium were relieved of their encephalopathy.

The etiologic role of thiamine in the Wernicke-Korsakoff syndrome is well recognized. Zieve et al. (1968b) demonstrated that magnesium deficiency interferes with the growth response to thiamine in the thiamine-deficient rats. These same authors (Zieve et al., 1968a) found that the activity of the thiamine-dependent enzyme, transketolase, increases to normal with thiamine treatment in rats that are only thiamine deficient, but requires both thiamine and magnesium if the animals are also magnesium deficient. This thiamine unresponsiveness in magnesium-deficient animals plus Stendig-Lindberg's observations raise the possibility that, although careful dietary management probably provides enough magnesium to cover any contribution of lack of this ion in the pathogenesis of delirium tremens, the prevention of chronic alcoholic encephalopathies may require more vigorous magnesium replacement. Based upon the evidence cited above, Flink (1978) indeed advocates such vigorous replacement in alcoholic patients.

Calcium

Hereditary Disorders

Idiopathic Hypercalcemia. This disorder may be due to an increased sensitivity to Vitamin D. It is observed in infancy and is characterized by mental retardation, elvin facies, high serum cholesterol, hypercalcemia, and failure to thrive. Successful treatment can be accomplished with cortisone and a Vitamin D and calcium-free diet (Harrison, 1970).

Acquired Calcium Toxicity. This is usually secondary to hyperparathyroidism which, in turn, is usually due to a parathyroid adenoma. Parathyroid hyperplasia or carcinoma seldom produces clinical hyperparathyroidism. Peterson (1968) studied 54 patients with hyperparathyroidism and found 65 percent to have one or more of a number of psychiatric disturbances. Most common were affective disturbance and disturbance of drives (36 patients each). Impairment of memory was seen in 12 and acute organic psychosis in 5. The onset of the personality change (affective disturbance) usually developed slowly over years or decades with typical symptoms of depression, including dysphoric mood, lack of interest, and suicidal thinking. The organic psychoses consisted of disorientation, delusions, and hallucinations.

Of particular interest is that the severity of the psychiatric symptoms directly paralleled the serum calcium levels with most of the unremarkable or moderate changes occurring between serum calcium levels of 10.5 and 14.5 mg%, severe changes clustered between 12.6 and 16.5 mg%, while psychotic changes occured at levels between 14.6 and 18.0 mg%. At levels higher than 19 mg%, stupor and coma result. The mental changes were independent of parathormone levels—dialysis improved the symptoms but produced no alteration of parathormone levels. Forty-six of the patients underwent parathyroid adenectomy with complete reversal of symptoms. Gatewood et al. (1975) reported five cases admitted to the hospital for neuropsychiatric complaints. Two patients were admitted with a diagnosis of depression; one with a diagnosis of catatonic schizophrenia; one with a confusional state; and one with a suspected stroke plus recent onset of syncope, progressive confusion, and drowsiness. One of the depressed patients experienced episodic confusion. None of these five patients was suspected of having hyperparathyroidism before admission. Diagnosis was made by serum calcium and phosphorus levels (SMA-12).

These two studies clearly illustrate that a psychiatric picture often precedes any other signs of the illness. In fact, Peterson (1968) states that hyperparathyroidism should be suspected in any patient who complains of gradually developing personality change with lack of drive and depression as major components of the change, and who complains of excessive thirst. Other symptoms and signs that may accompany the neuropsychiatric symptoms noted above are: polyuria and polydypsia, bone pain, renal colic, deafness, weight loss, and spontaneous fractures. Physical examination may reveal muscular weakness and hypotonia, bone deformities, subcutaneous and gingival tumors, and calcific keratitis. Radiographic examination may show a variety of skeletal abnormalities, such as generalized demineralization, "salt and pepper" appearance of the skull, cysts, tumors, fractures, and regression of the lamina dura of the teeth. Laboratory studies in hyperparathyroidism will reveal increased serum calcium, decreased serum phosphate, increased urinary calcium and phosphate, and sometimes anemia, leukopenia, and thrombocytopenia. Fecal calcium and phosphate are normal. Alkaline phosphatase may be normal or increased.

Other diseases that can cause elevated serum calcium are multiple myeloma, milk-alkali syndrome, vitamin D intoxication, metastic carcinoma, and sarcoidosis. It is important to keep in mind that serum magnesium may be decreased in hypercalcemic states. Both Peterson (1968) and Gatewood et al. (1975) recognize this possibility and that the hypomagnesemia may be contributing to the picture. Therefore, serum magnesium should also be measured in hypercalcemia and, if low, supplementation of magnesium should be part of the therapeutic regimen. Definitive treatment in hyperparathyroidism is usually parathyroid adenectomy. The prognosis is good if secondary renal disease is not too advanced.

Acquired Calcium Deficiency. Hypocalcemia can result from a variety of disorders, including renal failure, osteomalacia and rickets, hypoparathyroidism, pseudohypoparathyroidism, pseudo-pseudohypoparathyroidism, intestinal malabsorption of any cause, magnesium deficiency, renal tubular disorders, phosphate poisoning, malignant disease (especially leukemia), fluoride intoxication, and colchicine overdosage (Paterson, 1976). Hence, it is apparent that hypocalcemia may be present at any age from infancy to extreme old age. Psychiatric symptoms include anxiety, tiredness, weakness, irritability, depression, and psychosis. In osteomalacia, the combination of bone pain, muscular weakness and depression often leads to a misdiagnosis of neuroses (Paterson, 1976). These symptoms may persist for years before other signs and symptoms of hypocalcemia appear. These include neuromuscular irritability with positive Chvostek and Troussea signs, tetany, carpopedal spasm, muscular twitching and cramps, larangeal stridor (may result in death), and convulsions. Trophic changes of the skin, hair, and nails may occur. The skin may be dry, rough, and scaly, and various rashes occur including erythema, papules, vesicles, and bullae. There may be generalized hair loss; the nails may be brittle and transversely ridged; ridging and/or pitting of the enamel of the teeth may occur in children; cataracts occur when the hypocalcemia is prolonged. Also, prolonged hypocalcemia may result in progressive dementia with only partial return of function on correction of the deficiency.

Diagnosis of hypocalcemia depends on the clinical picture plus a low serum calcium level. Further diagnostic studies should be directed toward uncovering any one of the many possible underlying disorders listed above. Definitive treatment will, of course, be directed toward the underlying disorder when possible. Calcium replacement can be accomplished by intravenous calcium chloride, or calcium gluconate plus dihydrotachysterol, or Vitamin D orally in acute cases; or by oral calcium and dihydrotachysterol, or Vitamin D in more chronic cases. Paterson (1976) notes that antibodies develop to exogenous parathyroid hormone, so this agent should probably be avoided. Again, it must be kept in mind that magnesium deficiency can cause hypocalcemia and that when this is the case, the clinical picture will not respond to calcium but will to magnesium.

Zinc

Over the past 10 years, a great deal of study has been devoted to the physiological roles of this element and its probable clinical importance. Zinc has been reported to be essential for the function of more than 50 enzymes (Casper et al., 1978). Tuman and Doisy (1975) state that zinc is essential for the function of several enzymes, for protein synthesis, for carbohydrate metabolism, and for DNA and RNA synthesis. Adequate zinc levels appear to be necessary for the transport of Vitamin A from the liver presumably via a requirement for zinc in retinal binding protein (the serum transport protein for Vitamin A) (Smith et al., 1975).

Hereditary Disorders

Acrodermatitis Enteropathica. That zinc might play a role in the pathogenesis of acrodermatitis enteropathica (AE) was first postulated by Moynahan (1976). Lombeck et al. (1975b) demonstrated that patients with this disorder absorb significantly less zinc than normals and postulated a primary absorption defect. Oleske et al. (1978) characterized AE as an autosomal recessive disorder with intestinal malabsorption of zinc as the primary defect. The disorder begins in infancy, and until recently, was thought to be universally fatal. However, Olholm-Larsen (1978) discussed two cases of his own and six others found in a review of the literature surviving into adulthood without specific therapy, and postulated that the disorder may be underdiagnosed in adults. The incidence of the disease is unknown. AE in children characteristically presents with a bullous, exfoliative rash distributed distally and symmetrically on the extremities, periorally and perianally, and with alopecia and chronic, severe diarrhea. Mental symptoms in infancy are prominent and include tearfulness, irritability, a complete lack of smiling and laughing, and an avoidance of eye contact. Moynahan (1976) reported prompt reversal of all symptoms with zinc supplementation, with the gaze aversion disappearing first. Of the two adult patients reported by Olholm-Larsen (1978), one had periodic, typical, disabling depressions but the skin and intestinal disturbances disappeared at puberty; while the other retained only the typical skin lesions on the feet. Whether in the childhood or adult form, the diagnosis is established by very low serum zinc levels (normal is 80 micrograms/100 ml) and low hair zinc levels (normal is 125 micrograms/g of hair).

Acquired Zinc Toxicity. Zinc is a relatively nontoxic metal. Toxicities have been reported, and death can ensue with ingestion of huge quantities (Prasad, 1976). Mental symptoms have not been reported as a prominent feature of zinc toxicity.

Acquired Zinc Deficiency. Deficiency of this metal secondary to a wide variety of factors has been reported and has been well summarized by Prasad (1976), Sandstead et al. (1976), and Sandstead (1975). Some of these factors are: low dietary zinc; diets containing components leading to intestinal chelation of zinc (encountered with high phytate and fiber content in diets rich in whole grains, and in cultures that practice geophagia—clay eating); intestinal malabsorptive disorders; hemolytic anemias; prolonged blood loss; increased urinary excretion (diabetes mellitus, hepatic cirrhosis, and failure of renal tubular reabsorption); catabolic states; infections (zinc mobilized by leukocyte endogenous mediator); total parenteral alimentation without zinc supplementation; dialysis; and prolonged anorexia. Interestingly, the United States is not exempt from dietary zinc deficiency (Hambridge and Walravens, 1976).

The symptoms and signs of zinc deficiency are growth retardation, male hypogonadism, rough skin, poor appetite, mental lethargy, hypogeusia (impaired taste), hyposmia (impaired smell), poor wound healing, and susceptibility to infection. Caldwell et al. (1976) have shown decreased learning ability and increased emotionality in zinc-deficient female rats and their offspring. Kirscher (1978) found significantly lowered serum zinc levels in 12 children with learning disabilities and in 5 retarded children. These data suggest a possible role of zinc deficiency early in life (if not during intrauterine life) in the pathogenesis of some cases of learning disability and mental retardation. More data are needed to establish such a connection, but attention to proper zinc nutrition in pregnant mothers and young children would certainly not be unwarranted—animal proteins are high in zinc.

Casper et al. (1978) found significantly decreased serum zinc in 24 female anorexia nervosa patients. This deficiency was most certainly on a dietary basis, but it is interesting to speculate that the zinc deficiency may have aided in the perpetuation of the poor appetite via the hypogeusia and hyposmia caused by zinc deficiency. Moynahan (1976) has offered two insightful observations gleaned from his experience with AE: (1) the mood disturbances seen in AE are very reminiscent of those seen in Kwashiorkor; and (2) the gaze aversion in AE is very similar to that seen in infantile autism. It is again a provacative speculation that zinc deficiency may play a role in these two disorders, but this has not yet been demonstrated.

Zinc deficiency has also been demonstrated to be present in patients with Laennec's cirrhosis secondary to alcoholism (Smith et al., 1975; Hartoma et al., 1977). This occurs via increased urinary excretion, the mechanism of which is unexplained. What role this documented zinc deficiency may play in the mental disturbances of these chronic alcoholics is another thought-provoking, but speculative question.

Manganese

Although manganese is important in the function of several human enzymes, (Davies, 1972; Tuman and Doisy, 1975; Sandstead, 1975), neither genetic disorders nor acquired deficiency states have been documented. However, an interesting toxic disorder has been reported—"Manganic madness."

Manganic Madness

This disorder occurs almost exclusively in manganese miners and in workers in steel foundries and ore-crushing plants (Mena, 1974). The toxic state is caused by inhalation of manganese dust. In most foreign countries, a psychosis has been the presenting disorder and has been followed by a Parkinsonian syndrome. However, the initial psychosis was conspicuously absent in American steel foundry and ore-crushing plant workers (Mena, 1974). The syndrome has come on with as short an exposure as 5 months and as long as 25 years. The psychosis resembles schizophrenia, and consists of anxiety, emotional lability (with explosive and inappropriate laughter and crying), compulsive acts, hallucinations, and delusions. The onset may be acute or insidious. Abd El Naby and Hassanein (1965) have noted a less severe form of mental disturbance in patients with an insidious onset consisting of mental fatique, retardation of thought processes, and poor concentration. Some patients display an organic brain syndrome with impaired recent memory, impaired calculations, and disorientation (Cook et al., 1974; Banta and Markesberry, 1977). The Parkinsonian picture consists of masked facies, bradykinesia, rigidity, diminished reflexes, and dystonia. Sixteen of Abd El Naby and Hassanein's (1965) patients displayed pyramidal as well as extrapyramidal signs and six also had cerebellar signs. Psychiatric symptoms abate from 3 weeks to 10 months after removal from the source, but neurological signs persist. Diagnosis can be established by high serum levels (normal less than 0.05 ppm) and high hair manganese levels (normal is zero). Rosenstock et al. (1971) demonstrated a level of manganese in chest hair three times that in the patient's scalp hair. Treatment with chelating agents has been discouraging; L-Dopa has met with variable success.

Iron

The inherited disorders of iron metabolism (idiopathic hemochromatosis and the inherited hemoglobinopathies) produce psychiatric symptomatology largely from the complications of iron overload on the one hand, and poor oxygenation and intravascular thrombosis on the other. The reader is referred to the chapters discussing liver disease, diabetes (common sequelae of hemochromatosis), and the hemoglobinopathies. Exogenous iron overload (Bantusiderosis and hemochromatosis secondary to chronic, heavy intake of iron-rich wines in alcoholics) also occurs and produces complications similar to those seen in the idiopathic form.

Acquired Deficiency

A few words should be said about this entity, because some authors have found behavioral effects in iron-deficient subjects which seem to be independent of any concurrent anemia. Jacobs (1977) demonstrated significant impairment in work performance in iron-deficient subjects even when the hemoglobin was not less than 12 g/100 cc. Leibel (1977) found decreased attentiveness; narrow attention span; perceptual restriction; lower IQ; lower vocabulary scores; and worse scores on reading knowledge, arithmetic concepts, and problem solving in iron-deficient junior high school students than in controls. Leibel notes that changes of this type have not been reported in uncomplicated thallasemia and sickle cell anemia. He also points out that the changes seen in his subjects may be due to other deficiencies not measured. Oski and Honig (1978) demonstrated improved scores on the Bayley scales of infant development after iron-deficient infants were treated with intramuscular iron. Placebo treatment produced no improvement. Although the data are sparse and inconclusive, it would seem worthwhile to check serum iron levels in patients who present with poor work or school performance and fatique or lassitude even when anemia is not present, and that any deficiencies be corrected.

DISORDERS OF THE NONESSENTIAL METALS

As mentioned above, homeostatic mechanisms have not developed for the regulation of nonessential metals. Consequently, there exist no genetic disorders for these metals. Of course, if an organ that would ordinarily aid in the excretion of a metal is diseased, the individual will be rendered more susceptible to toxicity. This, however, is in no way specific and any such afflicted individual would be more vulnerable to the effects of any potentially toxic substance normally excreted by that organ.

Also, nonessential metals being nonessential, no deficiency states exist. The ensuing discussion, therefore, will deal with acquired toxic states only.

Lead

Lead is a heavily used metal in industry. Consequently, sources of intoxication are many and include lead-based paints (still present in many old houses); water that has stood in lead pipes; fumes from burning storage batteries, solder, lead-emitting smelters, and auto exhaust; illicit whiskey made in lead-pipe stills; and even lead bullets and buckshot embedded in a serious cavity. Lead is absorbed slowly and excreted even more slowly, excretion taking three times as long as absorption. Hence, lead is a cumulative poison. It is stored principally in bone from which it can be mobilized to toxic levels by intercurrent illness and alcohol abuse; often there is no apparent mobilizer. As a consequence of these peculiarities of lead metabolism, patients in whom toxicity has resolved may again become symptomatic at a later date due to toxic amounts of lead being mobilized from bone. Symptoms of toxicity can come on gradually, but often, as might be surmised from the above discussion, are dramatic in their appearance.

The effects of lead intoxication on both children and adults are well documented. Classically, children are more prone to develop an encephalopathy with lethargy and somnolence, persistent vomiting, ataxia, convulsions, manic behavior, delirium, stupor, and coma. In adults, abdominal cramping (painters' cramps) and peripheral neuropathy (often with wrist and/or ankle drop) are the more usual signs. Encephalitis is rare in adults, but when it does occur, the source is usually "moonshine" made in lead-pipe stills (Harrison, 1970).

The diagnosis of lead intoxication in suspected cases is established by a serum lead level greater than 60 micrograms per liter. A useful and simple screening test is the demonstration of the presence of increased coproporphyrin III in the urine, a consistent feature of the disorder. There may be an anemia and basophilic stippling of red cells, but neither is specific for lead toxicity.

Of perhaps more relevance than "classical toxicity" from a psychiatric point of view, are the delayed effects of lead exposure in documented toxic patients and in subclinical cases. The usual figure quoted for mental retardation following recognized lead toxicity in childhood is 25 percent (Harrison, 1970; Bryce-Smith, 1972). Bryce-Smith (1972) has stated that the incidence of permanent brain damage after two or more episodes of toxicity in childhood is probably close to 100 percent. Several authors have found elevated lead levels in serum or hair in children with learning disabilities, mental retardation, or hyperkinesis (Pihl and Parkes, 1977; Landujan et al., 1975; David et al., 1972; de la Burde and Choate, 1975; Moore et al., 1977; David et al., 1976). Silbergeld and Goldberg (1973) produced growth and developmental retardation and hyperactivity in mice fed lead acetate. In a later experiment (1974), these authors replicated these results and were able to produce the paradoxical responses to d- and l-amphetamine, methylphenidate, and phenobarbitol in these hyperactive animals, with which clinicians treating hyperactive children are so familiar. de la Burde and Choate (1975) also found only 35 percent of a group of 70 children with known lead exposure to show normal testing on all areas of a neuropsychological battery (IQ, fine motor development, gross motor development, concept formation, and behavior); while 65 percent of a control group (72 children) had normal results in all areas. Chisolm (1974) reported elevated blood lead levels in a 9-year-old psychotic child and in a child who had developed clinical autism after 3 years of normal development. Blood levels in patients who displayed behavioral disorders, mental retardation, or learning disabilities—but no symptoms of "classical toxicity" in most studies—have run in the range of 40 to 70 mg/dl. These levels have hitherto been considered nontoxic.

It is apparent that until recently, there is more to lead toxicity than meets the eye. It would behoove the careful clinician dealing with children who are hyperactive, learning disabled, retarded, or even autistic to obtain a careful history for possible lead exposure, to check urinary coproporphyrin III and blood and urine lead levels, and to not dismiss blood levels of 40 to 70 mg/dl as "normal".

Treatment of these nonclassical forms of lead intoxication has not been well outlined. However, since there has been fairly good success with calcium disodium versenote in more florid cases, this drug may also prove of benefit here. Most important in the treatment of any form of lead intoxication is removal of the source. It must be emphasized that even after apparently successful treatment, a patient may become toxic again especially if intercurrent illness or alcoholism ensues. Consequently, these patients must be followed closely and treatment reinstituted if lead is again mobilized.

Mercury

Mercury is toxic in its elemental form, and in organic and inorganic compounds. Sources of intoxication include: mercury vapor; mercury amalgam dental fillings; medicinal agents (douches, skin creams, diuretics, and laxatives); contamination by industry of food and water; and accidental, suicidal, or homicidal ingestion of mercuric chloride. Due to the various ways the body handles different forms of mercury, differing patterns of distribution occur resulting in differing clinical pictures (Gestner and Huff, 1977). Elemental mercury is converted slowly into the mercuric form in the blood. This allows time for accumulation in brain tissue, since elemental mercury readily crosses the blood-brain barrier where it is converted into the mercuric form. Elemental mercury exposure results in brain concentrations 10 times greater than does exposure to inorganic forms. Mercuric mercury is highly corrosive to the GI mucosa through which it is absorbed and is then concentrated in the kidneys where it is also highly destructive. Mercurus mercury is also readily absorbed, is immediately converted into the mercuric form, and is deposited in the tissues in a distribution identical to the mercuric; however, the accumulation of mercuric ions is usually slower, thus allowing time for the mercuric ion to play havoc upon the brain. Organic mercurials (usually methyl or ethyl mercury) are very stable compounds and are concentrated largely in the liver and kidney, but 10 percent can be found in brain tissue. Psychiatric manifestations are primarily associated with moderately prolonged exposure to the elemental form (massive exposure produces an acute pulmonary syndrome), prolonged ingestion of mercurous salts, and prolonged ingestion of organomercurials.

Elemental Mercury. A wide spectrum of clinical pictures can be seen ranging from very mild disturbances to complete incapacitation. Onset is insidious. Insomnia, loss of appetite, and diarrhea are often the earliest signs. Depression is a common complaint, complete with fatique, lassitude, loss of interests and social withdrawal. The patient often becomes increasingly irritable and, a peculiar oversensitivity and embarrassment is frequently present. A tendency for sweating and blushing (erethism') is a frequent finding. The emotional disorder may appear to be episodic, thus simulating manic depressive illness. These patients are often a suicidal risk. Hallucinations and delusions may occur. There may be an organic brain syndrome as well with the typical associated findings of poor memory and concentration and decline in intellectual functions. These symptoms may be admixed with various combinations of the following: fine intention tremor, which progressively becomes more coarse and generalized with continued exposure to mercury, eventually resulting in inability to talk, walk, or sit; the gingivae may be spongy and bleed easily, and a blue line may be present along the gingival margin; the teeth may become loose; there may be a foul breath odor; the lens usually shows a yellowish-brown discoloration, which does not interfere with vision.

Inorganic Mercury Salts. Ingestion of mercuric salts results in an acute fulminating oro-esophagogastroenteritis and often ends in renal failure. Ingestion of mercuric salts causes a gradual accumulation of mercuric ions in the brain resulting in personality changes similar to those seen in exposure to the elemental form. However, colitis and nephrosis, which can progress to renal failure, are frequent findings in mercurus mercury poisoning.

Organomercurials. These cross the blood-brain barrier and have a very long half life. There is, therefore, a gradual accumulation in the brain. Mental changes are similar to those seen in elemental mercury poisoning. Again, these can occur along with any of the following: tremor and ataxia progressing, as in elemental mercury poisoning; to coarse tremor and spasms; disturbances in sensation with numbness of fingers, toes, lips, and tonque (these tend to occur early); loss of peripheral vision leading to tunnel vision, multiple blind spots, or complete blindness in severe cases; auditory loss over the entire frequency range, which can progress to deafness; and loss of taste acuity.

Organomercurials readily cross the placenta and are even more toxic to the fetus than to the adult. Thus, fetal toxicity can occur when the mother is non-toxic. Disturbances in central nervous system (CNS) function are similar to, but more profound than, those seen in the adult. Mild forms of organomercurial toxicity resemble slow learners in children and presenile dementia in adults.

Diagnosis of mercury intoxication depends upon a combination of the clinical picture, a careful environmental history, and determinations of blood, urine, and hair mercury levels.

Treatment varies with the type of poisoning. Gestner and Huff (1977) recommend for elemental mercury poisoning, penicillamine; for inorganic mercury compounds, BAL, so as to avoid the renal excretion route along with dialysis when renal failure is present; and for organomercurials, removal from the source. Chelating agents do not remove organomercurials from the brain; hence, after removal from the source, the process is very much "wait-and-see". The prognosis in organomercurial poisoning is not good, and recovery, if it does occur, is very slow. The prognosis in prenatal intoxication is grave.

Thallium

Thallium poisoning in the past was a rather common event (Munch, 1934). In a review of the literature, Munch compiled 778 cases, 46 (6 percent) of which died. Most of these cases were due to the oral administration of thallium acetate in preparations for treatment of ringworm of the scalp: thallium is an effective depilatory agent, and this is a constant feature of the toxic state. After 1934, the medical use of thallium declined markedly with a consequent drop in toxic cases. However, cases continued to occur (Reed et al., 1963, reported 72 cases) and were primarily caused by thallium-containing insecticides and rodenticides (Greenfeld and Hinostroza, 1964; Reed et al., 1963; Banks et al., 1972). Legislation was enacted in the early 1970s limiting the use of thallium-containing pesticides in the United States to commercial use. However, poisoning from pesticides still occurs in other countries where similar legislation has not been passed (Kloppel and Weiler, 1978). Occasional cases will probably still occur in the United States, as in that reported in a clinical conference at the Johns Hopkins Hospital (1978) but, unless another industry chooses to use thallium in their processing or end products, the numbers should be small and will usually be the result of "creative" homicide or suicide attempts.

Psychiatric symptoms are the rule and include poor concentration, irritability, somnolence, fatique, anorexia, psychosis (with vivid auditory and visual hallucinations), and organic brain syndrome. Other nervous system symptoms are bulbar palsies, disturbances of vision, ataxia, tremor, peripheral neuropathy, chorea and athetosis, hypotonia, hypesthesia, convulsions, and coma. The peripheral neuropathy produces paresthesias, hypohypesthesia, pain, and motor weakness as prominent early symptoms with preservation of deep tendon reflexes until late. Irritation of the entire alimentary canal is also common with stomatitis, glossitis, and gastroenteritis (the last may be hemorrhagic). A blue line in the gum occurs in some cases. Sinus tachycardia, hypertension, chest pain, albuminuria, and hematuria may be present as well as dry skin, rashes, and dystrophic changes in the nails. Thallium accumulates in all tissue and produces damage in all. Death can occur secondary to renal failure, liver failure, CNS damage, cardiac arrhythmias, status epilepticus, or intercurrent infection during coma. Alopecia begins 1 to 3 weeks after exposure and, since most other symptoms begin immediately or a few days after exposure, it is not a useful early diagnostic sign. The clinical picture is highly variable; symptoms referable to any of the systems covered above may predominate, or there may be various mixtures. Diagnosis therefore depends on a careful environmental history and the demonstration of thallium in blood, urine, or stool. Neurological sequelae are common especially in children where they have been reported to be as high as 54 percent (Reed et al., 1963) and include reflex asymmetries, weakness, ataxia, tremor, seizures, dementia, and psychosis. Reed et al. (1963) found that coma, seizures, abnormal reflexes, tremor, muscle weakness, and movement disorders were prognostically unfavorable vis-á-vis the development of sequelae.

A promising treatment is the use of oral Prussian Blue (potassium ferric hexacyanoferrate), which firmly binds thallium secreted by the intestinal mucosa into the intestinal lumen and thus allows it to be passed in the stool (Kamerbeek et al., 1971). Chelating agents and potassium, which physiologically compete with thallium, may redistribute thallium with resultant higher brain levels, and are therefore probably more harm than good.

Bismuth

Toxicity due to bismuth is usually the result of the chronic ingestion of bismuth subgallate used in regulating colostomies (Burns et al., 1974); chronic ingestion of bismuth subnitrate, which is used in some constipation preparations (Loiseau et al., 1976); and from the chronic use of bismuth-containing skin lightening creams (Kruger and Thomas, 1976). The condition is characterized by irritability, antisocial behavior, organic brain syndrome (which may include hallucinations and delusions), intention tremor, ataxia, incoordination, myoclonic jerks, ataxia, astaxia-abasia, headaches, and seizures. The signs and symptoms may wax and wane. Diagnosis depends upon a careful medication history and the demonstration of bismuth in blood or urine. Removal from bismuth usually results in improvement, but death due to this toxicity has occurred.

Aluminum

Toxicity due to this metal has been implicated in dialysis dementia (Scheiber and Zeistat, 1976; Dunea et al., 1978; Elliott et al., 1978), in Alzheimer's disease (Duckett, 1976 and Crapper et al., 1975), and in a case of pulmonary fibrosis and encephalitis in an aluminum powder factory worker (McLaughlin et al, 1962). Whether or not the increased levels of aluminum in brain tissue of Alzheimer patients reported by Crapper et al. (1975) are of etiologic or pathogenetic significance, is at present a debatable issue, since McDermott et al. (1977) found no difference in aluminum levels of brain tissue between Alzheimer patients and age-matched controls. In dialysis dementia, however, the relationship appears more clear-cut. Dunea et al. (1978) reported an outbreak of the syndrome in dialysis patients (20 cases) between 1972 and 1976; in 1972, aluminum salts were substituted for a mixture of aluminum sulfate and ferrous sulfate for water clarification in the area studied. Elliott et al. (1978) found all cases of dialysis dementia in the west of Scotland to be restricted to areas where aluminum sulfate is added to the water. Also 8 of the 13 patients studied had markedly increased serum aluminum concentrations. The syndrome is characterized by insidious onset of behavioral alterations, organic brain syndrome, speech disturbance, myoclonus, and seizures. A majority of the patients in the report of Dunea et al. (1978) presented with dementia or behavioral disturbances, or both. All of the patients had frontal release signs as well (grasp, snout, and sucking reflexes). Untreated, the disease results in coma and death in virtually all patients. Diagnosis depends upon a high index of suspicion, knowledge of local water aluminum content, and demonstration of elevated serum aluminum levels. Treatment consists of passage of the water for dialysis through a deionizer.

Lithium

This metal is one of the more recent additions in the long list of metals used throughout medical history in the treatment of diverse illnesses. There seems to be little question that lithium is effective in the treatment of the acute manic state, in the prevention of future esisodes in bipolar affective disorder, and questionably for prophylaxis of unipolar affective disorder. The neuromuscular, gastrointestinal, renal, cardiovascular, endocrine, cutaneous, and hematological side effects and toxic signs have been well documented, and the reader is referred to several excellent sources for discussion of this information (Valcaflor, 1976; Davis, 1976; Baldessarini and Lipinski, 1975). Some less commonly appreciated side effects are worth noting, however. Some patients may develop an organic brain syndrome on lithium (Davis, 1976). This may be a difficult problem for the patient and his family to differentiate from mild symptoms of the basic illness, which they might otherwise not report to the doctor. This author has found elderly patients and patients with compensated organic brain syndrome to be particularly susceptible to this side effect and, in these types of patients, organic brain syndrome can occur at "normal" serum levels (0.8 to 1.2 mEq per liter). A small percentage of patients on lithium therapy may develop clinical hypothyroidism. This, again, is easily confused by patient and family with depression. Finally, this author has noted that some patients experience a "cognitive dulling" on the drug. From detailed conversations with more reliable patients, this does not appear to represent a mere desire to return to the euphoric state but, rather, is a genuine complaint. The physician must maintain a good relationship with patient and family, and consistent followup with the patient in order to catch these deceptive signs of lithium toxicity early. If toxic levels of lithium are present, the dose should be appropriately altered. In the elderly patient, or the patient with previously compensated organic brain syndrome, maintenance can be effectively achieved at serum levels below those usually considered adequate (as low as 0.4 mEq per liter). The thyroid deficient patient may require replacement. The patient who complains of mental dulling can often be effectively maintained at slightly lower serum levels with alleviation of this side effect, keeping the caveat firmly in mind that this kind of patient must be followed even more closely than others.

CONCLUSION

It is readily apparent that metals have not been innocent bystanders in the production of human illness, whether psychiatric or otherwise. With future research and clinical reporting in this area, a number of probable results come to mind. The essential metals will not change in the next millenium; however, our knowledge of them will. Barring a global accident resulting in mass amnesia (or worse), this change will be an increase in knowledge with consequent discovery of effective treatment for disorders previously not understood. Nonessential metals will continue to be mined, processed, used in manufacture of other products, and used as a part or total of a final product. As has been true in the past, when a metal is found to be highly toxic, its use will be limited (by the relatively slow legislative process). Industry, being as dependable as it is, will find new uses for others, some of which will be toxic. Besides research and environmental consciousness, the most effective process for quickly discovering these offenders is the acumen of the clinical diagnostician. This, combined with accurate reporting, will set the stage for the environmentalist and legislator.

REFERENCES

Abd El Naby, S., and Hassanein, M. Neuropsychiatric manifestations of chronic manganese poisoning. *J. Neurol. Neurosurg. Psychiat.* 28:282–288 (1965).

Baldessarini, R. J., and Lipinski, J. F. Lithium salts: 1970–1975. *Ann. Intern. Med.* 83:527–533 (1975).

Banks, W. J., Pleasure, D. E., Suzuki, K., Negio, M., and Katz, R. Thallium poisoning. *Arch. Neurol.* 26:456–564 (1972).

Banta, R. G., and Markesberry, W. R. Elevated manganese levels associated with dementia and extrapyramidal signs. *Neurol.* 27:3:213–216 (1977).

Bryce-Smith, D. Behavioral effects of lead and other heavy metal pollutants. *Chem. Br.* 8:240–243 (1972).

Burns, R., Thomas, D. W., and Barron, V. J. Reversible encephalopathy possibly associated with bismuth subgallate ingestion. *Brit. Med. J.* 1:220 (1974).

Caldwell, D. F., Oberleas, D., and Prasad, A. S. Psychobiological changes in zinc deficiency, in *Trace Elements in Human Health and Disease, 1* A. S. Prasad and D. Oberleas, eds. Academic Press, New York and London, England (1976), pp. 311–325.

Casper, R. C., Kirscher, B., and Jacob, R. A. Zinc and copper status in anorexia nervosa. *Psychopharm. Bull.* 14:3:53–55 (1978).

Chisolm, J. J., Jr. The susceptibility of the fetus and child to chemical pollutants. Heavy metal exposures: Toxicity from metal-metal interactions, and behavioral effects. *Pediat.* 53:5:841–843 (1974).

Cook, D. G., Fahn, S., and Bratt, K. A. Chronic manganese intoxication. *Arch. Neurol.* 30:1:52–58 (1974).

Crapper, D. R., Krishnan, S. S., De Boni, U., and Tomko, G. J. Aluminum: A possible agent in Alzheimer's disease. *Trans. Am. Neurol. Assn.* 100:154–156 (1975).

Danks, D. M., Campbell, P. E., Walker-Smith, J., Stevens, B. J., Gillespie, J. M., Blomfield, J., and Turner, B. Menkes' Kinky-Hair Syndrome. *Lancet.* 1:1100–1102 (1972).

David, O. J., Clark, J., and Voeller, K. Lead and hyperactivity. *Lancet.* 11:7783:900–903 (1972).

David, O. J., Hoffman, S., McGann, B., Sverd, J., and Clark, J. Low lead levels and mental retardation. *Lancet.* 11:8000:1376–1379 (1976).

Davies, I.J.T. *The Clinical significance of the Essential Biological Metals.* William Hunemen Medical Books Ltd., London, England (1972), pp. 105–119.

Davis, J. M. Overview: Maintenance therapy in psychiatry: II. Affective disorders. *Am. J. Psychiat.* 133:1:1–13 (1976).

Dekaban, A. S., and Steusing, J. K. Menkes' Kinky-Hair disease treated with subcutaneous copper sulfate (Letter). *Lancet.* 1:7918:1236 (1975).

de la Burde, B., and Choate, M. L. Early asymptomatic lead exposure and development at school age. *J. Pediat.* 87:4:638–642 (1975).

Duckett, S. Aluminum and Alzheimer's disease (Letter). *Arch. Neurol.* 33:10:730–731 (1976).

Dudrick, S. J. Personal communication (1978).

Dunea, G., Mahurkas, S. D., Mamdoni, B., and Smith, E. C. Role of aluminum in dialysis dementia. *Ann. Intern. Med.* 88:4:502–504 (1978).

Elliott, H. L., Dryburgh, F., Fell, G. S., Sabet, S., and Macdougall, A. I. Aluminum toxicity during regular haemodialysis. *Brit. Med. J.* 1:6120:101–103 (1978).

Estep, H., Shaw, W. A., Watlington, C., Jobe, R., Holland, W., and Tucker, St. G. Hypocalcemia due to hypomagnesemia and reversible parathyroid hormone unresponsiveness. *J. Clin. Endocrinol.* 29:842 (1969).

Faillace, L. A. Personal communication. (1978).

Fishman, R. A. Neurological aspects of magnesium metabolism. *Arch. Neurol.* 12:562–569 (1965).

Flink, E. B. Role of magnesium deficiency in Wernicke-Kossakoff syndrome (Letter). *N. Eng. J. Med.* 298:13:743–744 (1978).

Flink, E. B. Therapy of mangesium deficiency. *Ann. N. Y. Acad. Sci.* 162:901–905 (1969).

Flink, E. B., Stutzman, F. L., Anderson, A. R., Konig, T., and Fraser, R. Magnesium deficiency after prolonged parenteral fluid administration and after chronic alcoholism complicated by delerium tremens. *J. Lab. Clin. Med.* 43:2:169–183 (1954).

Gatewood, J. W., Organ, C. H., Jr., and Mead, B. T. Mental changes associated with hyperparathyroidism. *Am. J. Psychiat.* 132:2:129–132 (1975).

Gestner, H. B., and Huff, J. E. Clinical toxicology of mercury. *J. Toxic. Environ. Health* 2:3:491–526 (1977).

Graham, A. C., and Cordano, A. Copper deficiency in human subjects, in *Trace Elements in Human Health and Disease, I.* A. S. Prasad and D. Oberleas, eds. Academic Press, New York and London, England (1976), pp. 363–371.

Greenfeld, O., and Hinostroza, G. Thallium poisoning. *Arch. Int. Med.* 114:132–138 (1964).

Greiner, A. C., Chan, S. C., and Nicolson, G. A. Human brain concentrations of calcium, copper, magnesium, and zinc in some neurological pathologies. *Clin. Chim. Acta.* 64:2:211–213 (1975).

Hall, R.C.W., and Joffe, J. R. Hypomagnesemia: Physical and psychiatric symptoms. *J.A.M.A.* 224:13:1749–1751 (1973).

Hambridge, K. M., and Walravens, P. A. Zinc deficiency in infants and preadolescent children, in *Trace Elements in Human Health and Disease, I.* A. S. Prasad and D. Oberleas, eds. Academic Press, New York and London, England (1976), pp. 21–31.

Harrison's Principles of Internal Medicine, 6th ed. 659 McGraw-Hill Book Co. (1970).

Hartoma, T. R., Sotaniemi, E. A., Pelkonen, O., Ahlquist, J. Serum zinc and serum copper and indices of drug metabolism in alcoholics. *Eur. J. Phar.* 12:2:147–151 (1977).

Jacobs, A. The non-hemotological effects of iron deficiency. *Clin. Sci. Mol. Med.* 53:2:105–109 (1977).

Kamerbeek, H. H., Rauws, A. G., ten Ham, M., and van Heijst, A.N.P. Prussian Blue in therapy of thallotoxicosis: An experimental and clinical investigation. *ACTA. Med. Scand.* 189:321–324 (1971).

Kirscher, K. N. Copper and zinc in childhood behavior. *Psychopharm. Bull.* 14:3:58–59 (1978).

Klopper, A., and Weiler, G. –(On heavy-metal poisoning especially by thallium (author's translation)) *Deutsch Med. Wochenschr.* 103:2:75–76 (1978).

Kruger, G., and Thomas, D. J. Disturbed oxidative metabolism in organic brain syndrome caused by bismuth in skin creams. *Lancet.* 1:7984:485–487 (1976).

Landujan, P. J., Whiteworth, R. H., Balsh, R. W., Stachling, N. W., Barthel, W. E., and Rosenblum, B. F. Neuropsychological dysfunction in children with chronic low level lead absorption. *Lancet.* 1:7909:708–712 (1975).

Leibel, R. L. Behavioral and biochemical correlates of iron deficiency. *J. Am. Diet. Assn.* 71:4:398–404 (1977).

Loiseau, P., Henry, P., Jallon, P., and Legrouk, M. Iatrogenic myoclonic encephalopathies caused by bismuth salts. *J. Neurol. Sci.* 27:2:133–143 (1976).

Lombeck, I., Ritzl, F., Schnippering, H. G., Michael, H., and Bremer, H. J. Primary hypomagnesemia. *Z. Kinderheilk* 118:249 (1975a).

Lombeck, I., Schnippering, H. G., Ritzl, F., Feinendegen, L. E., and Bremer, H. J. Absorption of zinc in aerodermatitis enteropathica (Letter). *Lancet.* 1:7911:855 (1975b).

McDermott, J. R., Smith, A. I., Igbal, K., and Wisniewski, H. M. *Lancet.* 2:8040:710–711 (1977).

McLaughlin, A.I.G., Kajantzis, G., King, E., Teare, D., Porter, R. J., and Owen, R. Pulmonary fibrosis and encephalopathy associated with the inhalation of aluminum dust. *Brit. J. Indust. Med.* 19:253:–263 (1962).

Medalle, R., Waterhouse, C., and Hahn, T. J. Vitamin D resistance in magnesium deficiency. *Am. J. Clin. Nut.* 29:8:854–858 (1976).

Mena, I. The role of manganese in human disease. *Ann. Clin. Lab. Sci.* 4:6:487–491 (1974).

Menkes, J. H., Alter, M., Steigleder, G. K., Weakley, D. R., and Jvo Ho Sung. A sex-linked recessive disorder with retardation of growth, peculiar hair, and focal ceberal and cerebellar degeneration. *Pediat.* 29:764–779 (1962).

Moore, M. R., Meredith, P. A., and Goldberg, A. A retrospective analysis of blood-lead in mentally retarded children. *Lancet.* 1:8014:717–719 (1977).

Moynahan, E. J. Zinc deficiency and disturbances of mood and visual behavior (Letter). *Lancet.* 1:7950:91 (1976).

Munch, J. C. Human thalloxtoxicosis. *J.A.M.A.* 102:23:1929–1934 (1934).

Nordio, S., Donath, A., Macagno, F., and Gattis, R. Chronic hypomagnesemia with mangesium-dependent hypocalcemia. I. A. new syndrome with intestinal magnesium malabsorption. *ACTA Paediat. Scand.* 60:441 (1971).

O'Dell, B. L. Biochemistry and physiology of copper in vertebrates, in *Trace Elements in Human Health and Disease, I.* A. S. Prasad and D. Oberleas, eds. Academic Press, New York and London, England (1976), pp. 391–410.

Oleske, J. M., Caleb, M. H., and Starr, S. E. Acrodermatitis enteropathica, immunodeficiency, and zinc. *Cutis.* 21:3:297–298 (1978).

Olholm-Larsen, P. Untreated acrodermatitis enteropathica in adults. *Dermatologica.* 156:3:155–166 (1978).

Oski, F. A., and Honig, A. S. The effects of therapy on the developmental scores of iron-deficient infants. *J. Pediat.* 92:1:21–25 (1978).

Paterson, C. R. Hypocalcemia: Differential diagnosis and investigation. *Ann. Clin. Biochem.* 13:6:578–584 (1976).

eterson, P. Psychiatric disorders in primary hyperparathyroidism *J. Clin. Endocrinol.* 28:1491–1495 (1968).

Pfeiffer, C. C., and Iliev, V. A study of zinc deficiency and copper excess in the schizophrenics. *Int. Rev. Neurobiol* (Supp.) I (1972).

Pihl, R. O., and Parkes, M. Hair element content in learning disabled children. *Sci.* 198:4313:204–206 (1977).

Prasad, A. S. Deficiency of zinc in man and its toxicity, in *Trace Elements in Human Health and Disease, I.* A. S. Prasad and D. Oberleas, eds. Academic Press, New York and London, England (1976) pp. 1–17.

Rahman, B., Rahman, M. A., and Hassan, Z. Copper and ceruloplasmin in schizophrenia. *Biochem. Soc. Trans.* 4:6:1138–1139 (1976).

Reed, D., Crawley, J., Faro, S. N., Pieper, S. J., and Keerland, L. T. Thallotoxicosis: Acute manifestations and sequelae. *J.A.M.A.* 183:516–522 (1963).

Rosenstock, H. A., Simons, D. G., and Meyer, J. S. Chronic manganism: Neurologic and laboratory studies during treatment with levodopa. *J.A.M.A.* 217:1354–1358 (1971).

Sanstead, H. H. Some trace elements which are essential for human nutrition: Zinc, copper, maganese, and chromium. *Prog. Food Nut. Sci.* 1:6:371–391 (1975).

Sandstead, H. H., Vo-Khactu, K. P., and Solomons, N. Conditioned zinc deficiencies, in *Trace Elements in Human Health and Disease, I.* A. S. Prasad and D. Oberleas, eds. Academic Press, New York and London, England (1976), pp. 33–34.

Scheiber, S. C., and Zeistat, H. Jr. Dementia dialytica: A new psychotic organic brain syndrome. *Comp. Psychiat.* 17:6:781–785 (1976).

Scheinberg, I. H. A psychogenetic anecdote. *Psychosom. Med.* 37:4:368–371 (1975).

Scheinberg, I. H., and Sternlieb, I. Copper toxicity and Wilson's Disease, in *Trace Elements in Human Health and Disease, I.* A. S. Prasad and D. Oberleas, eds. Academic Press, New York and London, England (1976), pp. 415–431.

Shils, M. E. Magnesium deficiency and calcium and parathyroid hormone interrelations, in *Trace Elements in Human Health and Disease, II.* A. S. Prasad and D. Oberleas, eds. Academic Press, New York and London, England (1976), pp. 23–43.

Silbergeld, E. K., and Goldberg, A. M. Lead-induced behavioral dysfunction; An animal model of hyperactivity. *Exp. Neurol.* 42:146–157 (1974).

Silbergeld, E. K., and Goldberg, A. M. A lead-induced behavioral disorder. *Life Sci.* 13:1275–1283 (1973).

Smith, J. C., Jr., Brown, E. D., White, S. C., and Finklestein, J. D. Plasma vitamin A and zinc concentrations in patients with alcoholic cirrhosis (Letter). *Lancet.* 1:7918:1251–1252 (1975).

Solomons, N. W., Layden, T. J., Rosenberg, T. H., Vo-Khactu, K., and Sandstead, H. H. Plasma trace metals during total parenteral alimentation. *Gastroenterol.* 70:6:1022–1025 (1976).

Stendig-Lindberg, G. Hypomagnesemia in alcohol encephalopathies. *ACTA Psychiat. Scand. 50:465*–480 (1974).

Tarjan, R., and Morava, E. Nutritional importance of some trace elements and early signs of their deficiency. *Biblio. Nut. Dieta.,* No. 23, pp. 137–144, Karger, Baul (1976).

Tuman, R. W., and Doisy, R. J. The role of trace elements in human nutrition and metabolism, in *Physiological Effects of Food Carbohydrates*. A. Jeanes and J. Hodge, eds. Amer. Chem. Soc., Washington, D. C. (1975), pp. 156–177.

Valcaflor, L. Lithium side effects and toxicity: The clinical picture, in *Lithium Research and Therapy*. F. N. Johnson, ed. Academic Press, New York and London, England (1976), pp. 211–223.

Walker, S. III. They psychiatric presentation of Wilson's Disease (Hepatolenticular Degeneration) with an etiologic explanation. *Behav. Neuropsychiat.* 1:38–43 (1969).

Walshe, J. M. Missed Wilson's disease (Letter). *Lancet.* 2:7931:405 (1975).

Wilson, S.A.K. Progressive lenticular degeneration: A familial nervous disease associated with cirrhosis of the liver. *Brain.* 34:295 (1911–1912).

Zieve, L., Doizaki, W. M., and Stenroos, L. E. Effect of magnesium deficiency on blood and liver transketolase activity and on the recovery of enzyme activity in thiamine-deficient rats receiving thiamine. *J. Lab. Clin. Med.* 72:2:261–267 (1968).

Zieve, L., Doizaki, W. M., and Stenroos, L. E. Effect of magnesium deficiency on growth response to thiamine of thiamine-deficient rats. *J. Lab. Clin. Med.* 72:2:261–267 (1968).

Section IV
PHARMACOLOGICALLY RELATED PSYCHIATRIC DISORDERS

Psychiatric Presentations of Medical Illness

CHAPTER 18

Behavioral Toxicity of Psychiatric Drugs

MARK PERL, M.B.B.S.
RICHARD C. W. HALL, M.D.
EARL R. GARDNER, Ph.D.

Psychotropic drugs are prescribed for the express purpose of altering one or more components of the patient's mood, cognition, or gross behavior, which have become disturbed. Clinicians generally delineate a specific pharmacological action of a drug as its main therapeutic effect and regard other actions as side effects. While this determination may not always be as precise in psychiatry as in internal medicine, given the complexities of human behavior and of the target symptoms, one can usually designate specific drug actions as clinically beneficial and useful.

Modern psychotropic drugs are efficacious and valuable; nevertheless, their effects are not always those that were therapeutically desired. The patient may show adverse behavioral effects: " . . . a disruption of, or disturbance in, his behavior and emotions in areas where none had been present, or . . . an exacerbation of his present symptoms" (Shader and DiMascio, 1970: p. 37). His/her normal functioning may be interfered with by " . . . alterations in perceptual and cognitive functions, psychomotor performance, motivation, mood, interpersonal relationships, or intrapsychic processes . . . ." (Shader and DiMascio, 1970: p. 27).

Hollister (1972) and Caldwell (1976) have discussed the mechanisms by which psychotherapeutic drugs can exert adverse effects. These include:

1. Extension of the primary therapeutic action of the drug (e.g., oversedation with benzodiazepines; hypomanic response to antidepressant medications).

2. Undesired secondary pharmacologic actions of the drug (e.g., central anticholinergic effects of tricyclic antidepressants; extrapyramidal effects of phenothiazines).
3. Tolerance, dependence, and withdrawal effects (e.g., to benzodiazepines, barbiturates).
4. Drug interactions (e.g., alcohol potentiation of the psychomotor effects of many drugs).
5. Idiosyncratic "paradoxical" responses.
6. Simple toxicity, either through excessive self-administration (abuse of drug, suicidal overdose), or through an altered response to normal doses of the drug.

Relevant factors affecting a patient's response to a psychotropic drug include:

1. The dose of medication, the frequency of its administration, and the blood levels achieved in a particular patient. (These can now be determined for many drugs.) Obviously, toxic effects will be closely related to these variables.
2. Duration of administration of the drug; this is especially relevant to dependence and withdrawal effects.
3. The patient's age: Adverse reactions occur more often in the elderly and in children.
4. Intercurrent illness affecting the patient's metabolic state, and hepatic and renal functions; and consequently, the distribution, metabolism, and excretion of a drug.
5. Predisposing personality factors in the patient that might favor the emergence of particular untoward behavioral effects (Hollister, 1967.)

The following account describes adverse behavioral effects of the major classes of psychotropic drugs in clinical use today. Useful reference sources are: Shader and DiMascio (1970), Caldwell (1976), *Psychiatric Annals* (1975), Meyler and Herxheimer (1972), and Dukes (1975, 1977, 1978). A summary of the main effects appears in Table 8 at the end of the text.

ANTIPSYCHOTIC DRUGS

This group of drugs includes the phenothiazines, thioxanthenes, butyrophenones, and the newer dihydroindolones and dibenzoxazepines. (See Table 1 for a list of antipsychotic drugs currently in use in the USA and their roughly equivalent milligram potencies.) The major indication for these agents is schizophrenia. They are also very useful in the acute phase of mania and in some psychotic depressions; certain organic confusional states and other disorders respond to low doses of these medications.

TABLE 1. ANTIPSYCHOTIC MEDICATIONS

	APPROXIMATE EQUIVALENT ORAL DOSE (mg)
PHENOTHIAZINES	
Aliphatic	
Chlorpromazine (Thorazine)	100
Triflupromazine (Vesprin)	30
Piperidines	
Mesoridazine (Serentil)	50
Piperacetazine (Quide)	12
Thioridazine (Mellaril)	100
Piperazines	
Acetophenazine (Tindal)	20
Butaperazine (Repoise)	12
Carphenazine (Proketazine)	25
Fluphenazine (Prolixin)	2
Perphenazine (Trilafon)	10
Trifluperazine (Stelazine)	5
Thioxanthenes	
Aliphatic	
Chlorprothixene (Taractan)	65
Piperazine	
Thiothixene (Navane)	5
Dibenzoxazepines	
Loxapine (Loxitane)	15
BUTYROPHENONES	
Haloperidol (Haldol)	4
INDOLONES	
Molindone (Moban)	10

Adverse behavioral effects arise by most of the mechanisms outlined above. The central anticholinergic and extrapyramidal antidopaminergic properties of these agents are well known; tolerance to many of the resultant side effects develops within several weeks, but management in the acute phase requires close attention.

Oversedation is very common. Patients appear somnolent, lethargic, retarded, and depressed. Many complain of feeling heavy, sluggish, or weak. The "zombie"-like look of such patients is familiar to most people who have worked on inpatient wards; drug-induced Parkinsonian gait and facial expression may compound this picture.

Overmedication is the commonest cause of somnolence, and often the best remedy is simply to reduce the dose of the drug. Some antipsychotics are more sedating than others (see Table 2), the lower potency agents being the more sedating. Thus, the physician may choose to maintain antipsychotic effectiveness by switching to the equivalent dose of a less sedating drug. It has been observed, however, that even the "alerting" antipsychotics, for example, haloperidol (Murray et al., 1977), can lead to oversedation. The term "alerting" is therefore misleading, since all of these agents have a central nervous system (CNS) depressant effect.

TABLE 2. SEDATIVE PROPERTIES OF ANTIPSYCHOTIC AGENTS*

HEAVILY SEDATING
Chlorpromazine
Triflupromazine
Chlorprothixene
MODERATELY SEDATING
Thioridazine
Mesoridazine
Piperacetazine
SOME SEDATIVE PROPERTIES
Loxapine
LESS SEDATING
Trifluperazine
Perphenazine
Fluphenazine
Acetophenazine
Butaperazine
Carphenazine
Thiothixene
Haloperidol
Molindone

*Based on Shader and Jackson, (1975).

Emotional *depression* occurs in a variety of ways. Pre-existing primary endogenous depression may be worsened by the sedating antipsychotic compounds. Moreover, some schizophrenic patients will exhibit depression, either during the acute phase or in the recovery period ("postpsychotic depression"); this too can be exacerbated by many antipsychotics, particularly the aliphatics and other sedating compounds. The use of less sedating antipsychotics, with the judicious addition of a tricyclic antidepressant to the drug regimen, is the optimal management of these cases. Such combinations—for example, the perphenazine-amitriptyline preparations (Triavil, Etrafon)—may also be of value in primary, agitated, or psychotic depressions. Recent work suggests that akinesia, too, may present as depression, but patients with such manifestations should be managed somewhat differently. It has also been suggested, though not fully proven, that depression is a direct side effect of antipsychotic medications (Alarcon and Carney, 1969). In one study, 15 percent of patients developed severe depression while taking haloperidol or fluphenazine (Johnson, 1973). Depression can also be the result of overzealous "tranquilization" of acutely manic or hypomanic patients, causing a "switch" to the depressed phase. The patient's mood and mental state require daily monitoring, and the dose of medicine should be altered to match the clinical situation.

Four distinct extrapyramidal movement disorders are encountered with antipsychotic drugs: Parkinsonism, acute dystonia, akathisia, and tardive dyskinesia. Several of these may present as behavioral aberrations and may prompt the practitioner to increase the dose of medicine, thus inadvertently worsening the disorder. *Acute dystonia* occurs early in treatment, and is frequently seen with the more potent agents, such as haloperidol and the piperazine phenothiazines. Patients present dramatically with tonic contractions of the neck, mouth, pharynx, and muscles of the axial spine, and with oculogyric crisis. The syndrome is often misdiagnosed as hysteria, tetany, or even epilepsy. Dystonia may produce bizarre and unusual behavioral effects, e.g., contraction of one eyelid, opisthotonos ("arc de circle"). A trial of a specific anti-Parkinsonian medication is always indicated in such patients who are taking antipsychotics. Rapid relief is achieved with parenteral anti-Parkinsonian agents, (e.g., benztropine mesylate 2 mg intravenously (IV); diphenhydramine 25 to 50 mg intramuscularly (IM), or 25 mg IV). Follow-up oral anti-Parkinsonian therapy for several days may be indicated, e.g., benztropine mesylate 2 mg orally (p.o.), three times daily (TID).

Akathisia is a continuous motor restlessness, in which the patient fidgets; paces; cannot stand, sit still, or even lie in bed; and complains of "restless legs." Older patients are especially susceptible to this syndrome, which may come on several weeks after commencing treatment. In many patients, the akathisia is mild, so that the patient reports increased restless feelings, without necessarily becoming motorically more active. Obviously, this must be distinguished from true anxiety, stemming from an exacerbation of the psychotic process. The physician must entertain the diagnosis of akathisia in such "anxious" patients, and a trial of anti-Parkinsonian agents may be warranted. Most antipsychotic agents have been shown to cause akathisia, but haloperidol and the piperazine phenothiazines are again the worst offenders. In separate studies, 23 and 38 percent of patients on depot fluphenazine preparations developed akathisia (Johnson, 1973; Christodoulidis and Frangos, 1975). Recently, alcohol consumption has been reported to precipitate akathisia and dystonia in medicated patients (Lutz, 1976).

Treatment is to lower the dose of the antipsychotic. Anti-Parkinsonian agents and muscle relaxants, such as diazepam, may also be helpful. Other agents have been used in the management—citrated caffeine, caffeine sodium benzoate, calcium, paraldehyde—but these are not the treatments of choice.

Rifkin et al. (1977) have drawn attention to the prevalence of drug-induced Parkinsonian *akinesia*, claiming it is under-recognized; it was observed in 35 percent of depot fluphenazine patients in the study. High dose fluphenazine and haloperidol are the most likely causal agents, although others have been implicated. Patients are mute, immobile, and show reduced spontaneity and loss of interest in former activities. They may resemble depressed, withdrawn, or even catatonic patients (Behrman, 1972; Williams, 1972; Van Putten and May, 1978). Amytal interview is not helpful in distinguishing the syndrome from catatonia. Withdrawal of antipsychotic drugs and/or the addition of anti-Parkinsonian agents will relieve the syndrome.

Several of these drugs give rise to the *central anticholinergic toxic psychosis*, which will be discussed below. Table 3 lists some of the drugs and their relative anticholinergic activity.

TABLE 3. ANTIPSYCHOTIC DRUGS LISTED IN DECREASING ORDER OF ANTICHOLINERGIC EFFECT*

Strongly Anticholinergic	Clozapine (unavailable in USA)
	Thioridazine
Moderately Anticholinergic	Chlorpromazine
	Triflupromazine
Weakly Anticholinergic	Acetophenazine
	Perphenazine
	Fluphenazine
	Trifluoperazine
	Haloperidol

*Based on Snyder and Yamamura (1977).

Paradoxical reactions to antipsychotics may be observed, though infrequently. Increased anxiety, psychomotor agitation, or worsening of the psychotic manifestations may occur, especially with doses above 1500 mg/day of chlorpromazine, or the equivalent. These symptoms are relieved by lowering the drug dosage. The earlier reports may have included cases of the syndromes already discussed, but there does seem to be a small group of patients who exhibit a true idiosyncratic response (Angus et al., 1967; Chaffin, 1964). Personality factors may play a part in these responses (Heninger et al., 1965).

Withdrawal effects occur quite commonly, especially with abrupt cessation of medication (Gardos et al., 1978; Hall et al., 1978). Symptoms are nausea, vomiting, perspiration, restlessness, insomnia, and giddiness. They are usually mild, but are occasionally severe enough to require temporary antihistamine treatment. Gardos et al. (1978) have also reviewed the withdrawal dyskinetic syndromes, which resemble tardive dyskinesia.

Commonly, there is minimal impairment of hand-eye coordination and other laboratory tests of *psychomotor function* with the antipsychotic drugs (Penttila et al., 1975). These psychomotor effects are potentiated by alcohol, and are more likely to be found in chronic schizophrenics and in normals than in acutely psychotic individuals. Ballinger and Ramsay (1975) have implicated these agents in inpatient accidents in a psychiatric hospital. Patients are usually advised against driving, although Shader and DiMascio (1970) noted a paucity of hard data implicating these drugs in vehicle accidents "in vivo."

Hartmann and Spinweber (1976) have reviewed the literature on the effects of psychotropic medications on *sleep*, and conclude that antipsychotics slightly increase the duration of total sleep, without significantly altering the overall structure of sleep patterns; specifically, D-time (REM sleep) and delta-wave sleep are not greatly affected. Nighttime administration of the majority of the patient's dose of a sedating antipsychotic may be helpful if insomnia is a part of the symptom-complex, as is often the case in acute psychosis.

BENZODIAZEPINES AND OTHER SEDATIVE HYPNOTICS

The anti-anxiety agents in clinical use today are shown in Table 4 with their roughly equivalent daily dose ranges. The benzodiazepines are the most widely

TABLE 4. ANTI-ANXIETY (SEDATIVE-HYPNOTIC) DRUGS AND USUAL DAILY DOSE RANGES (AS IN TABLE 1)

BENZODIAZEPINES	
Chlordiazepoxide (Librium)	15 - 100
Chlorazepate (Tranxene)	15 - 60
Diazepam (Valium)	6 - 40
Oxazepam (Serax)	30 - 120
Lorazepam (Ativan)	2 - 10
Flurazepam (Dalmane)	15 - 30 (at h.s.)
ANTIHISTAMINES	
Hydroxyzine (Atarax) (Vistaril)	30 - 200
PROPANEDIOLS	
Tybamate (Solacen)	900 - 2100
Meprobamate (Equanil)	1200 - 2400

prescribed drugs in the USA and are among the safest. Their therapeutic index is high; and considering their widespread use, both for anticipatory anxiety and as hypnotics, the incidence of serious side effects is relatively low. Nevertheless, the physician should always consider the possibility of an adverse behavioral response, especially at higher dose levels.

Oversedation is a common complaint with all the anti-anxiety agents, and is dose-related. Patients on moderate to high daytime doses may be drowsy and exhibit ataxia on occasions. Other psychomotor effects may be evident (see below), and this syndrome is potentiated by alcohol. All the benzodiazepines cause somnolence, including the newer agent lorazepam (Gale and Galloon, 1976). Tolerance will eventually develop; but clearly, reduction of the dose will obviate the problem of oversedation simply and rapidly.

The benzodiazepines often *impair psychomotor skills* as measured in laboratory tests of reaction time, hand-eye coordination, and steadiness, and in simulated driving tests (Betts et al., 1972). These effects are compounded by alcohol, as was noted for the antipsychotic agents (Hollister, 1974). Lorazepam has similar effects. Although, as noted above, Shader and DiMascio (1970) question the validity of automatically extrapolating data from the laboratory to real driving situations, some data do show an increased correlation between road accidents and benzodiazepine ingestion (Murray, 1962).

Mild *impairment of alertness and concentration*, as measured by various tests of cognitive function (Kleinknecht and Donaldson, 1975), is common with these drugs and is a dose-related phenomenon. Minimal EEG changes may occur. These findings probably have little clinical significance.

The following *paradoxical reactions* to benzodiazepines are being increasingly recognized. As Hall and Kirkpatrick (1978) point out, their incidence is small, but not insignificant, considering the number of people taking these drugs:

1. A *disinhibition syndrome*, analogous to alcoholic disinhibition, is perhaps the most commonly encountered type of paradoxical reaction. Patients are motorically hyperactive, garrulous, and may either be euphoric, anxious; or more dramatically, they may exhibit hostility, "hatred," anger outbursts, and rage. Personality factors play a significant role in generating this response: With the depression of cortical control, previously learned impulsive or explosive behavior patterns can no longer be held in check (McDonald, 1967). Chlordiazepoxide and diazepam are more likely to produce this syndrome than oxazepam (Gardos et al., 1968; Greenblatt and Shader, 1974). Shader and DiMascio (1970) believe such responses to be quite common, and suggest that they be expected in patients with a history of poor impulse control.
2. *Severe depression with suicidal ideation* of sudden onset may occur in patients taking diazepam in doses greater than 30 mg daily for 1 week or more (Ryan et al., 1968; Hall and Joffe, 1972). Patients are apprehensive,

tremulous, and depressed, and experience the intrusion of ego-alien suicidal ideas. Symptoms disappear within a few days of ceasing the medication. Renal impairment may be a causal factor in some of these patients (Hall, 1978).

3. *Depersonalization or frank psychosis* occur rarely (Ayd, 1962; Viscott, 1968). Paranoid states, Korsakoff's syndrome, confusional states, feelings of intoxication and depersonalization, vivid bizarre dreams and nightmares, and toxic psychosis with vivid hallucinations have all been reported with chlordiazepoxide. Similar effects are cited for diazepam as well as meprobamate (Shader and DiMascio, 1970), and more recently, for lorazepam (Blitt and Petty, 1975). In Blitt and Petty's (1975) patients, physostigmine successfully reversed the psychotic symptoms, and this raises the interesting possibility of an anticholinergic mechanism for the syndrome.

It should be noted that *confusional states in elderly patients* taking anti-anxiety agents are not at all uncommon and deserve separate emphasis. They resemble the intoxications that were frequently seen with the barbiturates. Prominent symptoms are disorientation, oversedation, cognitive impairment, and agitation (Learoyd, 1972). Mild organic brain disease may be worsened by the administration of these agents to the elderly, and if this is not recognized, unnecessary—and sometimes dangerous—medical workup may be undertaken. Cessation of medication is the only treatment.

Withdrawal effects occur after prolonged intake of moderate to high doses of the benzodiazepines. Mild withdrawal effects are fairly common. Characteristic signs and symptoms are cramps, sweats, tremor, insomnia, anxiety, and depression (Hanna, 1972; Covi et al., 1973; Pevnick et al., 1978). Paulshock (1976) points out that some "withdrawal" symptoms may simply be a recurrence of the anxiety for which the drug was prescribed, but most authors describe withdrawal anxiety as all-pervasive and qualitatively different from the previous state. A more ominous, but fortunately rarer syndrome, has been reported; the cardinal features are delirium, with formication and visual hallucinations, and seizures (Preskorn and Denner, 1977). In some patients, convulsions and status epilepticus may occur, as with barbiturate withdrawal (Hall and Kirkpatrick, 1978). Meprobamate is more habituating than the benzodiazepines; hydroxyzine and tybamate are less so. Management of addiction is by slow rather than abrupt withdrawal.

The effects on *sleep* of all the benzodiazepines are similar, although certain agents (flurazepam, nitrazepam, flunitrazepam) have a more pronounced and prolonged hypnotic effect and are primarily used for this purpose. (Only flurazepam is currently in use in the USA). In addition to increasing the length of total sleep and decreasing sleep onset latency, these agents markedly reduce the amount of deeper delta-wave sleep (stages 3 and 4) (Hartmann, 1976). With most of these agents, no delta-sleep rebound occurs following withdrawal. D-sleep

(REM sleep) is also suppressed, but here, rebound does occur on withdrawal. However, some studies show no interference with D-sleep by flurazepam (Greenblatt et al., 1975; Greenblatt et al., 1977). "Hangover" effects—decreased intellectual and psychomotor skills—occur and may persist for 12 hours after waking.

Meprobamate also acts to reduce REM sleep.

ANTIDEPRESSANTS: TRICYCLICS

Tricyclic antidepressants in common clinical use are listed in Table 5, with their usual dose ranges. Hall et al. (1979c) have reviewed the pharmacology and clinical aspects of the tricyclic antidepressants. These drugs vary in their relative anticholinergic actions (see Table 6), and their relative sedating effects seem to correlate with this. Protriptyline is the least sedating tricyclic.

TABLE 5. TRICYCLIC ANTIDEPRESSANTS: USUAL DAILY DOSE RANGES (mg/day)

Imipramine (Tofranil)	50 - 300
Desipramine (Norpramin)	75 - 200
Amitriptyline (Elavil)	50 - 300
Nortriptyline (Aventyl)	50 - 150
Protriptyline (Vivactil)	15 - 60
Doxepin (Sinequan, Adapin)	75 - 300

TABLE 6. TRICYCLIC ANTIDEPRESSANTS (Listed in Order of Decreasing Anticholinergic Effects)*

Amitriptyline
Doxepin
Nortriptyline
Imipramine
Desipramine

*Based on Snyder and Yamamura (1977).

Fatique and somnolence are seen frequently, especially with doxepin and amitriptyline. Retarded, withdrawn patients are particularly prone to complain of these symptoms; consequently, a less sedating tricyclic may be indicated.

Conversely, increased *restlessness, nervousness, insomnia, and agitation* may result from the less sedating tricyclics (e.g., imipramine, desipramine). Patients especially at risk are those in whom anxiety or agitation are already a component of the depression. Here, a more sedating tricyclic may be indicated, with the possible addition of a nonsedating antipsychotic (e.g., perphenazine, thiothixene), as has already been discussed.

In depressed patients with severe agitation, or in those who exhibit delusional symptoms, tricyclic medications may precipitate a *schizophreniform psychosis*. At risk, too, are patients with a previous schizophrenic episode, those with a diagnosis of schizoaffective psychosis, or those with premorbid schizoid or paranoid personalities. Psychotic manifestations may include delusions, and auditory and visual hallucinations. Klein (1965) has termed this reaction an organic rather than a schizophrenic psychosis. Use of a nonsedating antipsychotic in combination with the tricyclic will be prophylactic in such cases. Treatment is to cease administration of the antidepressant and continue the antipsychotic alone.

Patients with bipolar affective illness, including depressed patients with a previous history of mania, or a family history of mania, are at high risk for developing a *hypomanic or manic reaction* to tricyclics, once the depression clears. The dose of drug should be lowered as the depression abates, and lithium or an antipsychotic agent may need to be added to the drug regimen.

The *central anticholinergic syndrome* can occur with any of the tricyclics, but is more likely with the more potent anticholinergic agents, especially in the elderly and at high doses (e.g., greater than 200 mg amitriptyline daily). The syndrome is discussed below.

In the past, a controversy existed as to whether the tricyclics could *paradoxically worsen depression* (DiMascio et al., 1968). DiMascio et al. found that truly depressed patients did not exhibit this syndrome, but that normal volunteers could (rarely) become depressed with imipramine. More recent work suggests that a "therapeutic window" exists for nortriptyline (but not clearly for amitriptyline, imipramine, or desipramine). Excessively high plasma levels—above the therapeutic range—can indeed worsen the depressed state (Asberg et al., 1971; Ziegler et al., 1976). Individuals vary markedly in the plasma level achieved with a given oral dose of tricyclic; so that in some patients, "normal" doses of nortriptyline will be sufficient to bring about these overly high plasma levels and the consequent increased depression.

Mild *withdrawal* effects may occur, uncommonly, with these medications, after prolonged use at high doses. Malaise, chills, coryza, and myalgia are experienced (Kramer et al., 1961). Minor *cognitive and psychomotor impairment*, similar to that produced by the benzodiazepines, is thought to be common; it is potentiated by alcohol.

All the tricyclics partially suppress D-sleep (REM sleep); and when the drug is ceased, rebound may occur, so that patients show an increase in D-sleep. This latter effect (REM rebound) only seems to occur at high doses and with prolonged administration. The sedating tricyclics (such as amitriptyline) may prolong overall sleep time, especially if insomnia was a problem initially (Hartmann and Cravens, 1973; Hartmann and Spinweber, 1976); however, tolerance usually develops to this hypnotic effect. Imipramine and desipramine increase restlessness during sleep, which correlates with the insomnia and nervousness mentioned above. Some tricyclics have been found to increase slow-wave (delta-wave) sleep, notably amitriptyline and desipramine. Speculatively, delta-wave deprivation has been thought to be causal in some depressions; thus, restoration of deep sleep may in itself be therapeutic.

ANTIDEPRESSANTS: MONO-AMINE OXIDASE INHIBITORS

Table 7 shows the currently used mono-amine oxidase inhibitors (MAOI's) and their usual daily dose ranges. They are thought to be useful in "atypical" depressions and in nonresponders to tricyclics. Because severe hypertensive crisis can be a side effect, their use is fairly limited, at least in the USA.

TABLE 7. MAO INHIBITORS

HYDRAZINES	
Penelzine (Nardil)	30 - 75 mg
Isocarboxazid (Marplan)	20 - 60 mg
Nialamide (Niamid)	50 - 200 mg
NON-HYDRAZINES	
Tranylcypromine (Parnate)	10 - 30 mg
Pargyline (Eutonyl)	25 - 75 mg

The behavioral side effects of MAOI's resemble many of the syndromes just discussed in connection with the tricyclic antidepressants. Tranylcypromine and phenelzine have an amphetamine-like "stimulant" effect, and may cause *restlessness, agitation, and insomnia*. The other MAOI's can also cause these symptoms, but to a lesser degree. MAOI's can *convert a retarded to an agitated depression*, and may precipitate a *manic or schizophrenic psychosis* in predisposed patients (Klein and Davis, 1969). Hypomanic or manic reactions may be a true pharmacologic effect of MAOI's, for procarbazine (an MAOI used only in the treatment of Hodgkin's disease) has produced these reactions in patients with no history of affective disorder (Mann and Hutchison, 1967).

The *effects on sleep* are similar to those of the tricyclics. D-sleep (REM sleep) is decreased, and with prolonged administration, may disappear totally (Wyatt et al., 1971). Nialamide has been reported to increase total sleep time, while phenelzine consistently decreases it. The amount of deep (delta-wave) sleep has been reported to increase with nialamide (Hartmann and Spinweber, 1976).

LITHIUM

Lithium carbonate is very useful in the treatment and prophylaxis of acute manic and hypomanic states. The drug may also prevent bipolar depressive episodes. Its use in acute depression and other conditions remains controversial, especially in view of recent findings of renal changes in many patients taking this medicine (Ayd, 1978). Schou (1968), Amdisen and Schou (1978), and Hall et al. (1979b) have reviewed the literature on this drug.

Since lithium has a low therapeutic index, serum levels must be carefully and frequently monitored, especially during the early phases of therapy. The accepted therapeutic range is 0.6 to 1.2 mEq per liter; serum levels greater than 1.5 mEq per liter are undesirable, and those above 2.0 mEq per liter should be considered toxic.

Lithium toxicity with a sudden rise in serum levels above 2.0 mEq per liter is often encountered unexpectedly in the course of normal maintenance; the mechanism is not clearly understood, but may be related to long-term lithium-induced renal toxicity and altered renal clearance of lithium. Toxic symptoms include anorexia, nausea, vomiting, diarrhea, dysarthria, muscle twitches, and muscle hypertonicity, with hyperreflexia. The cardinal manifestations, however, are those of central nervous system (CNS) depression, with apathy, inability to concentrate, sluggishness, lethargy, and drowsiness. These may progress to stupor and coma, possibly with agitation and convulsions. Death may ensue. Mild toxicity is managed by the temporary cessation of lithium administration. The management of severe toxicity is similar to that used in barbiturate poisoning and is outlined by Mielke (1975) and Hall et al. (1979b).

A separate *lithium neurotoxic syndrome* has been described (Shopsin et al., 1970; Agulnik et al., 1972; Rifkin et al., 1973; Strayhorn and Nash, 1977). Serum lithium levels are not necessarily in the toxic range, and gastrointestinal and neuromuscular symptoms may not occur. Patients exhibit confusion, disorientation, reduced comprehension, memory loss, agitation, delusions, and hallucinations. Reversible EEG-slowing with focal changes may be noted. Patients are often labeled "schizophrenic" or "schizoaffective." The etiology of the syndrome, though unclear, is thought to be via direct CNS cell toxicity in sensitive individuals. Cessation of the drug will reverse the disorder. In one report, concurrently administered methyldopa was suspected of facilitating lithium ion entry into nerve cells (Byrd, 1975). Lithium toxicity abated when the methyldopa was ceased.

Other minor behavioral effects of lithium have been reported, including slight *concentration and memory impairment* (Bajor, 1977), *psychomotor (driving) skill impairment* in the initial stages of therapy (Linnoila et al., 1974), and some *mood depression*, especially seen in normal volunteers (Judd et al., 1977).

Alarm was raised in 1974 over the possibility that a lithium-haloperidol interaction could produce an irreversible severe encephalopathy (Cohen and Cohen, 1974). Although other anecdotal reports appeared ascribing toxic effects to this combination (Marhold et al., 1974; Loudon and Waring, 1976), careful studies involving large numbers of patients failed to replicate these findings (Ayd, 1975; Shopsin et al., 1976; Baastrup et al., 1976; Juhl et al., 1977). While lithium and haloperidol continue to be a useful combination in the management of acute manic states, the clinician must maintain a vigilant and watchful attitude when prescribing this combination. Recently, Spring and Gould (1978) have drawn attention to the possible neurotoxicity of the thioridazine-lithium combination. Here too, caution and further investigation are needed.

THE CENTRAL ANTICHOLINERGIC SYNDROME

As mentioned above, many of the antipsychotic and tricyclic antidepressant drugs have anticholinergic properties. Anti-Parkinsonian agents, often used to counteract the extrapyramidal effects of the antipsychotics, are also anticholinergic in their action (e.g., benztropine, trihexyphenidyl). Many antihistamines (e.g., promethazine, diphenhydramine) also have these properties, as do a number of proprietary sleep medications and many other agents listed in the previous chapter.

Peripheral effects include dry mouth, mydriasis, tachycardia, and decreased gastrointestinal motility. More severe peripheral toxicity may lead to urinary retention, glaucoma in susceptible individuals, and cardiac arrhythmias (especially with tricyclics).

Central toxicity produces a *delirium*, whose features are disorientation, anxiety, illusions, visual and auditory hallucinations, confusion, incoherence, and agitation (Granacher et al., 1976; Hall et al., 1977). Dysarthria, seizures, stupor, and coma may supervene, with possible cardiac and respiratory arrest.

The syndrome must be differentiated from the functional psychoses. It will often follow an overdose with any of the above medications, but may occur with doses in the therapeutic range, especially when combinations of drugs having anticholinergic properties are used. The elderly are particularly at risk.

Management of the delirium is with physostigmine, 1 to 2 mg IM or slow IV, repeated as necessary every ½ to 2 hours (Granacher and Baldessarini, 1975; Hall et al., 1979a). This anticholinesterase agent crosses the blood-brain barrier and reverses the anticholinergic effects. Medical management of tricyclic overdose is outlined by Mielke (1975) and Hall et al. (1979a).

CONCLUSION

When a psychiatric patient's behavior suddenly changes, the clinician must consider the psychotropic medications that are being administered as a potential cause of such change. A summary of the major classes of psychiatric drugs and their known behavioral side effects are given in Table 8.

TABLE 8. BEHAVIORAL TOXICITY OF PSYCHIATRIC DRUGS

DRUG CLASS	SIDE EFFECT	RELATIVE INCIDENCE	MAJOR MANIFESTATIONS	TREATMENT
Antipsychotics	**Oversedation**	Very common	Somnolence. Lethargy.	1. Reduce dosage, or 2. Switch to a less sedating drug.
	Emotional Depression	Fairly common	Dysphoric, sad mood.	1. Switch to another antipsychotic, or reduce dose. 2. Possibly add a tricyclic antidepressant.
	Acute Dystonia	Fairly common	Tonic contractions of neck, mouth, pharynx, axial spine muscles. Oculogyric crisis. Dramatic presentation, sometimes bizarre.	1. Parenteral anti-Parkinsonian agents (Diphenhydramine 25–50 mgm IM or 25 mgm IV; or Benztropine Mesylate 2. Followup oral anti-Parkinsonian therapy (e.g., Benztropine Mesylate 2 mgm p.o., TID).
	Akathisia	Common	Motor restlessness, fidgeting. "Internal restlessness."	1. Reduce dose of antipsychotic. 2. Anti-Parkinsonian agents.

TABLE 8. BEHAVIORAL TOXICITY OF PSYCHIATRIC DRUGS (Cont.)

DRUG CLASS	SIDE EFFECT	RELATIVE INCIDENCE	MAJOR MANIFESTATIONS	TREATMENT
Antipsychotics (Cont.)	**Central Anti-cholinergic Toxic Psychosis**	Fairly common in high doses of certain antipsychotics and in combination with other anticholinergic medications	See Below	See Below
	Paradoxical Reaction	Rare	Increased anxiety. Agitation. Worsening of the psychosis.	Reduce dose, or cease medication.
	Withdrawal Effects	Fairly common	Nausea, vomiting, perspiration, restlessness, insomnia, giddiness. "Latent" dyskinesia, like tardive dyskinesia.	Occasionally require brief antihistamine therapy.
	Impaired Psycho-motor Function	Common	Minimally impaired hand-eye coordination, lab psychomotor tests, (?) driving skills. Potentiation of effect by alcohol.	
	Sleep Effects	Very common	Increased total sleep. Basic structure of sleep preserved.	
Anti-Anxiety Agents	**Oversedation**	Very common	Drowsiness. Ataxia.	Reduce dose.

TABLE 8. BEHAVIORAL TOXICITY OF PSYCHIATRIC DRUGS (Cont.)

DRUG CLASS	SIDE EFFECT	RELATIVE INCIDENCE	MAJOR MANIFESTATIONS	TREATMENT
Anti-Anxiety Agents (Cont.)	**Impaired Psychomotor Function**	Common	Impaired reaction time, hand-eye coordination, steadiness, driving skills (in lab). Effect compounded by alcohol. (?) Increased risk of motor vehicle accidents.	
	Cognitive Impairment	Common	Mildly impaired alertness and concentration. Minimal EEG changes.	
	Paradoxical Reactions			
	1. Disinhibition syndrome	1. Uncommon, but not rare	Hyperactivity, garrulousness, euphoria, or anxiety. In some cases, rage and "hatred."	Cease medication.
	2. Severe suicidal depression	2. Rare	Dysphoria, depression. Apprehensive tremulousness. Ego-alien suicidal ideas.	Cease medication.
	3. Depersonalization, psychosis	3. Rare	Paranoid state, confusion, depersonalization, confabulation. Visual hallucinations.	Cease medication
	Confusion in the elderly	Common	Disorientation, somnolence, confusion, agitation. Worsened O.B.S.	Cease medication.

TABLE 8. BEHAVIORAL TOXICITY OF PSYCHIATRIC DRUGS (Cont.)

DRUG CLASS	SIDE EFFECT	RELATIVE INCIDENCE	MAJOR MANIFESTATIONS	TREATMENT
Anti-Anxiety Agents (Cont.)	**Withdrawal Effects**			
	1. Mild	Common	Cramps, sweats, tremor, insomnia, anxiety, depression.	Slow withdrawal.
	2. Severe	Rare	Delirium, visual and tactile hallucinations. Seizures, status epilepticus.	Slow withdrawal.
	Sleep Effects	Very common	Increased total sleep, decreased sleep-onset latency. Reduced delta-wave sleep. Reduced REM-sleep (except (?) Flurazepam). "Hangover" effects.	
Antidepressants: Tricyclics	**Oversedation**	Common	Fatigue. Somnolence.	Switch to a less sedating compound.
	Overstimulation	Common	Restlessness, nervousness. Insomnia. Agitation.	1. Switch to a more sedating compound. 2. Possibly, add an anti-psychotic, e.g., Perphenazine, Thiothixene).
	Schizophreniform Psychosis	Uncommon, but not rare.	Delusions. Hallucinations – visual and auditory.	Substitute a nonsedating antipsychotic agent.

TABLE 8. BEHAVIORAL TOXICITY OF PSYCHIATRIC DRUGS (Cont.)

DRUG CLASS	SIDE EFFECT	RELATIVE INCIDENCE	MAJOR MANIFESTATIONS	TREATMENT
Antidepressants: Tricyclics (Cont.)	**Manic or Hypomanic Reaction**	Fairly common	Typical manic or hypomanic presentation in bipolar patient.	1. Reduce tricyclic. 2. Antipsychotic agent. 3. Possibly lithium carbonate.
	Central Anti-cholinergic Syndrome	Fairly common with high doses, and in combination with other anticholinergic medications	See Below	See Below
	Paradoxical Depression	Common with certain tricyclics – Nortriptyline	Increased depression.	Adjust tricyclic dose to bring plasma level within therapeutic range.
	Withdrawal Effects	Uncommon	Malaise, chills, coryza, myalgia – clinically probably unimportant.	
	Cognitive, psychomotor Impairment	Common	Similar to Benzodiazepine effects; mild. Potentiated by alcohol.	
	Sleep Effects	Common	REM-sleep suppression with rebound. Doxepin, Amitriptyline increase sleep time. Desipramine, imipramine increase restlessness, insomnia. Increased slow-wave sleep.	If insomnia is a problem, switch to more sedating tricyclic, or give drug in daytime not at night.

TABLE 8. BEHAVIORAL TOXICITY OF PSYCHIATRIC DRUGS (Cont.)

DRUG CLASS	SIDE EFFECT	RELATIVE INCIDENCE	MAJOR MANIFESTATIONS	TREATMENT
Antidepressants: MAOI's	**Overstimulation**	Fairly common	Restlessness, insomnia. Agitation. Convert retarded to agitated depression.	Lower dose, or change to another antidepressant or cease medication.
	Manic or Hypomanic Reaction	Fairly common	Typical manic or hypomanic symptoms.	1. Cease medication. 2. Antipsychotic drug. 3. Possibly lithium.
	Schizophrenic Reaction	Uncommon, but not rare	Schizophreniform psychosis.	1. Cease medication. 2. Antipsychotic agents.
	Sleep Effects	Very common	REM-sleep decreases or disappears. Nialamide increases total sleep, deep sleep. Phenelzine decreases total sleep.	
Lithium	**Toxicity**	Common – depends on high serum level above 2.0 mEq/l	Anorexia, nausea, vomiting, diarrhea, dysarthria, hypertonicity, fasciculations. CNS depression: apathy, poor concentration, drowsiness. Convulsion, coma, death.	1. Cease medication. 2. Gastric lavage, forced diuresis, dialysis, etc. (See text for detailed references.)

TABLE 8. BEHAVIORAL TOXICITY OF PSYCHIATRIC DRUGS (Cont.)

DRUG CLASS	SIDE EFFECT	RELATIVE INCIDENCE	MAJOR MANIFESTATIONS	TREATMENT
Lithium	**Neurotoxicity**	Uncommon	Absent G-1 and neuromuscular symptoms. Possible serum levels in therapeutic range. Confusion, disorientation, memory loss. Agitation. Delusions, hallucinations. EEG-slowing, focal changes.	Cease drug.
	Cognitive Impairment	Common	Minor cognitive psychomotor and mood effect; memory loss, concentration impairment. Possible impaired driving skills.	
	(?) Lithium-Haldol Encephalopathy	Very rare – existence controversial. Follow-up studies have not confirmed early reports.	Permanent severe deficits in mental functioning.	
	(?) Lithium-Thioridazine Neurotoxicity	Very rare – existence controversial – only 2 cases reported.	Convulsive disorder. Encephalopathy.	

TABLE 8. BEHAVIORAL TOXICITY OF PSYCHIATRIC DRUGS (Cont.)

DRUG CLASS	SIDE EFFECT	RELATIVE INCIDENCE	MAJOR MANIFESTATIONS	TREATMENT
Certain Anti-psychotics Tricyclic Anti-depressants Anti-Parkinsonian Agents Many other drugs	**Central Anti-cholinergic Syndrome**	Fairly common, depending on the dosages of drugs and the combinations used.	*Peripherally:* dry mouth mydriasis, tachycardia, decreased G-1 motility. Urinary retention, glaucoma, arrhythmias. *Centrally:* Delirium: Disorientation, anxiety, visual and auditory hallucinations, confusion, agitation, dysarthria, seizures, stupor, coma.	Physostigmine 1–2 mgm IM or slow IV, every ½ – 2 hrs.

Unless recognized, these behavioral changes may prompt the use of increased amounts of medication, thus further worsening the patient's condition. Patients' functioning may even deteriorate to the point where they are relegated to chronic care facilities as "back ward" cases. In other cases, toxic effects can do irreparable harm, and may be life-threatening.

As more drugs are added to the clinical armamentarium, the physician must continue to be aware of currently known side effects and drug interactions, as well as being alert to the possibility that hitherto unrecognized effects may occur.

REFERENCES

Agulnik, P. L., DiMascio, A., and Moore, P. Acute brain syndrome associated with lithium therapy. *Am. J. Psychiat.* 129:621–623 (1972).

Alarcon, R. De, and Carney, M.W.P. Severe depressive mood changes following slow-release intramuscular fluphenazine injection. *Brit. Med. J.* 3:564–567 (1969).

Amdisen, A., and Schou, M. Lithium, in *Side Effects of Drugs: Annual 2,* M.N.G. Dukes, ed. Exerpta Medica, Amsterdam, Holland (1978), pp. 17–29.

Angus, J.W.S., Iqbal, F., Iqbal, J., and Simpson, G. M. A year's trial of thiothixene in chronic schizophrenia. *Int. J. Neuropsychiat.* 3:408–412 (1967).

Asberg, M., Cronholm, B., Sjoqvist, F., and Tuck, D. Relationship between plasma level and therapeutic effect on nortriptyline. *Brit. Med. J.* 3:331–334 (1971).

Ayd, F. J. Lithium-induced nephrotoxicity: A further report. *Int. Drug Ther. Newsletter.* 13:25–28 (1978).

Ayd, F. J. Lithium-haloperidol for mania: Is it safe or hazardous? *Int. Drug Ther. Newsletter.* 10:29–36 (1975).

Ayd, F. J. Critical appraisal of chlordiazepoxide. *J. Neuropsychiat.* 3:177–180 (1962).

Baastrup, P. C., Hollnagel, P., Sorensen, R., and Schou, M. Adverse reactions in treatment with lithium carbonate and haloperidol. *J.A.M.A.* 236:2645–2646 (1976).

Bajor, G. F. Memory loss with lithium (Letter). *Am. J. Psychiat.* 134:588 (1977).

Ballinger, B. R., and Ramsay, A. C. Accidents and drug treatment in a psychiatric hospital. *Brit. J. Psychiat.* 126:462–463 (1975).

Behrman, S. Mutism induced by phenothiazines. *Brit. J. Psychiat.* 121:599–604 (1972).

Betts, T. A., Clayton, A. B., and Mackay, G. M. Effects of four commonly used tranquillizers on low-speed driving performance tests. *Brit. Med. J.* 4:580–584 (1972).

Blitt, C. D., and Petty, W. C. Reversal of lorazepam delirium by physostigmine. *Anesth. Anal. Curr. Res.* 54:607–608 (1975).

Byrd, G. Methyldopa and lithium carbonate: Suspected interaction (Letter). *J.A.M.A.* 233:320 (1975).

Caldwell, J. Toxic effects of psychotherapeutic agents, in *Psychotherapeutic Drugs. Part 1: Principles,* E. Usdin and I. S. Forrest, eds. Psychopharmacology Series, Volume 2. Marcel Dekker, Inc. New York and Basel, Switzerland (1976), pp. 437–481.

Chaffin, D. S. Phenothiazine-induced acute psychotic reaction: The psychotoxicity of a drug. *Am. J. Psychiat.* 121:26–32 (1964).

Christodoulidis, H., and Frangos, H. Clinical experience with fluphenazine decanoate in the treatment of patients with long-standing chronic schizophrenia. *Curr. Ther. Res.* 18:193–198 (1975).

Cohen, W. J., and Cohen, N. H. Lithium carbonate, haloperidol, and irreversible brain damage. *J.A.M.A.* 230:1283–1287 (1974).

Covi, L., Lipman, R. S., Pattison, J. H., Derogatis, L. R., and Uhlenhuth, E. H. Length of treatment with anxiolytic sedatives and response to their sudden withdrawal. *ACTA Psychiat. Scand.* 49:51–64 (1973).

DiMascio, A., Meyer, R. E., and Stifler, L. Effects of imipramine on individuals varying in level of depression. *Am. J. Psychiat.* 124:S:55–S:58 (Feb. 1968).

Dukes, M.N.G., ed. *Side Effects of Drugs. Annual 1; Annual 2.* Exerpta Medica, Amsterdam, Holland (1977, 1978).

Dukes, M.N.G., ed. *Meyler's Side Effects of Drugs.* Vol. 8. Exerpta Medica, Amsterdam, Holland (1975).

Gale, G., and Galloon, S. Lorazepam as a premedication. *Canad. Anesth. Soc. J.* 23:22–29 (1976).

Gardos, G., Cole, J. O., and Tarsy, D. Withdrawal syndromes associated with antipsychotic drugs. *Am. J. Psychiat.* 135:1321–1324 (1978).

Gardos, G., DiMascio, A., Salzman, C., and Shader, R. I. Differential actions of chlordiazepoxide and oxazepam on hostility. *Arch. Gen. Psychiat.* 18:757–760 (1968).

Granacher, R. P., and Baldessarini, R. J. Physostigmine—its use in acute anticholinergic syndrome with antidepressant and antiparkinson drugs. *Arch. Gen. Psychiat.* 32:375–380 (1975).

Granacher, R. P., Baldessarini, R. J., and Messner, E. Physostigmine treatment of delirium induced by anticholinergics. *Am. Fam. Phys.* 13:99–103 (1976).

Greenblatt, D. J., Allen, M. D., and Shader, R. I. Toxicity of high-dose flurazepam in the elderly. *Clin. Pharm. Ther.* 21:355–361 (1977).

Greenblatt, D. J., and Shader, R. I. *Benzodiazepines in Clinical Practice.* Raven Press, New York (1974), pp. 83–86.

Greenblatt, D. J., Shader, R. I., and Koch-Weser, J. Flurazepam hydrochloride, a benzodiazepine hypnotic. *Ann. Int. Med.* 83:237–241 (1975).

Hall, R.C.W., Fox, J., Stickney, S. K., Gardner, E. R., and Perl, M. Anticholinergic delirium. Etiology, presentations, diagnosis, and management. *J. Psychedel. Drugs.* 10:237–241 (1979).

Hall, R.C.W., Perl, M., and Pfefferbaum, B. Clinical pharmacology of lithium therapy and toxicity. *Am. Fam. Phys.* 19:133–139 (1979).

Hall, R.C.W., Robbins, J., and Perl, M. Tricyclic antidepressants: Pharmacology and clinical considerations. *Tex. Med. J.* 75:1–4 (1979).

Hall, R.C.W. Personal communication (1978).

Hall, R.C.W., and Kirkpatrick, B. The Benzodiazepines. *Am. Fam. Phys.* 17:131–134 (1978).

Hall, R.C.W., Perl, M., Gardner, E. R., and Stickney, S. K. Phenothiazine withdrawal syndromes (In preparation) (1979).

Hall, R.C.W., Strong, P. L., Popkin, M. K., and Stickney, S. K. Psychosis induced by datura suaveolens: Hallucinosis and anticholinergic delirium. *World J. Psychosynth.* 9:3:19–22 (1977).

Hall, R.C.W., and Joffe, J. R. Aberrant response to diazepam: A new syndrome. *Am. J. Psychiat.* 129:738–742 (1972).

Hanna, S. M. A case of oxazepam (Serenid D) dependence. *Brit. J. Psychiat.* 120:443–445 (1972).

Hartmann, E., and Cravens, J. The effects of long-term administration of psychotropic drugs on human sleep: III. The effects of amitriptyline. *Psychopharmacologia.* (Berlin) 33:185–202 (1973).

Hartmann, E., and Spinweber, C. The effects of psychotropic medication on sleep, in *Psychotherapeutic Drugs. Part 1: Principles.* E. Usdin and I. S. Forrest, eds. Psychopharmacology Series, Vol. 2. Marcel Dekker, Inc., New York and Basel, Switzerland (1976), pp. 665–698.

Heninger, G., DiMascio, A., and Klerman, G. L. Personality factors in variability of response to phenothiazines. *Am. J. Psychiat.* 121:1091–1094 (1965).

Hollister, L. E. Psychotherapeutic drugs and driving (Letter). *Ann. Int. Med.* 80:413 (1974).

Hollister, L. E. Psychiatric syndromes due to drugs, in *Drug-Induced Diseases,* Volume 4, L. Meyler and H. M. Peck, eds. Exerpta Medica, Amsterdam, Holland (1972), pp. 561–570.

Hollister, L. E. Newer complications of psychotherapeutic drugs. *Int. J. Neuropsychiat.*, Suppl. 1. 3:141–145 (1967).

Johnson, D.A.W. The side-effects of fluphenazine decanoate. *Brit. J. Psychiat.* 123:519–522 (1973).
Judd, L. L., Hubbard, B., Janowsky, D. S., Huey, L. Y., and Attewell, P. A. The effect of lithium carbonate on affect, mood, and personality of normal subjects. *Arch. Gen. Psychiat.* 34:346–351 (1977).
Juhl, R. P., Tsuang, M. T., and Perry, P. J. Concomitant administration of haloperidol and lithium carbonate in acute mania. *Dis. Nerv. Syst.* 38:675–676 (1977).
Klein, D. F. Visual hallucinations with imipramine. *Am. J. Psychiat.* 121:911–914 (1965).
Klein, D. F., and Davis, J. M. *Diagnosis and Drug Treatment of Psychiatric Disorders.* Williams & Wilkins, Baltimore, Maryland (1969) p. 234.
Kleinknecht, R. A., and Donaldson, D. A review of the effects of diazepam on cognitive and psychomotor performance. *J. Nerv. Ment. Dis.* 161:399–411 (1975).
Kramer, J. C., Klein, D. F., and Fink, M. Withdrawal symptoms following discontinuation of imipramine therapy. *Am. J. Psychiat.* 118:549–550 (1961).
Learoyd, B. M. Psychotropic drugs and the elderly patient. *Med. J. Aust.* 1:1131–1133 (1972).
Linnoila, M., Saario, I., and Maki, M. Effect of treatment with diazepam or lithium and alcohol on psychomotor skills related to driving. *Eur. J. Clin. Pharm.* 7:337–342 (1974).
Loudon, J. B., and Waring, H. Toxic reactions to lithium and haloperidol (Letter). *Lancet.* 2:1088 (1976).
Lutz, E. G. Neuroleptic-induced akathisia and dystonia triggered by alcohol. *J.A.M.A.* 236:2422–2423 (1976).
Mann, A. M., and Hutchison, J. L. Manic reaction associated with procarbazine hydrochloride therapy of Hodgkin's disease. *Canad. Med. Assn. J.* 97:1350–1353 (1967).
Marhold, J., Zimanova, J., Lachman, M., Kral, J., and Vojtechovsky, M. To the imcompatibility of haloperidol with lithium salts. *Activ. Nerv. Sup.* (Praha) 16:3:199–200 (1974).
McDonald, R. L. The effects of personality type on drug response. *Arch. Gen. Psychiat.* 17:680–686 (1967).
Meyler, L., and Herxheimer, A. *Side Effects of Drugs.* Vol. 7. Exerpta Medica, Amsterdam, Holland (1972).
Mielke, D. H. Adverse reactions associated with mood-altering drugs. *Psychiat. Ann.* 5:11:71–89 (1975).
Murray, N. Covert effects of chlordiazepoxide therapy. *J. Neuropsychiat.* 3:168–170 (1962).
Murray, T. J., Kelly, P., Campbell, L., and Stefanik, K. Haloperidol in the treatment of stuttering. *Brit. J. Psychiat.* 130:370–373 (1977).
Paulshock, B. Z. Withdrawal of diazepam (Letter). *J.A.M.A.* 235:597 (1976).
Penttila, A., Lehti, H., and Lonnqvist, J. Psychotropic drugs and impairment of psychomotor function. *Psychopharmacologia* (Berlin) 43:75–80 (1975).
Pevnick, J. S., Jasinski, D. R., and Haertzen, C. A. Abrupt withdrawal from therapeutically administered diazepam. *Arch. Gen. Psychiat.* 35:995–998 (1978).
Preskorn, S. H., and Denner, L. J. Benzodiazepines and withdrawal psychosis: Report of three cases. *J.A.M.A.* 237:36–38 (1977).
Psychiatric Annals. Psychotropic drugs: Side effects. 5:11 (November, 1975).
Rifkin, A., Klein, D. F., and Quitkin, F. Organic brain syndrome during lithium carbonate treatment. *Comp. Psychiat.* 14:251–254 (1973).
Rifkin, A., Quitkin, F., Rabiner, C. J., and Klein, D. F. Fluphenazine decanoate, fluphenazine hydrochloride given orally, and placebo in remitted schizophrenics. *Arch. Gen Psychiat.* 34:43–47 (1977).
Ryan, H. F., Merrill, F. B., Scott, G. E. Krebs, R., and Thompson, B. L. Increase in suicidal thoughts and tendencies—Association with diazepam therapy. *J.A.M.A.* 203:1137–1139 (1968).
Schou, M. Lithium in psychiatric therapy and prophylaxis. *J. Psychiat. Res.* 6:67–95 (1968).
Shader, R. I., and Jackson, A. H. Approaches to schizophrenia, in *Manual of Psychiatric Therapeutics.* R. I. Shader, ed. Little, Brown and Co., Boston, Massachusetts (1975), p. 90.

Shader, R. I., DiMascio, A., (eds.). *Psychotropic Drug Side Effects*. Chapters 14–16. Williams & Wilkins, Baltimore, Maryland (1970), pp. 124–148.

Shopsin, B., Johnson, G., and Gershon, S. Neurotoxicity with lithium; differential drug responsiveness. *Int. Pharm.* 5:170–182 (1970).

Shopsin, B., Small, J. G., Kellams, J. J., Milstein, V., and Moore, J. E. Combining lithium and neuroleptics (Letter). *Am. J. Psychiat.* 133:980–981 (1976).

Snyder, S., and Yamamura, H. I. Antidepressants and the muscarinic acetylcholine receptor. *Arch. Gen. Psychiat.* 34:236–239 (1977).

Spring, G. K., and Gould, D. J. Hazards of combined lithium and thioridazine use. Presented at 131st Annual Meeting, A.P.A., Atlanta, Ga., May 8–12, 1978. Abstract in "CME Syllabus and Scientific Proceedings of 131st Ann. Meet. of the A.P.A." American Psychiatric Association (April 1978).

Strayhorn, J.M., and Nash, J.L. Severe neurotoxicity despite "therapeutic" serium lithium levels. *Dis. Nerv. Syst.* (38 (2): 107–111 (1977).

Van Putten, T., and May, P.R.A. "Akinetic depression" in schizophrenia. *Arch. Gen. Psychiat.* 35:1101–1107 (1978).

Viscott, D. S. Chlordiazepoxide and hallucinations. *Arch. Gen. Psychiat.* 19:370–376 (1968)

Williams, P. An unusual response to chlorpromazine therapy. *Brit. J. Psychiat.* 121:439–440 (1972).

Wyatt, R. J., Fram, D. H., Kupfer, D. J., and Snyder, F. Total prolonged drug-induced REM sleep suppression in anxious-depressed patients. *Arch. Gen. Psychiat.* 24:145–155 (1971).

Ziegler, V. E., Clayton, P. A., Taylor, J. R., Co, B. T., and Biggs, J. T. Nortriptyline plasma levels and therapeutic response. *Clin. Pharm. Ther.* 20:458–463 (1976).

Psychiatric Presentations of Medical Illness

CHAPTER 19

Behavioral Toxicity of Nonpsychiatric Drugs

RICHARD C. W. HALL, M.D.
SONDRA K. STICKNEY, R.N.
EARL R. GARDNER, Ph.D.

Pharmacologic advances provide the physician with a two-edged sword, for while the efficacy of his treatment increases, the iatrogenic illnesses produced by his therapeutics also increase. Adverse drug reactions represent a major cause of iatrogenic illness. It is estimated that one-and-one-half million patients experience a significant adverse drug reaction, at a cost of $3,000,000,000 annually. Such patients represent 5 percent of all hospital admissions and account for 14.3 percent of all hospital days. Of the individuals requiring hospitalization for an adverse drug reaction, 30 percent will experience a second such reaction while hospitalized. Of patients hospitalized for other reasons, 18 to 30 percent will develop an adverse drug reaction during their hospital stay. If such a reaction occurs, the patients's hospital days will double. Five percent of all hospital deaths are directly attributable to adverse drug reactions (Cluff, 1971; Cluff, 1967; Melmon, 1971).

Several factors increase the incidence of adverse drug reactions. These include: patient's age; number of illnesses present; use of over-the-counter medications and alcohol; telephone prescription; and polypharmacy. In a survey of outpatients, Freidman (1971) found that 25 percent were receiving two drugs, while an additional 20 percent received three or more medications. The problem of drug-induced illness has become so severe that Cluff (1971) suggests, "Whenever a sick person is seen, irrespective of the nature of the illness, the doctor should ask himself, 'could this be drug-related'?"

In a study of over 90,000 drug exposures in approximately 9,000 patients, the Boston Collaborative Drug Related Programs (1971) concluded that,

"Psychological disturbance, directly attributable to drugs commonly used in medical inpatient populations, can justifiably be regarded as an important and common problem." Of the 9,000 patients seen, 50 developed severe psychiatric disorders, which included hallucinations, delusions, and/or the development of florid psychoses. An additional 200 patients experienced moderately severe symptoms, such as agitation, bizarre and unusual feelings, depersonalization, anxiety, depression, fatigue, nervousness, malaise, and nightmares. The two agents most apt to produce psychiatric disturbance were prednisone, where 1/6 of the reactions that occurred were psychiatric in nature, and Isoniazid, where nearly 1/3 were neuropsychiatric.

In the limited space available, one cannot describe all drugs known to produce psychiatric disorders; however, the more common or major reactions to particular drugs will be mentioned. The reader is provided with a table at the end of the chapter which lists drugs producing psychiatric reactions by both brand and generic name. It is hoped that this table will provide a useful reference for agents not mentioned in the body of the chapter.

ANTICHOLINERGIC AGENTS

These compounds are responsible for more drug-induced psychiatric disorders than any other class of drugs, because of the large number available, their extensive prescription, and the ease of over-the-counter accessibility. Anticholinergic agents, such as scopolamine, are included in many proprietary sleep preparations (i.e., Sominex), cough syrups, decongestants and over-the-counter tranquilizers (Hall et al., 1978c). Substance abuse for hallucinogenic effect is becoming more frequent, particularly with plants containing belladonna alkaloids, such as jimson weed, devil's trumpet, and angel's trumpet (Hall et al., 1977a, 1977b; McHenry and Hall, 1978). Street abuse of asmador has increased (DerMarderosian and Tramontana, 1967; Gibson, 1961; Haddon, 1954).

Medications with potent anticholinergic effects include such drugs as atropine, scopolamine, homatropine, benzotropine (Cogentin), methantheline (Banthine), cyclopentolate, (Cyclogyl), dicyclomine (Bentyl), trihexyphenidyl (Artane), procyclidine (Kemadrin), biperiden (Akineton), diphenhydramine (Benadryl), dimenhydrinate (Dramamine), cyclizine (Marezine), and mexlizine (Bonine).

Anticholinergics are used as preanesthetics (i.e., atropine and scopolamine) for their drying, sedative, amnestic, and antiemetic effects when coadministered with narcotics. These agents may produce paradoxical excitement, agitation, or delirium during the pre- or post-operative period (Eckenhoff et al., 1961). Such reactions occur in up to 10 percent of obstetrical cases where scopolamine is administered (Mundy and Zeller, 1958). Although much speculation has been offered concerning the effect of psychiatric illness on the development of anticholinergic delirium, current evidence suggests that prior or concurrent psychiatric illness does not increase the incidence of atropine or scopolamine psychosis.

The psychiatric picture of *central anticholinergic syndrome*, ranges from unusual and stereotyped behavior through agitation with hallucinosis simulating a functional psychosis, to the development of delirium with disorientation, incoherence, memory impairment, and fluctuations in the level of awareness. Physical examination reveals dilated, unreactive pupils; flushed face; dry, warm skin; foul breath; dry mouth; diminished or absent bowel sounds; tachycardia; and fever. Widening of pulse pressure is a useful differential sign. Treatment is with physostigmine, 1 to 4 mg intravenously (IV). Readministration every 20 to 40 minutes until the patient is stable, may be necessary due to the short half-life of the drug (Hall et al., 1977a, 1977b; McHenry and Hall, 1978; Hall et al., 1978c; Crowell and Ketchum, 1967; Duvoisin and Katz, 1968).

ANTIHYPERTENSIVES

Reserpine, a major antihypertensive, is the agent most classically associated with the production of depression (Goodwin et al., 1972). This agent depletes serotonin, norepinephrine, and dopamine from storage sites in brain and other tissues, thereby disrupting the uptake and storage functions of presynaptic vesicles (Shore et al., 1955; Carlsson et al., 1957).

The incidence of Reserpine-induced depression is approximately 20 percent. Seven percent of patients develop psychotic depression, manifested by severe mood disruption, psychomotor retardation or agitation, and diurnal variability with worsening of symptoms in the morning. Other symptoms include sleep continuity disorder, early morning awakening, weight loss, self reproach, guilt, and a lack of environmental reactivity.

In a controlled study of 296 patients attending a hypertensive clinic, 30 (15 percent) of the 195 patients treated with Reserpine developed depression, while none of the 101 patients treated with other antihypertensives (hydralazine, hexamethonium, or pentolinium) experienced depressive symptoms. Presenting symptoms in the depressed population included: feelings of sadness, worthlessness, and discouragement; loss of energy and ambition; spontaneous weeping; loss of interest; and cyclical thinking. Ten of the 30 cases (5 percent of the total sample) required admission to hospital; 2.5 percent required electro-convulsive therapy (ECT). The remaining patients improved when Reserpine was reduced or discontinued (Lemieux et al., 1956).

A Reserpine psychosis manifested by a prodrome of increasing nervousness; agitation; diminished frustration tolerance; sleep continuity disorder; and difficulty falling asleep, associated with mild initial depression, may also develop. Prodromal symptoms are followed by recurring bouts of emotional lability, paranoid ideation, and suicidal thoughts. Lucid intervals, where the patient has clear insight into the nature of his condition, characteristically punctuate the course.

Other patients present with an admixture of organic brain syndrome and mood disturbance (Schroeder and Perry, 1955). The majority of these episodes resolve with discontinuation of the drug. Although ECT has been used to treat Reserpine-induced depression, one must be cautious in administering ECT to patients undergoing Reserpine treatment, as irreversible cardiovascular collapse may occur. It is recommended that a period of 2 weeks elapse after discontinuing the medication before administering ECT (Ban, 1969).

In addition to depression and psychosis, Reserpine may produce organic brain syndromes with disturbances of the sensorium, visual hallucinations (Kass and Brown, 1955), anxiety (Muller et al., 1955), and phobias (Freis, 1954). The drug may impair higher cognitive functions without producing other symptoms. Such changes include diminished auditory and visual reaction time, flicker fusion threshold, and paired associate learning (Ban, 1969).

Reserpine-treated patients may experience an increased number of nightmares, which are thought to be related to the drug's ability to increase REM sleep while diminishing slow-wave sleep. Some investigators feel that the incidence of depression is increased in patients who experience nightmares (Jensen, 1959; Hoffman and Domino, 1969).

METHYLDOPA (ALDOMET) AND GUANETHIDINE (ISMELIN)

Both of these drugs can produce depression. Guanethidine characteristically produces depression of mild to moderate intensity, while methyldopa is more apt to produce a severe depression. Pritchard et al. (1968) suggested that 75 percent of patients receiving alpha methyldopa experienced tiredness and lassitude; 10 percent developed mild to moderate depression, and 7 percent became severely depressed. Complaints of tiredness were virtually absent in patients treated with guanethidine, but 20 percent of these patients developed mild to moderate depressive symptoms. No psychotic depressions occurred in patients treated with guanethidine, perhaps because of its inability to cross the blood-brain barrier.

PROPRANOLOL (INDERAL)

The most frequent psychiatric disorder produced by this potent beta adrenergic blocker is depression, which has been reported in 30 to 50 percent of patients taking significant doses over time (Waal, 1967; Greenblatt and Koch-Weser, 1973). Depression abates rapidly upon discontinuation of the drug. Other psychiatric symptoms produced by propranolol include weakness, lassitude, auditory and visual hallucinations, and the development of a frank organic brain syndrome. Many of the nonspecific symptoms seen may be related to the drug's tendency to reduce cardiac output.

DIGITALIS

Psychiatric symptoms occur in from 3 to 8 percent of patients treated with digitalis (*Lancet*, 1971; Burwell and Hendrix, 1950; Carr, 1921; Fisch, 1971; Gotsman and Schrire, 1966; Marriott, 1968; Ogilvie and Ruedy, 1967; Seidl et al., 1966; Shrager, 1957; Smith et al., 1966; Sodeman, 1965). Digitalis intoxication may present with a wide variety of symptoms, including headache, trigeminal neuralgia, visual disturbances, hallucinations, delirium, depression, weakness, apathy, nausea, vomiting, and diarrhea (Ellis and Dimond, 1966). A characteristic 3-per-second spike wave occurs on the electroencephalogram (EEG) (Douglas et al., 1971) of patients with digitalis neurotoxicity.

Controversy has existed for some time concerning whether or not digitalis has specific neuropsychiatric toxicity, since the major condition for which it is administered, cardiac failure, may produce psychiatric findings. The current evidence seems overwhelming that the psychiatric symptoms associated with digitalis are a result of the drug rather than of anoxia or electrolyte shift. (Andrus and Padget, 1933; Cassem and Hackett, 1971; Hamburger, 1923; Chung, 1971; Parker and Hodge, 1967). The spectrum of neuropsychiatric symptoms produced by digitalis includes: weakness, lassitude, fatigue, drowsiness, somnolence, apathy, depression, personality and affective change, memory loss, confusion, disorientation, aphasia, irritability, restlessness, nervousness, euphoria, excitement, combativeness, agitation, belligerence, delusions, hallucinations, schizophreniform psychosis, classical delirium, manic-like episodes, terminal insomnia, nightmares, and pavor nocturnus. The sudden occurrence of any of these symptoms in a patient taking digitalis and complaining of visual changes, where fundiscopic examination is negative, should alert to central nervous system (CNS) toxicity. The reported visual changes may include blurring or dimness of vision, scotomata, flickering or flashing of lights, diplopia, blindness or colored vision (yellow, green, red, or white).

Age per se does not influence either the incidence or severity of digitalis psychosis. Psychotic reactions are however, increased in both frequency of occurrence and severity by potassium and magnesium depletion, hyperaldosteronism, hypercalcemia, cor pulmonale, hypothyroidism, and the simultaneous administration of reserpine (Cohen, 1952; DeGraff and Lyon, 1967; Dreifus et al., 1963).

CORTICOSTEROIDS

A great deal of confusion has existed concerning the nature of the psychiatric reactions produced by corticosteroids. Current evidence suggests that the incidence of psychiatric side effects produced by these drugs is dose-related. Seventy-five percent of patients who experience significant psychiatric reactions have received more than 40 mg of prednisone a day. The incidence of adverse psychiatric effects in patients taking less than 40 mg a day is 1 percent, as compared to 18 percent in patients taking 80 mg a day, or more (Boston Collaborative Drug Surveillance, 1972; Hall et al.,. 1978a; Hall et al., 1978b). The majority of steroid psychoses develop within 6 days of the onset of therapy (2:1 ratio). Pre-existing personality disturbance, or a history of previous psychiatric disorder or steroid psychosis, do not increase the risk for the development of a subsequent steroid psychosis during any given course of treatment (Hall et al., 1978a).

The only thing characteristic of steroid psychoses are their variability (Hall et al., 1978a). The symptom course shifts from one configuration to another and at any given time, may appear as a manic reaction, endogenous depression, schizophreniform psychosis, or delirium. During the course of a given psychotic episode, the most frequently seen symptoms include emotional lability, severe anxiety, marked distractability, pressured speech, sensory flooding, insomnia, depression, perplexity, agitation, auditory and visual hallucinations, mutism, intermittent memory impairment, disturbances of bodily image, delusions, and apathy. Prior to the availability of phenothiazine treatment, it was noted that steroid psychosis cleared within 4 to 6 weeks following discontinuation of steroids and was not associated with an increased incidence of subsequent depression or psychosis.

Treatment consists of tapering or eliminating steroids where possible, administration of 50 to 250 mg per day of chlorpromazine or thiorizidine and environmental control. Tricyclic antidepressants may exacerbate symptoms in some patients (Hall et al., 1978b).

ANTITUBERCULAR AGENTS

The antitubercular drugs most frequently producing psychiatric symptoms include isoniazid (INH), iproniazid, cycloserine, and ethambutol. The Boston Collaborative Drug-Related Programs (1971) suggest that isoniazid is one of the most frequent causes of drug-induced psychiatric disorders. It is capable of producing a wide variety of psychiatric disturbances, including visual and auditory hallucinations, disorientation, agitation verging on mania, structured and persistent delusions, paranoid states, schizophreniform psychosis, psychotic depression, and acute brain syndromes associated with peripheral neurological signs. Its interference with pyridoxine absorption necessitates simultaneous administration of this vitamin for patients receiving long-term therapy. Treatment of INH-induced psychiatric disorders consists of the administration of nicotinamide and pyridoxine and discontinuation of the drug (Jackson, 1967).

Three specific psychiatric presentations may occur following INH administration. The first consists of excitation, violence, interpersonal abuse uncharacteristic of the individual, suspiciousness, and persecutory delusions followed by apathy (Chu, 1953). If the medication is not discontinued, agitation worsens and auditory and visual hallucinations become prominent. Some authors have reported a symptom presentation such as that described above in the absence of disorientation, or where disorientation occurred only after the onset of hallucinations and paranoia, suggesting that the condition is not a variant of organic brain syndrome (OBS) (Wiedorn and Ervin, 1954).

The second presentation is one of acute organic brain syndrome. Such conditions, when caused by a toxin, usually clear rapidly following its elimination. However, several cases have been reported where patients with isoniazid-induced OBS failed to clear for periods of several weeks or longer after the drug was discontinued (Vysniauskas and Brueckner, 1954).

The third type of INH reaction consists of a mixed depressive-schizophreniform psychosis with catatonic features. Symptoms include inappropriate affect; thought blocking; ambivalence; loosening of associations; irrational thoughts; and pacing and impulsive movements, followed by memory impairment. Such symptoms may represent a pellagra psychosis caused by an associated niacin deficiency.

Ipronazid has a marked tendency to produce psychiatric symptoms. Most characteristically, it induces a paranoid confusional state, acute brain syndrome, or manic-like episode (O'Connor et al., 1953; Bloch et al., 1954; Crane, 1956). This agent is a monoamine oxidase inhibitor that inactivates both catecholamines and serotonin. Because of these properties, the drug may activate a latent schizophrenia or exacerbate already existing schizophrenic symptoms (Freymuth et al., 1959). Iproniazid has been reported to decrease the incidence of catatonic behavior in catatonic schizophrenics (Breitner, 1958). A withdrawal syndrome consisting of severe, repetitive, and terrifying nightmares, associated with daytime anxiety, restlessness, nervousness, mild to moderate depression, and nausea, may occur following its sudden discontinuation (O'Connor et al., 1953).

Ethionamide may produce: depression (Poole and Schewiss, 1961); emotional lability associated with alternating periods of somnolence and agitation; an inebriated-like state; anxiety; diminished attention span; suicidal ideation; or manic-like excitement (Ono et al., 1969).

Cycloserine has marked psychiatric toxicity. When used with other antitubercular agents, its psychotomimetic effects are increased. The drug may produce: (1) an acute organic brain syndrome; (2) a schizophreniform psychosis; (3) a psychotic depressive disorder; or (4) a hypomanic or manic state (Epstein et al., 1955; Murray, 1956; Kanaya et al., 1965; Mitchell and Lester, 1970). The agent increases agitation, hallucinations, and confusion in schizophrenics (Simeon et al., 1970).

Lewis et al. (1957) defined three types of cycloserine toxicity consisting of: (1) hyperirritability, diminished frustration tolerance, socially inappropriate language, drowsiness, and dizziness; (2) personality change, confusional states, and central nervous system hyperirritability, progressing in some patients to convulsion and the development of what they defined as a "borderline psychosis"; (3) either convulsions, or florid psychosis. Fifty percent of all patients receiving 1.0 gm of cycloserine per day developed some toxicity; 20 percent of such patients had a type 3 response.

HORMONES

The effects of hormones are covered in other sections of this text. In summary, both androgens and estrogens may produce agitation, organic brain syndrome, schizophreniform psychoses, hallucinations, and acute confusional states.

ORAL CONTRACEPTIVES

Depression is the most frequent significant psychiatric side effect of oral contraceptives. Estimates as to the frequency of occurrence range as high as 34 percent. Large population surveys suggest an incidence of 7 percent (Herzberg, 1970).

Women with significant premenstrual tension associated with marked lability of mood and those with previous histories of depression, are at greatest risk. Although the issue is not finally settled, it appears that the higher the estrogen to progesterone ratio of a particular contraceptive, the greater the probability is that a patient will experience an adverse mental effect. Women taking pills high in progesterone are more likely to experience anxiety, depression, and chronic tension states (Cullberg, 1972). Depression may also occur in some women as a result of a fall of estrogen level prior to menstruation, or due to estrogen decline during menopause. Psychotic depression has been reported following withdrawal of oral contraceptives. No direct cause-and-effect relationship exists linking depression to specific levels of estrogen or progesterone.

The marked differences in the incidence figures of depression related to use of the pill and the fact that women with a previous history of depression are more subject to affective disorder, suggests biologically distinct and separate depressogenic mechanisms, with some women being more susceptible to the hypothalamic norepinephrine-depleting effects of estrogen, while others respond with a lowering of serotonin (Price and Toseland, 1969; Winston, 1969).

DISULFIRAM (ANTABUSE)

This agent, a behavioral modifier for alcoholics, produces an accumulation of acetaldehyde following alcohol ingestion. It blocks crucial enzyme systems including dopamine-beta-hydroxylase, which is responsible for the conversion of dopamine to norepinephrine. The incidence of psychiatric toxicity from this drug has diminished from the 20 percent initially reported to about 5 percent, because of more cautious administration and the use of lower maintenance dosages. Three characteristic antabuse psychoses have been reported. The first, a classic delirium, occurs in approximately 39 percent of patients who become psychotic. Group two psychoses represent a combination of delirium with depression, manic, paranoid or delusional states, and occur in approximately 37 percent of psychotic patients. Group three patients present with psychotic depression or schizophreniform psychoses without signs of delirium; 24 percent of all antabuse psychoses fall into this category (Liddon and Satran, 1967). It is noteworthy that in one study, 17 percent of patients with antabuse psychosis attempted suicide, and that over half of these attempts were successful (Liddon and Satran, 1967). Treatment consists of discontinuation of the drug, careful patient monitoring, and observation. Treatment with antipsychotic medication may be contraindicated since these agents may worsen delirium and have little specific salutory effect (Knee and Razani, 1974). Following discontinuation of antabuse, group one patients recover within a week. Groups two and three patients require 1 to 3 weeks to clear. Less than one third of group one or two patients experienced a similar psychotic episode when rechallenged.

L-DOPA

Because of its salutory effect in the treatment of Parkinson's disease, the frequency of use of this agent is increasing. The drug represents the immediate precursor of dopamine and is thought to increase its concentration. L-dopa has been estimated to produce psychosis in up to 20 percent of the Parkinsonian patients to whom it is administered. Incidence figures range from 10 to 50 percent (Celesia and Barr, 1970; Jenkins and Grok, 1970). The large, collaborative studies involving totals of over 17,000 patients, suggest that mental effects represent the third most common group of side effects, following only gastrointestinal and movement disorders (Keenan, 1970; Langrall, 1970). The major psychiatric constellations seen include: confusion and delirium (4.4 percent of patients); significant depression (4.2 percent); overactivity, restlessness, and agitation (3.6 percent); florid psychosis with delusions and paranoia (3.6 percent); hypomania (1.5 percent); hypersexual behavior (0.9 percent); and other miscellaneous conditions (1.5 percent) (Goodwin, 1972).

AMPHETAMINES

Recent national attention has been focused on the overproduction and overprescription of these agents as mood elevators and anorexics. They normally produce either a dysphoric, jittery state, or a sensation of well-being. Prolonged use is associated with the development of paranoid reactions, lability of mood, paranoid psychoses, and psychotic depression, particularly when discontinued. Insomnia characteristically occurs following use. The suppression of both REM and total sleep time by these agents, may contribute to the development of psychosis. Although not conclusively proven at this time, there is evidence to suggest that long-term use may be associated with neurohistological damage (Lemere, 1966).

The amphetamine psychoses usually simulate paranoid schizophrenia, where hallucinations and delusions occur in a setting of clear consciousness. The condition may be indistinguishable from acute or chronic paranoid schizophrenia, with ideas of reference, delusions of persecution, and hallucinations. Slater (1959), however, believes that the presence of psychopathic personality traits, the rapidity of onset, the dream-like quality of the experience, the tendency toward visual hallucinations, and the presence of brisk emotional reactions with anxiety differentiate the amphetamine psychosis from a true paranoid schizophrenia. Other authors disagree, feeling that the symptomatology of paranoid schizophrenia may be completely replicated, including such symptoms as thought insertion, control, broadcasting, and blunted affect (Angrist and Gershon, 1969; Angrist et al., 1969).

The recommended treatment for amphetamine psychosis is the administration of a psychotropic drug, such as haloperidol, in conjunction with a structured, supportive, and safe environment. Haldol is specifically preferrable to chlorpromazine, since the latter has been reported to significantly increase the half-life of amphetamine in the brain and raise its blood level (Davis, 1970).

CONCLUSION

Polypharmacy places patients at risk and, as has been discussed, increases the incidence of drug-induced psychiatric symptoms, which may mimic many primary psychiatric disorders. Whenever psychiatric symptoms appear in a patient taking medical agents known to be associated with the production of psychiatric symptoms, the physician's safest posture is to consider the syndrome as drug-related until proven otherwise. In the majority of instances, discontinuation of as many medications as possible is the most specific and salutory intervention that can be made. An awareness of the specific constellation of symptoms produced by various agents may be of great value in determining their influence on a patient's mental state.

REFERENCES

Andrus, E. C., and Padget, P. Delirium in association with myocardial insufficiency. *Trans. Am. Clin. Climatol. Assn.* 49:100–121 (1933).

Angrist, B., and Gershon, S. Amphetamine abuse in New York City—1966–1968. *Sem. Psychiat.* 1:195–207 (1969).

Angrist, B., Schweitzer, J., Friedhoff, A. J., Gershon, S. Hekimian, L. J., and Floyd, A. The clinical symptomatology of amphetamine psychosis and its relationship to amphetamine levels in urine. *Int. Pharmaco-Psychiat.* 2:125–139 (1969).

Ban, T. A. *Psychopharmacology*. Williams & Wilkins, Baltimore, Maryland (1969).

Bloch, R. G., Dooneief, A. S., Buchberg, A. S., and Spellman, S. The clinical effects of isoniazid and iproniazid in the treatment of pulmonary tuberculosis. *Ann. Intern. Med.* 40:881–900 (1954).

Boston Collaborative Drug-Related Programs. Psychiatric side effects of non-psychiatric drugs. *Sem. Psychiat.* 3:406–420 (1971).
Boston Collaborative Drug Surveillance. Acute adverse reactions to prednisone in relation to dosage. *Clin. Pharm. Ther.* 13:694–698 (1972).
Breitner, C. Marsilid in catatonic schizophrenia. *Am. J. Psychiat.* 114:941 (1958).
Burwell, W. B., and Hendrix, J. P. Digitalis poisoning. *Am. J. Med.* 8:640–657 (1950).
Carlsson, A., Rosengren, E., Bertler, A., and Nilsson, J. *Effect of Reserpine on the Metabolism of Catecholamines in Psychotropic Drugs.* S. Garaltini and V. Ghetti, eds. Elsevier, Amsterdam, Holland (1957), pp. 363–372.
Carr, J. G. The toxic effects of digitalis. *Ann. Med.* 1:548–552 (1921).
Cassem, N. H., and Hackett, T. P. Psychiatric consultations in a coronary care unit. *Ann. Intern. Med.* 75:9–14 (1971).
Celesia, G. G., and Barr, A. N. Psychosis and other psychiatric manifestations of levodopa therapy. *Arch. Neurol.* 23:193–200 (1970).
Chu, J. Toxic psychosis due to overdosage of isonicotinic acid hydrazide. *W. Va. Med. J.* 49:125–127 (1953).
Chung, E. K. Guide to managing digitalis intoxication. *Postgrad. Med.* 49:99–103 (1971).
Cluff, L. E. Diagnosing adverse drug reactions in outpatients. *Hosp. Phys.* 5:56–59 (1971).
Cluff, L. E. Studies on the epidemiology of adverse drug reactions: I Methods of surveillance. *J.A.M.A.* 188:976–983 (1967).
Cohen, B. M. Digitalis poisoning and its treatment. *N. Eng. J. Med.* 246:225–232; 254–259 (1952).
Crane, G. E. The psychiatric side effects of iproniazid. *Am. J. Psychiat.* 112:494–501 (1956).
Crowell, E. B., and Ketchum, J. S. The treatment of scopolamine-induced delirium with physostigmine. *Clin. Pharm. Ther.* 8:409–414 (1967).
Cullberg, J. Mood changes and menstrual symptoms with different gestagen/estrogen combinations. *ACTA Psychiat. Scand.*, Suppl. 236:1–86 (1972).
Davis, J. Presentation, Callegium International Neuropsychopharmacologicum. Prague, Czechoslovakia (August, 1970).
DeGraff, A. C., and Lyon, A. F. Reappraisal of digitalis. Part IX: Digitalis toxicity. *Am. Heart J.* 73:710–712 (1967).
DerMarderosian, A. H., and Tramontana, J. A. Antiasthmatics as hallucinogens. *Penn. Med.* 70:58–60 (1967).
Douglas, E. F., White, P. T., and Nelson, J. W. Three per second spike wave in digitalis toxicity. *Arch. Neurol.* 25:373–375 (1971).
Dreifus, L. S., McNight, E. H., Katz, M., and Likoff, W. Digitalis intolerance. *Geriat.* 18:494–502 (1963).
Duvoisin, R. C., and Katz, R. Reversal of central anticholinergic syndrome in man by physostigmine. *J.A.M.A.* 206:1963–1965 (1968).
Eckenhoff, J. E., Kneale, D. H., and Dripps, R. D. The incidence and etiology of postanesthetic excitement. *Anesth.* 22:667–673 (1961).
Ellis, J. G.,. and Dimond, E. G. Newer concepts of digitalis. *Am. J. Cardiol.* 17:759–767 (1966).
Epstein, I. G., Nair, K.G.S., and Boyd, L. J. Cycloserine. A new antibiotic in the treatment of human pulmonary tuberculosis: A preliminary report. *Antib. Med.* 1:80–93 (1955).
Fisch, C. Digitalis intoxication. *J.A.M.A.* 216:1770–1775 (1971).
Freis, E. D. Mental depression in hypertensive patients treated for long periods with large doses of reserpine. *N. Eng. J. Med.* 251:1006–1008 (1954).
Freymuth, H. W., Waller, H., Baumecker, P., and Stein, H. Effects of iproniazid on chronic and regressed schizophrenics. *Dis. Nerv. Syst.* 20:123–125 (1959).
Friedman, G. D., Collen, M. F., Harris, L. E., Van Brunt, E. E., and Davis, L. S. Experience in monitoring drug reactions in outpatients. *J.A.M.A.* 217:567–572 (1971).
Gibson, R. K. Jimson weed poisoning in children. *J. Ind. St. Med. Assn.* 54:1018–1020 (1961).

Goodwin, F. K. Behavioral effects of l-dopa in man, in *Psychiatric Complications of Medical Drugs*. R.I. Shader ed. Raven Press, New York (1972), pp. 149–174.

Goodwin, F. K., Ebert, M. H., and Bunney, W. E., Jr. Mental effects of reserpine in man: A review, in *Psychiatric Complications of Medical Drugs*. R.I. Shader, ed. Raven Press, New York (1972), pp. 73–101.

Gotsman, M. S., and Schrire, V. Toxicity—A frequent complication of digitalis therapy. *S. Afr. Med. J.* 40:590–593 (1966).

Greenblatt, D. J., and Koch-Weser, J. Adverse reactions to propranolol in hospitalized medical patients: A report from the Boston Collaborative Drug Surveillance Program. *Am. Heart J.* 86:478–483 (1973).

Haddon, W., and Delaplaine, R. P., Stramonium poisoning. *J.A.M.A.* 154:855 (1954).

Hall, R.C.W., Popkin, M. K., Stickney, S.K., and Gardner, E. R. Presentation of the "Steroid Psychosis." *J. Nerv. Ment. Dis.* 167:229–236 (1979).

Hall, R.C.W., Popkin, M. K., and Kirkpatrick, B. Tricyclic exacerbation of steroid psychosis. *J. Nerv. Ment. Dis.* 166:10:738–742 (1978).

Hall, R.C.W., and Stickney, S. K. Rapidly developing psychosis as complication of innocent over-the-counter drug use. Program and Summary Book of the National Drug Abuse Conference. Seattle, Washington. (1978), p. 86, No. 23

Hall, R.C.W., McHenry, L., and Popkin, M. K. Angel's Trumpet Psychosis. *Am. J. Psychiat.* 134:3:313–314 (1977).

Hall, R.C.W., Strong, P., Popkin, M. K., and Stickney, S. K. Psychosis induced by datura suaveolens: Hallucinosis and anticholinergic delirium. *World J. Psychosynth.* 9:3:19–22 (1977).

Hamburger, W. W. Acute cardiac psychoses: Analysis of toxic and circulatory factors in 5 cases of acute confusion. *Med. Clin. N. Am.* 7:465–475 (1923).

Herzberg, B., and Coppen, A. Change in psychological symptoms in women taking oral contraceptives. *Brit. J. Psychiat.* 116:161–164 (1970).

Hoffman, J. S., and Domino, E. Comparative effects of reserpine on the sleep cycle of man and cat. *J. Pharm. Exp. Ther.* 170:190–198 (1969).

Jackson, S.L.O. Psychosis due to isoniazid. *Brit. Med. J.* 1:743–746 (1967).

Jenkins, R. B., and Grok, R. H. Mental symptoms in Parkinsonian patients treated with l-dopa. *Lancet.* 2:177–179 (1970).

Jensen, K. Depressions in patients treated with reserpine for arterial hypertension. *ACTA Psychiat. Neurol. Scand.* 34:195–204 (1959).

Kanaya T., Ohta, Y., and Nabeshnia, Y. Psychoneurotic symptoms due to cycloserine. *Jap. J. Chest. Dis.* 24:889–893 (1965).

Kass, I., and Brown, E. C. Treatment of hypertensive patients with rauwolfia compounds and reserpine. *J.A.M.A.* 159:1513–1516 (1955).

Keenan, R. E. The Eaton collaborative study of levodopa therapy in Parkinsonism: A summary. *Neurol.* 20:46–59 (1970).

Knee, S. T., and Razani, J. Acute organic brain syndrome: A complication of disulfiram therapy. *Am. J. Psychiat.* 131:1281–1282 (1974).

Lancet, Digitalis intoxication. edit. 2:7720:362–363 (1971).

Langrall, H. M. The Roche collaborative study of levodopa. Second Roche Symposium on Levodopa. Nutley, New York (June, 1970).

Lemere, F. The danger of amphetamine dependency. *Am. J. Psychiat.* 123:569–571 (1966).

Lemieux, G., Davignon, A., and Genest, J. Depressive states during rauwolfia therapy for arterial hypertension. A report of 30 cases. *Canad. Med. Assn. J.* 74:522–526 (1956).

Lewis, W. C., Calden, G., Thurston, J. R., and Gilson, W. E. Psychiatric and neurologic reactions to cycloserine in the treatment of tuberculosis. *Dis. Chest.* 32:172–182 (1957).

Liddon, S. C., and Satran, R. Disulfiram (Antabuse) psychosis. *Am. J. Psychiat.* 123:1284–1289 (1967).

Marriott, H.J.L. Delirium from digitalis toxicity. *J.A.M.A.* 203:156 (1968).

McConnell, R. B., and Cheetham, H. D. Acute pellagra during isoniazid therapy. *Lancet*. 2:959–960 (1952).
McHenry, L., and Hall, R.C.W. Angel's trumpet: Lethal and psychogenic aspects. *J. Fla. Med. Assn.* 65:3:192–196 (1978).
Melmon, K. L. Preventable drug reactions: Causes and cures. *N. Eng. J. Med.* 284:1361–1368 (1971).
Mitchell, R. S., and Lester, W. Clinical experience with cycloserine in the treatment of tuberculosis. *Scand. J. Resp. Dis.*, (Supp). 51:94–108 (1970).
Muller, J. C., Pryor, W. W., Gibbons, J. E., and Orgain, E. S. Depression and anxiety occurring during rauwolfia therapy. *J.A.M.A.* 159:836–839 (1955).
Mundy, L. R., and Zeller, W. W. Acute toxic psychoses due to scopolamine. *Dis. Nerv. Syst.* 19:423–424 (1958).
Murray, F. J. A pilot study of cycloserine toxicity. *Am. Rev. Tuberc.* 74:196–209 (1956).
O'Connor, J. B., Howlett, K. S., Jr., and Wagner, R. R. Side effects accompanying the use of iproniazid. *Am. Rev. Tuberc.* 68:270–272 (1953).
Ogilvie, R. I., and Ruedy, J. Adverse drug reactions during hospitalization. *Canad. Med. Assn. J.* 97:1450–1457 (1967).
Ono, K., Hashigami, Y., Itonaga, K., Aida, Y., Fujino, S., and Tsuchiy, A.I. Mental disorders induced by cycloserine and ethionamide. Joint study unit on side effects of secondary antituberculosis drugs. *IRYO*. 23:85–91 (1969).
Parker, D. L., and Hodge, J. R. Delirium in a coronary care unit. *J.A.M.A.* 201:702–703 (1967).
Poole, G. W., and Schewiss, J. Peripheral neuropathy due to ethioniamide. *Am. Rev. Resp. Dis.* 84:890–892 (1961).
Price, S. A., and Toseland, P. A. Oral contraceptives and depression. *Lancet*. 2:158–159 (1969).
Pritchard, N. C., Johnston, A. W., Hill, I. D., and Rosenheim M. L. Bethanidine, guanethidine, and methyldopa in treatment of hypertension: a within-patient comparison. *Brit. Med. J.* 1:135–144 (1968).
Schroeder, H. A., and Perry, H. M. Psychosis apparently produced by reserpine. *J.A.M.A.* 159:839–840 (1955).
Seidl, L. G. Thornton, G. F., Smith, J. W., and Cluff, L. E. Studies on the epidemiology of adverse drug reactions III: Reactions in patients on a general medical service. *Bull. Johns Hopkins Hosp.* 119:299–315 (1966).
Shore, P. A., Silver, S. L., and Brodie, B. B. Interaction of reserpine, serotonin, and lysergic acid diethylamide in brain. *Sci.* 122:284–285 (1955).
Shrager, M. W. Digitalis intoxication, a review and report of 40 cases with emphasis on etiology. *Arch. Int. Med.* 100:881–893 (1957).
Simeon, J., Fink, M., Itil, T. M., and Ponce, D. d-cycloserine therapy of psychosis by symptom provocation. *Comp. Psychiat.* 11:80–88 (1970).
Slater, E. Review of amphetamine psychosis by P. H. Connell. *Brit. Med. J.* 1:488 (1959).
Smith, J. W., Seidl, L. G., and Cluff, L. E. Studies on the epidemiology of adverse drug reactions. V.: Clinical factors influencing susceptibility. *Ann. Intern. Med.* 65:629–640 (1966).
Sodeman, W. A. Diagnosis and treatment of digitalis toxicity. *N. Eng. J. Med.* 273:35–37; 93–95 (1965).
Verbist, L., Prignot, J., Cosemans, J., and Gyselen, A. Tolerance to ethionamid and PAS in original treatment of tuberculosis. *Scand. J. Resp. Dis.* 47:225–235 (1966).
Vysniauskas, G., and Brueckner, H. H. Severe reactions of the central nervous system following isoniazid treatment. *Am. Rev. Tuberc.* 69:759–765 (1954).
Waal, H. J. Propranolol-induced depression. *Brit. Med. J.* 2:50 (1967).
Wiedorn, W. S., and Ervin, F. Schizophrenic-like psychotic reactions with administration of isoniazid. *Arch. Neurol. Psychiat.* 72:321–324 (1954).
Winston, F. Oral contraceptives and depression. *Lancet*. 1:1209 (1969).

Appendix
PSYCHIATRIC SIDE EFFECTS OF MEDICAL DRUGS

PSYCHIATRIC SIDE EFFECTS OF MEDICAL DRUGS

General Classification	Generic	Trade Name	Psychiatric Side Effects
Sulfonamides*	Mafenide acetate	Sulfamylon	General statement regarding sulfonamides:
	Phthelylsulfathiazole		depression
	Salicylazosulfapyridine		psychosis
	Sulfacetamide sodium	Sultrin Triple Sulfa	restlessness
	Sulfachlorpyridazine		irritability
	Sulfadiazine	Suladyne	
	Sulfamerazine		
	Sulfameter	Sulla	
	Sulfamethazine		
	Sulfamethizole	Azotrex	
		Microsul	
		Microsul-A	*May cause retardation if given during 3rd trimester, to nursing mothers, or to children less than 2 months old
		Suladyne	
		Thiosulfil	
		Thiosulfil Forte	
		Thiosulfil-A Forte	
		Urobiotic-250	
	Sulfamethoxazole	Azo Gantanol	
		Bactrim DS	
		Bactrim	
		Gantanol	
		Gantanol DS	
		Septra DS	
		Septra	
	Sulfaphenasole		
	Sulfisoxazole	Azo Gantrisin	
		Gantrisin	
		SK-Soxazole	
		Sulfisoxazole	
		Vagilia	

PSYCHIATRIC SIDE EFFECTS OF MEDICAL DRUGS (Cont.)

General Classification	Generic	Trade Name	Psychiatric Side Effects
Sulfones	Dapsone Sulfoxone sodium		General statement regarding sulfones: nervousness insomnia psychosis
Anthelmintics	Aspidium oleoresin Quinacrime HCl Tetrachloroethylene	Male Fern Oleoresin Atabrine HCl	Delirium Psychosis Inebriation
Antitubercular Agents	Cycloserine	Seromycin	Confusion Lethargy Psychosis
	Ethionamide Isoniazid	Trecator-SC INH Isonicotinic Acid Hydrazine Hyzyd Laniazid Niconyl Nydrazid Teebaconin	Depression Toxic psychosis Parasthesia Excitement Euphoria
	Rifampin	Rifadin Rimactane	Confusion
Antimalarials	Chloroquine HCl Chloroquine phosphate	Aralen HCl Aralen Phosphate	General statement regarding antimalarials: fatigue lassitude nervousness irritability psychosis
	Amodiaquin HCl	Camoquin HCl	Spasticity

PSYCHIATRIC SIDE EFFECTS OF MEDICAL DRUGS (Cont.)

General Classification	Generic	Trade Name	Psychiatric Side Effects
Amebicides and Trichomonacides	Metronidazole	Flagyl	Confusion Irritability Depression Insomnia
Antineoplastic Agents	Fluorouracil	Efudex 5-Fluorouracil 5-FU Fluoroplex	Euphoria Insomnia Irritability
	Procarbazine HCl	Matulane	Depression Psychosis Manic reactions Nervousness Insomnia Nightmares Disorientation Delirium
	Vinblastine sulfate	Velban VLB	Depression
Cardiac Glycosides	Acetyldigitoxin	Acylanid	General statement regarding cardiac glycosides: disorientation confusion depression aphasia delirium hallucinations especially in the elderly or arteriosclerotic
	Deslanoside	Cedilanid-D	
	Digitalis glycoside	Crystodigin	
	Digitalis leaf		
	Digitoxin	Digitoxin	
	Digoxin	Digoxin Lanoxin SK-Digoxin	
	Gitalin	Gitaligin	
	Lanatoside C	Cedilanid	
	Ouabain	Ouabain	

PSYCHIATRIC SIDE EFFECTS OF MEDICAL DRUGS (Cont.)

General Classification	Generic	Trade Name	Psychiatric Side Effects
Peripheral Vasodilators	Nylidrin HCl	Nylidrin	Nervousness
		Arlidin	
Antihypertensive Agents			
Rauwolfia Alkaloids	Alseroxylon		General statement regarding
	Deserpidine	Enduronyl	Rauwolfia alkaloids:
		Harmonyl	nightmares
		Oreticyl	depression (to point of
	Rauwolfia serpentina	Raudixin	suicide attempt)
		Rauzide	Rare: nervousness, paradoxical
		Rauwolfia Serpentine	anxiety, decreased libido,
	Rescinnamine	Moderil	Parkinson-like syndrome
	Reserpine	Butiserpazide-25/50 Prestabs	
		Demi-Regroton	
		Diupres	
		Diutensen-R	
		Dralserp	
		Exna-R	
		Hydromox R	
		Hydropres	
		Hydrotensin-50	
		Hydrotensin-Plus	
		Metatensin	
		Naquival	
		Ran-Sed	
		Regroton	
		Renese-R	
		Reserpine	
		Ruhexatal with reserpine	
		SK-Reserpine	

PSYCHIATRIC SIDE EFFECTS OF MEDICAL DRUGS (Cont.)

General Classification	Generic	Trade Name	Psychiatric Side Effects
Rauwolfia Alkaloids (Cont.)	Reserpine (Cont.)	Salutensin	
		Sandril	
		Ser-Ap-Es	
		Serpasil	
		Serpasil-Apresoline	
		Serpasil-Esidrix	
	Syrosingopine	Singoserp-Esidrix	
Ganglionic Blocking Agents	Mecamylamine HCl		General statement regarding ganglionic blocking agents:
	Pentolinium tartrate		
	Trimethaphan camsylate	Arfonad	tremor
			confusion
Sympathetic Nervous System Depressants	Guanethidine sulfate	Ismelin Sulfate	Depression
	Methyldopate HCl	Aldomet HCl	Parkinsonism
			Diminished cognition
			Choreoathetotic movements
			Nightmares
			Depression
			Psychosis
	Methyldopa	Aldomet	Parkinsonism
		Aldoclor	Diminished cognition
		Aldoril	Choreoathetotic movements
			Nightmares
			Depression
			Psychosis
Agents that Act Directly on Vascular Smooth Muscle	Hydralazine HCl	Apresazide	Depression
		Apresoline HCl	Disorientation
		Apresoline-Esidrix	Anxiety

PSYCHIATRIC SIDE EFFECTS OF MEDICAL DRUGS (Cont.)

General Classification	Generic	Trade Name	Psychiatric Side Effects
Agents that Act Directly on Vascular Smooth Muscle (Cont.)	Hydralazine HCl (Cont.)	Dralserp Dralzine Hydralazine HCl Hydrotensin-Plus Ser-Ap-Es Serpasil-Apresoline Unipres	
Antiarrhythmic Agents	Lidocaine HCl	Anestacon LTA 11 Lidocaine HCl Lidosporin Xylocaine HCl	Transient excitement Depression Restlessness Euphoria Apprehension Hallucinations Insomnia Incoordination
	Propranolol HCl	Inderal	
Hypocholesterolemic and Antilipemic Agents	Nicotinic acid	Cerebro-Nicin Diacin Lipo-Nicin Menic Niac Niacin Nicalex Nicobid Nicocap Nico-400 Nicolar Nico-Metrazol	Nervousness Panic reactions

PSYCHIATRIC SIDE EFFECTS OF MEDICAL DRUGS (Cont.)

General Classification	Generic	Trade Name	Psychiatric Side Effects
Hypocholesterolemic and Antilipemic Agents (Cont.)	Nicotinic acid (Cont.)	Nico-Span	
		Nicotinex Elixir	
		Nicozol	
		Progiatric	
		Ragus	
		Tega-Span	
		Tinic	
		Wampocap	
	Dextrothyroxine sodium	Choloxin	Insomnia Nervousness Changes in libido (> or <) Bizarre subjective complaints
Barbiturates	Amobarbital	Amesec	General statement regarding barbiturates:
		Amytal	excitement
		Dexamyl	euphoria
		Ectasule	restlessness
	Amobarbital sodium	Amytal Sodium	delirium
		Tuinal	psychological dependence
	Aprobarbital	A.P.B.	nervousness
		Alurate Elixir	
		Alurate Elixir Verdum	
	Butabarbital	Broncomar	
		Butabarbital Sodium Elixir	
		Butiserpazide-25/50	
		Cystospaz-SR	
		Dolonil	
		Quibron Plus	
		Sedapap-10	
		Sidonna	
		Tedral-25	

PSYCHIATRIC SIDE EFFECTS OF MEDICAL DRUGS (Cont.)

General Classification	Generic	Trade Name	Psychiatric Side Effects
Barbiturates (Cont.)	Butabarbital sodium	Buticaps	
		Butisol	
		Dularin-TH	
		Gaysal	
		Minotal	
		Phrenilin	
	Hexobarbital		
	Mephobarbital	Mebaral	
	Metharbital	Gemonil	
	Methhexital sodium		
	Pentobarbital	Eme-Nil Inserts	
		Emesert Inserts	
		Matropinal	
		Matropinal Forte	
		Nembutal Elixir	
		Pentobarbital Sodium	
	Phenobarbital	A.P.B.	
		Antrocol	
		Arco-Lase Plus	
		Belap	
		Bentyl with Phenobarbital	
		Bronkolixir	
		Bronkotabs	
		Bronkotabs-Hafs	
		Cantil with Phenobarbital	
		Cardilate-P	
		Donphen	
		Eskabarb	
		Gaysal	
		Gustase-Plus	
		Isordil	

PSYCHIATRIC SIDE EFFECTS OF MEDICAL DRUGS (Cont.)

General Classification	Generic	Trade Name	Psychiatric Side Effects
Barbiturates (Cont.)	Phenobarbital (Cont.)	Levsin/Phenobarbital	
		Levsinex/Phenobarbital	
		Lufyllin-EPG	
		Luminal	
		Matropinal	
		Mundrane GG	
		Oxoids	
		Pamine PB	
		Peritrate with Phenobarbital	
		Phazyme-PB	
		Phenobarbital	
		Pro-Banthine with Phenobarbital	
		Proval	
		Quadrinal	
		Robinul with Phenobarbital	
		SK-Phenobarbital	
		Solfoton	
		Trasentine with Phenobarbital	
		Valpin	
		Verequad	
	Phenobarbital sodium	Luminal Sodium	
	Secobarbital	Antora-B	
		Secobarbital	
		Seconal Elixir	
	Secobarbital sodium	Seconal Sodium	
	Talbutal	Lotusate	
	Thiamylal sodium	Surital Sodium	
	Thiopental sodium	Pentothal Sodium	

PSYCHIATRIC SIDE EFFECTS OF MEDICAL DRUGS (Cont.)

General Classification	Generic	Trade Name	Psychiatric Side Effects
Nonbarbiturate sedatives and hypnotics	Bromide salts	Sodium Potassium Ammonium	Bromide psychosis Depression
	Bromide salts, mixed	Neurosine	Depression Bromide psychosis
	Bromisovalum	Bromural	Bromide psychosis
	Chloral hydrate	Aquachloral Chloral Hydrate Cohydrate Felsules Kessodrate Lycoral Noctec Oradrate Rectules SK-Chloral Hydrate Somnos	Paranoid reactions Chloral delirium Somnambulism
	Ethinamate	Valmid	Paradoxical excitement in children
	Glutethimide	Doriden Glutethimide, NF	Psychosis Confusion Delirium Hallucinations
	Methyprylon	Noludar	Paradoxical excitement Confusion

PSYCHIATRIC SIDE EFFECTS OF MEDICAL DRUGS (Cont.)

General Classification	Generic	Trade Name	Psychiatric Side Effects
Anticonvulsants			
Hydantoins	Diphenylhydantoin	Dihycon Dilantin DPH Ekko Phenytoin Toin Unicelles	General statement regarding hydantoins: hallucinations delusions extrapyramidal reactions
	Diphenylhydantoin sodium	Dilantin Sodium Kessodanten Phenytoin Sodium	
	Ethotoin	Peganone	
	Mephenytoin	Mesantoin	Confusion Psychosis Irritability Depression
Succinimides	Ethosuximide Phensuximide	Zarontin Milontin	General statement regarding succinimides: nervousness apathy euphoria depression personality change confusion severe depression
	Methsuximide	Celontin	
Miscellaneous	Phenacemide	Phenurone	Psychosis with suicidal tendencies Depression Aggressiveness

PSYCHIATRIC SIDE EFFECTS OF MEDICAL DRUGS (Cont.)

General Classification	Generic	Trade Name	Psychiatric Side Effects
Miscellaneous (Cont.)	Primidone	Mysoline	Irritability Hyperexcitability (particularly in children)
Narcotic analgesics			
Morphine and Congeners	Codeine	Calcidrine Syrup Empracet with Codeine Promethazine HCl Expectorant with Codeine Pyribenzamine Expectorant with Codeine & Ephedrine SK-APAP with Codeine	General statement regarding morphine and congeners: mental clouding euphoria excitement restlessness delirium insomnia
	Codeine phosphate	APC with Codeine Actifed-C Ascodeen-30 Ascriptin with Codeine Bancap with Codeine Capital with Codeine Chlor-Trimeton Expectorant with Codeine Codalan Codimal PH Colrex Compound Dimetane Expectorant-DC Empirin Compound with Codeine Emprazil-C Fiorinal with Codeine Isoclor Expectorant Novahistine DH Novahistine Expectorant	

PSYCHIATRIC SIDE EFFECTS OF MEDICAL DRUGS (Cont.)

General Classification	Generic	Trade Name	Psychiatric Side Effects
Morphine and Congeners (Cont.)	Codeine phosphate (Cont.)	Nucofed Syrup	
		Pediacof	
		Phenaphen with Codeine	
		Phenergan Expectorant with Codeine	
		Proval #3	
		Robitussin A-C	
		Robitussin DAC	
		Ryna-C Syrup	
		Ryna-CX Syrup	
		Sinutab with Codeine	
		Soma Compound with Codeine	
		Triaminic Expectorant with Codeine	
		Tussi-Organidin	
		Tylenol with Codeine	
	Codeine Sulfate	Copavin	
	Fentanyl	Innovar	
		Sublimaze	
	Hydromorphone	Dilaudid	
	Levorphanol tartrate	Levo-Dromoran	
	Methadone HCl	Dolophine HCl	
		Vitarine	
		Westadone	
	Morphine sulfate		
	Opium preparations	B&O Supprettes No. 15A & 16A	
		BPP-Lemmon	
		Donnagel PG	
		Pantopon	
		Parepectolin	

PSYCHIATRIC SIDE EFFECTS OF MEDICAL DRUGS (Cont.)

General Classification	Generic	Trade Name	Psychiatric Side Effects
Morphine and Congeners (Cont.)	Oxycodone	Percocet-5 Percodan Tylox	
	Oxymorphone	Numorphan HCl	
	Pentazocaine	Talwin	Dysphoria Nightmares Hallucinations Psychological dependence
Meperidine and Congeners	Alphaprodine HCl Anileridine Meperidine HCl	Nisentil HCl Leritine Demerol	General statement regarding Meperidine and Congeners: dysphoria agitation euphoria transient hallucinations disorientation
Miscellaneous Analgesics	Methotrimeprazine	Levoprome	Delirium Extrapyramidal symptoms
Narcotic Antagonists	Levallorphan tartrate	Lorfan	Dysphoria Bizarre or unusual dreams Visual hallucinations Disorientation Derealization
	Nalorphine HCl	Nalline HCl	Dysphoria Psychotomimetic manifestations

PSYCHIATRIC SIDE EFFECTS OF MEDICAL DRUGS (Cont.)

General Classification	Generic	Trade Name	Psychiatric Side Effects
Cerebral and Respiratory Stimulants			
Amphetamines and Derivatives	Amphetamine sulfate	Delcobese Fetamin Obetrol	General statement regarding amphetamines and derivatives: paradoxical increased depression & agitation in depressed patients depression disorientation hallucinations Psychic dependence Paranoia Schizophreniform psychosis
	Benzphetamine HCl	Didrex	
	Chlorphentermine HCl	Pre-Sate	
	Dextroamphetamine sulfate	Dexamyl Dexedrine Dextro-Amphetamine Eskatrol	
	Dextroamphetamine tannate	Obotan Obotan Forte	
	Diethylpropion HCl	Tenuate Dospan Tenuate 25 Tepanil Tepanil Ten-Tab	
	Methamphetamine HCl	Desoxyn Fetamin	
	Phendimetrazine tartrate	Bacarate Banobese Bontril PDM Melfiat Phendiet Plegine	

PSYCHIATRIC SIDE EFFECTS OF MEDICAL DRUGS (Cont.)

General Classification	Generic	Trade Name	Psychiatric Side Effects
Amphetamines and Derivatives (Cont.)			
	Phendimetrazine tartrate (Cont.)	Statobex	
		Statobex-G	
		Trimstat	
		Trimtabs	
	Phenmetrazine HCl	Phendimetrazine bitartrate	
		Preludin Endurets	
		Preludin	
	Phentermine HCl	Adipex 8	
		Adipex-P	
		Fastin	
		Phentercot T.D.	
	Phentermine resin	Ionamin	
Miscellaneous Agents	Methylphenidate HCl	Ritalin HCl	Nervousness
			Insomnia
			Psychological dependence
Nonnarcotic Analgesics and Antipyretics			
Salicylates	Acetylsalicyclic acid		General statement regarding salicylates:
	Calcium carbaspirin	Fiogesic	emotional disturbances that mimic alcohol inebriation.
		Ursinus Inlay-Tabs	
	Choline salicylate	Arthropan	
		Trilisate	hyperventilation
	Magnesium salicylate	Hyalex	agitation
		Lorisal	confusion
		Magan	
		Mobidin	
		Trilisate	

PSYCHIATRIC SIDE EFFECTS OF MEDICAL DRUGS (Cont.)

General Classification	Generic	Trade Name	Psychiatric Side Effects
Salicylates (Cont.)	Methylsalicylate		
	Salicylamide	Arthralgen	
		Bancap	
		Bancap with Codeine	
		Codalan	
		Coriforte	
		Excedrin	
		Excedrin P.M.	
		Os-Cal-Gesic	
		Rhinex D·Lay	
		Sinulin	
	Sodium salicylate	Corilin	
		Gaysal	
		Gaysal-S	
		Pabalate	
Para-Aminophenol Derivatives	Acetaminophen	APAP	General statement regarding para-aminophenol:
		Acetaminophen	confusion
		Anuphen Suppositories	excitement
		Arthralgen	delirium
		Bancap	psychological dependence
		Bancap with Codeine	
		Capital	
		Capital with Codeine	
		Codalan	
		Colrex	
		CoTylenol	
		Darvocet	
		Datril	
		Demerol APAP	
		Dialog	

PSYCHIATRIC SIDE EFFECTS OF MEDICAL DRUGS (Cont.)

General Classification	Generic	Trade Name	Psychiatric Side Effects
Para-Aminophenol Derivatives (Cont.)	Acetaminophen (Cont.)	Dularin-TH	
		Duradyne DHC	
		Empracet with Codeine	
		Esgic	
		Excedrin	
		Excedrin P.M.	
		Febrigesic	
		Gaysal	
		Gaysal-S	
		Liquiprin	
		Midrin	
		Minotal	
		Nebs Analgesic	
		Ornex	
		Parafon Forte	
		Percocet-5	
		Percogesic	
		Phenaphen	
		Phenaphen with Codeine	
		Phrenilin	
		Proval #3	
		Repan	
		Rhinex D·Lay	
		SK = APAP	
		SK = APAP with Codeine	
		SK = 65 APAP	
		Sedapap-10	
		Sinarest	
		Singlet	
		Sinubid	
		Sinulin	

PSYCHIATRIC SIDE EFFECTS OF MEDICAL DRUGS (Cont.)

General Classification	Generic	Trade Name	Psychiatric Side Effects
Para-Aminophenol Derivatives (Cont.)	Acetaminophen (Cont.)	Sinutab	
		Sinutab II	
		Sinutab with Codeine	
		Sunril	
		Supac	
		Tempra	
		Trind	
		Trind-DM	
		Tussagesic	
		Tylenol	
		Tylenol Extra Strength	
		Tylenol with Codeine	
		Tylox	
		Valadol	
		Vanquish	
		Wygesic	
	Phenacetin (acetophenetidin)	A.P.C.	
		A.P.C. with Codeine	
		A.P.C. with Butalbital	
		Buff-A Comp	
		Buffadyne-Lemmon	
		Empirin	
		Empirin with Codeine	
		Emprazil	
		Emprazil-C	
		Fiorinal	
		Fiorinal with Codeine	
		Monacet (APC) with Codeine	
		Norgesic	
		SK-65 Compound	

PSYCHIATRIC SIDE EFFECTS OF MEDICAL DRUGS (Cont.)

General Classification	Generic	Trade Name	Psychiatric Side Effects
Para-Aminophenol Derivatives (Cont.)	Phenacetin (acetophenetidin) (Cont.)	Soma Soma with Codeine Synalgos Synalgos-DC	
Miscellaneous Agents	Fenoprofen calcium	Nalfon	Confusion Nervousness Insomnia
	Indomethacin	Indocin	Confusion Depression Psychosis
	Naproxen	Naprosyn	Depression Decreased concentration
	Propoxyphene HCl	Darvon Darvon-ASA Dolene Harmar Progesic-65 Propoxychel Propoxyphene Compound 65 Propoxyphene HCl APAP Propoxyphene HCl with APC Proxagesic SK-65 Stero-Darvon with ASA Unigesic-A Wygesic	Euphoria Dysphoria Psychological dependence
	Tolmetin sodium	Tolectin	Tension Nervousness

PSYCHIATRIC SIDE EFFECTS OF MEDICAL DRUGS (Cont.)

General Classification	Generic	Trade Name	Psychiatric Side Effects
Adrenergic (Sympathomimetic) Drugs	Dopamine HCl	Intropin	General statement regarding
	Ephedrine	Amesec	adrenergic drugs:
		Bronkolixir	excess stimulation
		Bronkotabs	insomnia
		Bronkotabs-Hafs	restlessness
		I-Sedrin Plain	nervousness
		Pyribenzamine with Codeine and Ephedrine	tremor
		Pyribenzamine with Ephedrine	
		Quibron Plus	
	Ephedrine HCl	Bronchobid Duracap	
		Calcidrine Syrup	
		Derma Medicone-HC	
		KIE	
		Lufyllin-EPG	
		Mudrane GG	
		Mudrane	
		Quadrinal	
		Quelidrine Syrup	
		Tedral	
		Tedral SA	
		Tedral-25	
		Verequad	
	Ephedrine lactate	Gluco-Fedrin	
	Ephedrine sulfate	Ectasule Minus	
		Ephed-Organidin	
		Isuprel Compound	
		Marax	
		Pazo Ointment	
		Slo-Fedrin	

PSYCHIATRIC SIDE EFFECTS OF MEDICAL DRUGS (Cont.)

General Classification	Generic	Trade Name	Psychiatric Side Effects
Adrenergic (Sympathomimetic) Drugs (Cont.)	Epinephrine	Adrenalin Chloride	
		Asmolin	
		Asthma-meter	
		Primatene Mist	
		Sus-phrine	
	Epinephrine bitartrate	Asmatane	
		Medihaler-Epi	
		Epitrate Opthalmic	
		Lyophrin Opthalmic	
		Mytrate Opthalmic	
	Ephinephrine borate	Epinal Opthalmic	
		Eppy Opthalmic	
	Ephinephrine HCl	Adrenaline HCl	
		Vaponefrin	
		Epifrin Opthalmic	
		Glaucon Opthalmic	
		Mistura E Opthalmic	
	Ethylnorepinephrine HCl	Bronkephrine	
	Hydroxyamphetamine hydrobromide	Paredrine	
	Isoproterenol HCl	Aerolone Compound	
		Duo-Medihaler	
		Iprenol	
		Isuprel	
		Norisodrine Aerotrol	
		Norisodrine with Calcium Iodide	
		Vapo-N-Iso	

PSYCHIATRIC SIDE EFFECTS OF MEDICAL DRUGS (Cont.)

General Classification	Generic	Trade Name	Psychiatric Side Effects
Adrenergic (Sympathomimetic) Drugs (Cont.)	Isoproterenol sulfate	Iso-Autohaler	
		Luf-Iso	
		Medihaler-Iso	
		Norisodrine Sulfate	
	Levarterenol bitartrate	Levophed Bitartrate	
		Norepinephrine Bitartrate	
	Mephentermine sulfate	Wyamine Sulfate	
	Metaraminol bitartrate	Aramine Bitartrate	
		Pressonex Bitartrate	
	Methoxamine HCl	Vasoxyl	
	Methoxyphenamine HCl	Orthoxine	
	Nylidrin HCl	Arlidin HCl	
	Phenylephrine HCl	Chlor-Trimeton	
		Chlor-Trimeton with Codeine	
		Citra	
		Citra Forte	
		Codimal DH	
		Codimal DM	
		Codimal PH	
		Colrex Compound	
		Congespirin	
		Coricidin	
		Coricidin Demilets	
		Coryban-D	
		Dallergy	
		Demazin	
		Dimetane	
		Dimetane DC	
		Dimetapp	
		Dimetapp Extentabs	
		Entex	

PSYCHIATRIC SIDE EFFECTS OF MEDICAL DRUGS (Cont.)

General Classification	Generic	Trade Name	Psychiatric Side Effects
Adrenergic (Sympathomimetic) Drugs (Cont.)	Phenylephrine HCl (Cont.)	Extendryl	
		4-Way Nasal Spray	
		Guistrey Fortis	
		Histalet Forte	
		Histaspan-D	
		Histaspan-Plus	
		Histatapp	
		Histatapp TD	
		NTZ	
		Naldecon	
		Napril Plateau Caps	
		Narine Gyrocaps	
		Neo-Synephrine	
		Ocusol Opthalmic	
		Oraminic Spancap	
		Pediacof	
		Phenergan VC	
		Phenergan VC with Codeine	
		Puretapp	
		Puretapp PA	
		Quelidrine	
		Respinol-G	
		Rhinex	
		Ryna-Tussadine	
		S-T Forte	
		Singlet	
		Trind	
		Trind-DM	
		Tussanil DH	
		Tympagesic	

PSYCHIATRIC SIDE EFFECTS OF MEDICAL DRUGS (Cont.)

General Classification	Generic	Trade Name	Psychiatric Side Effects
Adrenergic (Sympathomimetic) Drugs (Cont.)	Phenylpropanolamine HCl	Allerest	
		Allerest Timed Release	
		Anorexin	
		Bayer Children's Cold Tablets	
		Codimal	
		Coricidin	
		Coricidin "D"	
		Coryban-D	
		Cotofed	
		Decongest TD	
		Dibron	
		Dimetane	
		Dimetane-DC	
		Dimetapp	
		Dimetapp Extentabs	
		Dorcol	
		Entex	
		Fiogesic	
		Histabid Duracap	
		Histalet Forte	
		Histatapp	
		Histatapp T.D.	
		Hycomine	
		Korigesic	
		Kronohist Kronocaps	
		MSC Triaminic	
		Naldecon	
		Napril Plateau	
		Nolamine	
		Novahistine	
		Novahistine DH	

PSYCHIATRIC SIDE EFFECTS OF MEDICAL DRUGS (Cont.)

General Classification	Generic	Trade Name	Psychiatric Side Effects
Adrenergic (Sympathomimetic) Drugs (Cont.)	Phenylpropanolamine HCl (Cont.)	Ornacol	
		Ornade	
		Ornex	
		Puretapp	
		Puretapp-PA	
		Respinol-G	
		Rhinex D·Lay	
		Rhinex DM	
		Robitussin-CF	
		Ryna-Tussadine	
		S-T Forte	
		Sinarest	
		Sinubid	
		Sinulin	
		Sinutab	
		Sinutab-II	
		Sinutab with Codeine	
		Triaminic	
		Triaminic DH	
		Triaminic with Codeine	
		Triaminicin	
		Triaminicol	
		Tussagesic	
		Tussaminic	
		Tussanil DH	
		Tuss-Ornade	
		Ursinus Inlay-Tabs	
	Protokylol HCl	Ventaire	
	Pseudoephedrine HCl	Actifed-C	
		Brexin	
		Broncomar	

PSYCHIATRIC SIDE EFFECTS OF MEDICAL DRUGS (Cont.)

General Classification	Generic	Trade Name	Psychiatric Side Effects
Adrenergic (Sympathomimetic) Drugs (Cont.)	Pseudoephedrine HCl (Cont.)	Codimal-L.A.	
		Cotofed	
		CoTylenol	
		D-Feda Gyrocaps	
		Dimacol	
		Emprazil	
		Emprazil-C	
		Fedahist	
		Fedrazil	
		Histalet DM	
		Histalet	
		Histalet X	
		Isoclor	
		Novafed	
		Novafed A	
		Novahistine DMX	
		Nucofed	
		Pseudo-Bid	
		Pseudocot-G Laytabs	
		Pseudo-Hist	
		Rhinosyn	
		Rhinosyn-DM	
		Robitussin-DAC	
		Robitussin-PE	
		Ryna-C	
		Ryna-Cx	
		Sudachlor T.D.	
		Tussend	
Theophylline Derivatives	Aminophylline	Amesec	
		Aminodur Dura-Tabs	
		Mudrane GG	
		Mudrane GG-2	

PSYCHIATRIC SIDE EFFECTS OF MEDICAL DRUGS (Cont.)

General Classification	Generic	Trade Name	Psychiatric Side Effects
Theophylline Derivatives (Cont.)			
	Aminophylline (Cont.)	Mudrane	
		Mudrane-2	
		Quinamm	
		Somophyllin	
	Dyphylline	Airet	
		Airet L.A.	
		Dilor	
		Dilor-G	
		Emfaseem	
		Lufyllin	
		Lufyllin-EPG	
		Lufyllin-GG	
		Neothylline	
		Neothylline-G	
	Oxtriphylline		
	Theophylline	Aerolate	
		Bronchobid Duracap	
		Broncomar	
		Bronkodyl	
		Bronkolixir	
		Bronkotabs	
		Bronkotabs-Hafs	
		Dibron	
		Elixicon	
		Elixophyllin	
		Elixophyllin SR	
		Elixophyllin-Kl	
		Fleet Theophyllin	
		Hylate	
		Isofil	
		Isuprel	

PSYCHIATRIC SIDE EFFECTS OF MEDICAL DRUGS (Cont.)

General Classification	Generic	Trade Name	Psychiatric Side Effects
Theophylline Derivatives (Cont.)	Theophylline (Cont.)	Marax	
		Mudrane	
		Quibron	
		Quibron Plus	
		Slo-Phyllin GG	
		Slo-phyllin GG	
		Slo-phyllin Gyrocaps	
		Synophylate	
		Synophylate-GG	
		Synophylate-L.A.	
		Tedral	
		Tedral SA	
		Tedral-25	
		Theobid	
		Theo-Dur	
		Theolair	
		Theo-Organidin	
		Theophyl-225	
		Theospan	
	Theophylline monoethanolamine	Fleet Theophylline	
	Theophylline sodium glycinate	Asbron G Inlay-Tabs	
		Synophylate	
		Synophylate-GG	
Adrenergic-Blocking (Sympatholytic) Drugs	Methysergide maleate	Sansert	Depersonalization
			Depression
			Confusion

PSYCHIATRIC SIDE EFFECTS OF MEDICAL DRUGS (Cont.)

General Classification	Generic	Trade Name	Psychiatric Side Effects
Cholinergic-Blocking (Parasympatholytic) Agents*			General statement regarding cholinergic-blocking agents: agitation nervousness hallucinations disorientation psychosis *Symptoms often may be mistaken for senility or mental deterioration caused by progression of the disease in Parkinsonism patients.
	Adiphenine HCl	Transentine Transentine-Phenobarbital	
	Alverine citrate	Spacolin	
	Anisotropine methylbromide	Valpin 50 Valpin 50-PB	
	Atropine sulfate	Antispasmodic Antrocol Arco-Lace Plus Diphenoxylate with atropine Donphen Hybephen Oraminic Spancap Prosed Prydon Trac Tabs Trac Tabs 2x Urised Uristat	Restlessness Irritability Disorientation Incoherence Depression

PSYCHIATRIC SIDE EFFECTS OF MEDICAL DRUGS (Cont.)

General Classification	Generic	Trade Name	Psychiatric Side Effects
Cholinergic-Blocking (Parasympatholytic) Agents (Cont.)	Belladonna extract	Belap	
		Oxoids	
		Ro-Bile	
	Belladonna leaf		
	Belladonna leaf fluid extract		
	Belladonna preparations	Barbidonna	
		Belap	
		Belladenal	
		Belladonna Tincture	
		Donnagel	
		Donnagel-PG	
		Donnatal	
		Donnatal Extentabs	
		Donnatal No. 2	
		Donnazyme	
		Donphen	
		Kinesed	
		Prydon Spansule	
		Sidonna	
		Trac Tabs	
		Trac Tabs 2x	
		Uristat	
	Benztropine mesylate	Cogentin	
	Biperiden	Akineton	
	Chlorphenoxamine HCl	Phenoxene HCl	
	Cycrimine HCl	Pagitane HCl	
	Dicyclomine HCl	Bentyl	
		Bentyl with Phenobarbital	
		Dyspas	

PSYCHIATRIC SIDE EFFECTS OF MEDICAL DRUGS (Cont.)

General Classification	Generic	Trade Name	Psychiatric Side Effects
Cholinergic-Blocking (Parasympatholytic) Agents (Cont.)	Diphemanil methylsulfate	Prantal	
	Ethopropazine HCl	Parsidol HCl	Restlessness Delirium Hallucinations Paranoid psychosis
	Glycopyrrolate	Robinul Robinul forte Robinul with Phenobarbital Robinul Forte with Phenobarbital	
	Hexocyclium methylsulfate	Tral Filmtab Tral Gradumet	
	Homatrophine methylbromide	Gustase-Plus Homapin Liquitab Homapin-5 Homapin-10 Matropinal Metropinal Forte Sed-Tens SE Sinulin	
	Hyoscyamine	Cystospaz Kutrase Levsin Levsin with Phenobarbital Levsinex Timecaps Levsinex with Pehnobarbital Prosed Urised	

PSYCHIATRIC SIDE EFFECTS OF MEDICAL DRUGS (Cont.)

General Classification	Generic	Trade Name	Psychiatric Side Effects
Cholinergic-Blocking (Parasympatholytic) Agents (Cont.)			
	Hyoscyamine sulfate	Anaspaz	
		Anaspaz PB	
		Antispasmodic Elixir	
		Antispasmodic	
		Arco-Lase Plus	
		Cytospaz-M	
		Cytospaz-SR	
		Donphen	
		Hybephen	
		Hybephen Elixir	
		Levsin	
		Levsin/Phenobarbital Timecaps	
		Prydon Spansule	
		Sidonna	
		Uristat	
	Isometheptene HCl	Octin Hcl	
	Isometheptene mucate	Midrin	
		Octin Mucate	
	Isopropamide iodide	Combid Spansule	
		Darbid	
		Ornade Spansule	
		Tuss-Ornade	
	Mepenzolate bromide	Cantil	
		Cantil with Phenobarbital	
	Methantheline bromide	Bantine Bromide	
	Methixene HCl	Trest	
	Methscopolamine bromide	Hyoscine Methylbromide	
		Pamine Bromide	
		Pamine PB	
		Scopolamine Methylbromide	

PSYCHIATRIC SIDE EFFECTS OF MEDICAL DRUGS (Cont.)

General Classification	Generic	Trade Name	Psychiatric Side Effects
Cholinergic-Blocking (Parasympatholytic) Agents (Cont.)	Methscopolamine nitrate	Extendryl	
		Histaspan-D	
		MSC Triaminic	
		Narine Gyrocaps	
		Paraspan	
		Sinovan Timed	
	Methylatropine nitrate	Atropine Methylnitrate	
		Metropine	
	Orphenadrine citrate	Norflex	
		Norgesic	
		Orforine	
		Orphengesic	
	Orphenadrine HCl	Disipal	
	Oxyphencyclimine HCl	Daricon	
		Daricon PB	
		Enarax	
		Gastrix	
	Oxyphenonium bromide	Antrenyl Bromide	
	Pipenzolate bromide	Piptal	
	Piperidolate HCl	Dactil	
	Poldine methylsulfate	Nacton	
	Procyclidine HCl	Kemadrin	
	Propantheline bromide	Giquel	
		Pro-Banthine	
		Pro-Banthine PA	
		Pro-Banthine with Dartal	
		Probanthine with Phenobarbital	
		Propantheline Bromide with Phenobarbital	

PSYCHIATRIC SIDE EFFECTS OF MEDICAL DRUGS (Cont.)

General Classification	Generic	Trade Name	Psychiatric Side Effects
Cholinergic-Blocking (Parasympatholytic) Agents (Cont.)			
	Scopolamine hydrobromide	Donphen	Disorientation
		Hyoscine Hydrobromide	Delirium
		Prydon	
		Scopolamine Hydrobromide	
		Sidonna	
	Thiphenamil HCl	Trocinate	
	Tridihexethyl chloride	Milpath	
		Pathibamate	
		Pathilon	
	Trihexyphenidyl HCl	Antitrem	Psychosis
		Artane	
		Artane Sequels	
		Hexyphen 5	
		Pipanol	
		Tremin	
Mydriatics and Cycloplegics	Atropine sulfate	Atropisol	General statement regarding mydriatics and cycloplegics:
		BufOpto Atropine	
		Isopto Atropine	irritability
	Cyclopentolate HCl	Cyclogyl	hyperactivity
	Homatropine hydrobromide	BufOpto Homatrocel	confusion
		Isopto Homatropine	hallucinations
	Scopolamine	Isopto Hyoscine	delirium
	Tropicamide	Mydriacyl	

PSYCHIATRIC SIDE EFFECTS OF MEDICAL DRUGS (Cont.)

General Classification	Generic	Trade Name	Psychiatric Side Effects
Insulin and Oral Antidiabetics			
Insulins	Extended insulin zinc suspension	Ultralente Iletin Ultralente Insulin	General statement regarding insulins: nervousness confusion diminished coordination psychosis
	Globin zinc insulin injection		
	Insulin injection	Crystalline Zinc Insulin Regular Iletin Regular Insulin	
	Insulin zinc suspension	Iletin, Lente Iletin, Semilente Iletin, Ultralente Insulin, Lente Insulin, Protamine Zinc Insulin, Semilente Insulin, Ultralente Protamine, Zinc, & Iletin	
	Isophane insulin suspension	NPH Iletin NPH Insulin	
Oral Antidiabetic Agents	Acetohexamide	Dymelor	General statement regarding oral antidiabetic agents: confusion paresthesia
	Chlorpropamide	Diabinese	
	Phenformin HCl	DBI DBI-TD Meltrol	
	Tolazamide	Tolinase	
	Tolbutamide	Ornase	

PSYCHIATRIC SIDE EFFECTS OF MEDICAL DRUGS (Cont.)

General Classification	Generic	Trade Name	Psychiatric Side Effects
Thyroid and Antithyroid Drugs			
Thyroid Preparations	Levothyroxine sodium	Cytolen	General statement regarding thyroid preparations:
		Letter	nervousness
		Levoid	agitation
		Ro-Thyroxin	hyperirritability
		Synthroid	insomnia
		I-Thyroxine Sodium	twitching
	Liothyronine sodium	Cytomel	tremor
		Ro-thyronine	
		Sodium-I-Triiodothyronine	
	Thyroglobulin	Proloid	
	Thyroid	Armour Thyroid	
		Euthroid	
		Thyrolar	
	Thyroid desiccated	Dried Thyroid	
		S-P-T	
		Thyrar	
		Thyrocrine	
		Thyroglandular	
		Thyroid Extract ThyroTeric	
	Thyrotropin	Thytropar	
Adrenocorticosteroids and Analogs*	Betamethasone	Celestone	General statement regarding adrenocorticosteroids and analogs:
	Betamethasone benzoate	Benisone	euphoria
		Flurobate	manic-depressive states
		Uticort	psychosis
	Betamethasone valerate	Valisone	*Aggravation of existing emotional instability or psychotic tendencies
	Corticotropin	ACTH	
		Acthar	

PSYCHIATRIC SIDE EFFECTS OF MEDICAL DRUGS (Cont.)

General Classification	Generic	Trade Name	Psychiatric Side Effects
Adrenocorticosteroids and Analogs (Cont.)	Corticotropin (Cont.)	Adrenocorticotropic Hormone	
		Cortigel	
		Cortrophin	
	Cortisone acetate	Compound E	
		Cortone Acetate	
	Desoxycorticosterone acetate	DOCA Acetate	
		Percorten	
		Percorten Pellets	
	Desoxycorticosterone pivalate	Percorten Pivalate	
	Dexamethasone	Aeroseb-Dex	
		Decaderm in Estergel	
		Decadron	
		Deronil	
		Dexone	
		Gammacorten	
		Hexodrol	
		SK-Dexamethasone	
	Dexamethasone acetate	Decadron-La	
		Delladec	
	Dexamethasone sodium phosphate	Decadron Phosphate	
		Deksone	
		Delladec	
		Dexasone	
		Dezone	
		Hexadrol Phosphate	

PSYCHIATRIC SIDE EFFECTS OF MEDICAL DRUGS (Cont.)

General Classification	Generic	Trade Name	Psychiatric Side Effects
Adrenocorticosteroids and Analogs (Cont.)	Fludrocortisone acetate	Florinef	
	Flumethasone pivalate	Locorten	
	Fluocinolone acetonide	Fluonid	
		Neo-Synalar	
		Synalar	
		Synalar-HP	
		Synemol	
	Fluocinonide	Lidex	
		Lidex-E	
		Topsyn	
	Fluorometholone	Neo-Oxylone	
		Oxylone	
	Fluprednisolone	Alphadrol	
	Hydrocortisone	Aeroseb-HC	
		Allersone	
		Alphosyl-HC	
		Biocort Otic	
		Carmol HC	
		Cort-Dome	
		Cortef	
		Cortenema	
		Corticaine	
		Cortisporin	
		Cortril	
		Cotacort	
		Dek-Quin	
		Dermacort	
		Formtone-HC	
		Hydrocortisone	
		Hytone	
		Loroxide-HC	

General Classification	Generic	Trade Name	Psychiatric Side Effects
Adrenocorticosteroids and Analogs (Cont.)	Hydrocortisone (Cont.)	Orlex HC	
		Otic Neo-Cort-Dome	
		Otobione	
		Otocort	
		Proctocort	
		Pyocidin-Otic	
		Racet	
		Racet LCD	
		Rectoid	
		Terra-Cortril Spray with Polymyxin B Sulfate	
		Texacort Scalp Lotion	
		Vanoxide-HC	
		Vioform-Hydrocortisone	
		Vosol HC Otic	
		Vytone	
		Ze-Tar-Quin	
		Zetone	
	Hydrocortisone acetate	Anusol-HC	
		Carmol HC	
		Coly-Mycin S Otic with Neomycin and Hydrocortisone	
		Cort-Dome	
		Cortef Acetate Ointment	
		Cortisporin	
		Derma Medicone-HC	
		Komed HC	
		Mantadil	
		Neo-Cortef	
		Orabase HCA	

PSYCHIATRIC SIDE EFFECTS OF MEDICAL DRUGS (Cont.)

General Classification	Generic	Trade Name	Psychiatric Side Effects
Adrenocorticosteroids and Analogs (Cont.)	Hydrocortisone acetate (Cont.)	Pramosone	
		Protofoam-HC	
		Rectal Medicone-HC	
		Terra-Cortril	
	Hydrocortisone cypionate	Cortef Fluid	
	Hydrocortisone sodium phosphate	Hydrocortone Phosphate	
	Hydrocortisone sodium succinate	A-hydro Cort	
		Solu-Cortef	
	Hydrocortamate HCl	Ulcort	
	Methylprednisolone	Medrol	
		Neo-Medrol	
	Methylprednisolone acetate	Depo-Medrol	
		Medrol Acetate	
		Medrol Enpak	
		Neo-Medrol Acetate	
	Methylprednisolone sodium succinate	A-MethaPred	
		Solu-Medrol	
	Paramethasone acetate	Haldrone	
		Stemex	
		Stero-Darvon with ASA	
	Prednisolone	Delta-Cortef	
		Meticortelone	
		Meti-Derm	
		Prednisolone	
		Sterale	
		Sterane	

PSYCHIATRIC SIDE EFFECTS OF MEDICAL DRUGS (Cont.)

General Classification	Generic	Trade Name	Psychiatric Side Effects
Adrenocorticosteroids and Analogs (Cont.)	Prednisolone acetate	Meticortelone Acetate	
		Metimyd	
		Neo-Delta-Cortef	
		Nisolone	
		Savacort	
		Sterane	
	Prednisolone sodium phosphate	Hydeltrasol	
		Metreton	
		Optimyd	
		PSP-IV	
		Savacort-S	
		Sodasone	
	Prednisolone sodium succinate	Meticortelone Soluble	
	Prednisolone tebutate	Hydeltra-TBA	
	Prednisone	Delta-Dome	
		Deltasone	
		Meticorten	
		Paracort	
		Prednisone	
		Servisone	
		SK-Prednisone	
		Sterapred Uni-Pak	
	Triamcinolone	Aristocort	
		Kenacort	
		Rocinolone	
	Triamcinolone acetonide	Aristocort A	
		Aristoderm	
		Kenalog	
		Mycolog	
	Triamcinolone diacetate	Aristocort Diacetate	
		Cenocort Forte	

PSYCHIATRIC SIDE EFFECTS OF MEDICAL DRUGS (Cont.)

General Classification	Generic	Trade Name	Psychiatric Side Effects
Adrenocorticosteroids and Analogs (Cont.)	Triamcinolone diacetate (Cont.)	Cino-40 Kenacort	
	Triamcinolone hexacetonide	Aristospan	
Estrogens, Progestins and Oral Contraceptives			
Estrogens	Benzestrol Chlorotrianisene Dienestrol Diethylstilbestrol	Chemestrogen Tace AVC/Dienestrol DES Stilbestrol Tylosterone	General statement regarding estrogens: irritabiltiy depression paresthesia lassitude anxiety insomnia
	Diethylstilbestrol diphosphate	Stilphostrol	
	Diethylstilbestrol diproprionate		
	Estradiol	Aquadiol Estrace Progynon Pellets Test-Estrin	
	Estradiol benzoate		
	Estradiol cypionate	Depa-Estradiol Cypionate E-Ionate Femogen	
	Estradiol dipropionate		
	Estradiol valerate	Delestrogen Ditate-DS Duratrad Estate Estraval PA Femogen LA Rep-Estra	

PSYCHIATRIC SIDE EFFECTS OF MEDICAL DRUGS (Cont.)

General Classification	Generic	Trade Name	Psychiatric Side Effects
Estrogens (Cont.)	Estrogens conjugated	Milprem	
		Premarin	
	Esterified estrogens	Amnestrogen	
		Estratab	
		Evex	
		Femogen	
		Menest	
		Menrium	
		SK-Estrogens	
	Estrone	Estrusol	
		Menformin (A)	
		Theelin	
		Wynestron	
	Estrone piperazine sulfate	Ogen	
	Estrone potassium sulfate	Fernspan	
		Spanestrin P	
		Theelin R-P	
	Ethinyl estradiol	Brevicon	
		Demulen	
		Estinyl	
		Feminone	
		Gevrine	
		Gynetone	
		Loestrin	
		Lo/Ovral	
		Lynoral	
		Modicon	
		Nolestrin	
		Os-Cal Mone	
		Ovcon	
		Ovral	

PSYCHIATRIC SIDE EFFECTS OF MEDICAL DRUGS (Cont.)

General Classification	Generic	Trade Name	Psychiatric Side Effects
Estrogens (Cont.)	Ethinyl estradiol (Cont.)	Testand-B	
		Zorane	
	Hexestrol		
	Methallenestril	Vallestril	
	Polyestradiol phosphate	Estradurin	
	Promethestrol dipropionate	Meprane Dipropionate	
Estrogen-Progestin Combinations (Oral Contraceptives)		Brevicon	General statement regarding estrogen-progestin combinations: marked mood swings
		Demulen	
		Envoid	
		Loestrin	
		Lo/Ovral	
		Modicon	
		Norinyl	
		Norlestrin	
		Ortho-Novum	
		Ovulen	
		Ovral	
		Zorane	
Progestin Only (Contraceptives)		Micronor	
		Nor QD	
		Ovrette	

PSYCHIATRIC SIDE EFFECTS OF MEDICAL DRUGS (Cont.)

General Classification	Generic	Trade Name	Psychiatric Side Effects
Diuretics			
Carbonic Anhydrase Inhibitor Diuretics	Acetazolamide	Diamox	General statement regarding carbonic anhydrase inhibitor diuretics:
		Hydrazol	
	Dichlorphenamide	Daranid	
		Oratrol	irritability
	Ethoxzolamide	Cardrase	disorientation
		Ethamide	
	Methazolamide	Neptazane	
Xanthines	Theobromine calcium salicylate	Theocalcin	General statement regarding Xanthines:
	Theobromine magnesium oleate	Athemol	
		Athemol-N	nervousness
			insomnia
			restlessness
			irritability
			delirium
Miscellaneous Agents	Ethacrynic acid	Edecrin	Confusion
			Apprehension
	Spironolactone	Aldactazide	Confusion
		Aldactone	
Histamine/Antihistamines			
Antihistamines	Bromodiphenhydramine	Ambodryl	General statement regarding antihistamines:
	Brompheniramine maleate	Brocon C.R.	
		Dimetane	decreased coordination
		Dimetane-Ten	paradoxical excitation—
		Dimetapp	expecially in children:
		Dimetapp Extentabs	restlessness
		Histatapp	insomnia
		Histatapp T.D.	tremor

PSYCHIATRIC SIDE EFFECTS OF MEDICAL DRUGS (Cont.)

General Classification	Generic	Trade Name	Psychiatric Side Effects
Antihistamines (Cont.)	Brompheniramine maleate (Cont.)	Puretane	euphoria
		Puretapp	nervousness
		Puretapp-PA	delirium
	Carbinoxamine maleate	Clistin	epileptiform seizures
		Rondec	personality changes
		Rondec-DM	hallucinations
	Chlorpheniramine maleate	Alka-Seltzer Plus	
		Allerest	
		Chlor-Trimeton	
		Chlor-Trimeton with Codeine	
		Chlor-Trimeton Repetabs	
		Codimal L.A.	
		Colrex	
		Coricidin	
		Coricidin D	
		Coriforte	
		Corilin	
		CoTylenol	
		Deconamine	
		Decongest T.D.	
		Demazin Repetabs	
		Extendryl	
		Fedahist	
		Guistrey Fortis	
		Histabid Duracap	
		Histalet DM	
		Histalet Forte	
		Histaspan	
		Histaspan-D	
		Histaspan-Plus	
		Isoclor	

PSYCHIATRIC SIDE EFFECTS OF MEDICAL DRUGS (Cont.)

General Classification	Generic	Trade Name	Psychiatric Side Effects
Antihistamines (Cont.)	Chlorpheniramine maleate (Cont.)	Korigesic	
		Kronohist Kronocaps	
		Matropinal	
		Naldecon	
		Napril Plateau Caps	
		Narine Gyrocaps	
		Neotep Granucaps	
		Nolamine	
		Novafed	
		Novahistine	
		Oraminic	
		Ornade	
		Pediacof	
		Pseudo-Hist	
		Quelidrine	
		Rhinex D-Lay	
		Rhinex	
		Rhinex DM	
		Rhinosyn	
		Rhinosyn-DM	
		Ryna-C	
		Ryna-Tussadine	
		Sinarest	
		Singlet	
		Sinovan Timed	
		Sinulin	
		Sudachlor T.D.	
		Teldrin	
		Triaminicin	
		Tusquelin	

PSYCHIATRIC SIDE EFFECTS OF MEDICAL DRUGS (Cont.)

General Classification	Generic	Trade Name	Psychiatric Side Effects
Antihistamines (Cont.)	Chlorpheniramine maleate (Cont.)	Tussanil DH	
		Tussi-Organidin	
		Tussi-Organidin DM	
		Tuss-Ornade	
	Cyclizine HCl	Marezine Hydrochloride	
		Migral	
	Cyclizine lactate	Marezine Lactate	
	Cyproheptadine HCL	Periactin	
	Dexbrompheniramine maleate	Disomer	
		Disophrol Chronotab	
		Drixoral	
	Dexchlorpheniramine maleate	Polaramine	
	Dimenhydrinate	Dimenest	
		Dramamine	
		Meni-D	
		Reidamine	
	Dimethindene maleate	Forhistal Maleate	
		Triten	
	Diphenhydramine HCl	Bax	
		Benadryl	
		Benylin	
		Diphenadril	
		Fenylhist	
		Rohydra	
		SK-Diphenhydramine	
		Valdrene	
	Diphenylpyraline HCl	Diafen	
		Hispril	
	Doxylamine succinate	Bendectin	
		Decapryn	

PSYCHIATRIC SIDE EFFECTS OF MEDICAL DRUGS (Cont.)

General Classification	Generic	Trade Name	Psychiatric Side Effects
Antihistamines (Cont.)	Meclizine HCl	Antivert	
		Bonine	
		Meclizine	
	Methapyrilene HCl	Brexin	
		Citra	
		Citra Forte	
		Co-Pyronil	
		Ephed-Organidin	
		Hista-Clopane	
		Histadyl	
		Histadyl Pulvules	
	Methdilazine HCl	Tacaryl HCl	
	Promethazine HCl	Lemprometh	
		Phenergan	
		Phenergan with Codeine	
		Phenergan with Dextro-methorphan	
		Phenergan VC	
		Phenergan VC with Codeine	
		Promethazine with Codeine	
		Quadnite	
		Remsed	
		Synalgos	
		Synalgos-DC	
		ZiPan	
	Pyrilamine maleate	Allerest	
		Citra	
		Citra Forte	
		Codimal DH	
		Codimal DM	
		Codimal PH	

PSYCHIATRIC SIDE EFFECTS OF MEDICAL DRUGS (Cont.)

General Classification	Generic	Trade Name	Psychiatric Side Effects
Antihistamines (Cont.)	Pyrilamine maleate (Cont.)	Eme-Nil	
		Emesert	
		4-Way Nasal Spray	
		Fiogesic	
		Histalet Forte	
		Kronohist Kronocaps	
		MSC Triaminic	
		Matropinal	
		Matropinal Forte	
		Napril Plateau Caps	
		Ryna-Tussadine	
		Sunril	
		Triaminic	
		Triaminic DH	
		Triaminic with Codeine	
		Tussagesic	
		Tussaminic	
		Tussanil DH	
		Ursinus	
		Wans	
	Trimeprazine tartrate	Temaril	
	Tripelennamine citrate	Pyribenzamine Citrate	
	Tripelennamine HCl	PBZ-SR	
		Pyribenzamine Hcl	
		Rhulihist	
	Triprolidine HCl	Actidil	
		Actifed-C	

PSYCHIATRIC SIDE EFFECTS OF MEDICAL DRUGS (Cont.)

General Classification	Generic	Trade Name	Psychiatric Side Effects
Vitamins			
Vitamin B Complex	Leucovorin	Calcium Leucovorin Folinic Acid	Diminished concentration Altered sleep patterns Irritability Hyperactivity Excitement Depression Confusion Impaired judgment
Antitussives and Expectorants			
Nonnarcotic antitussives	Chlophedianol HCl	Ulo	Excitation Hyperirritability Nightmares Hallucinations
Expectorants	Ammonium chloride	Benylin Coricidin Diphenadril Quelidrine Rhinex DM Triaminicol Zypan	Confusion Excitement Hyperventilation
Antidiarrheal Agents			
Systemic Agents	Diphenoxylate	Lomotil	Euphoria Depression

PSYCHIATRIC SIDE EFFECTS OF MEDICAL DRUGS (Cont.)

General Classification	Generic	Trade Name	Psychiatric Side Effects
Emetics/Antiemetics			
Antiemetics	Diphenidol hcl	Vontrol	Hallucinations Disorientation Confusion
Miscellaneous Agents	Carbidopa/levodopa	Sinemet	Twisting of tongue Grimacing Waving of hands, neck and feet Bruxism Jerky and involuntary movements Dyskinesia Agitation Anxiety Confusion Depression Antisocial behavior Suicidal tendencies Increased libido Mood swings
	Levodopa	Bendopa Bio/Dopa Dopar Larodopa L-dopa	Grimacing Bruxism Twisting of tongue Waving of neck, hands and feet Jerky and involuntary movements

TABLE 1. PSYCHIATRIC SIDE EFFECTS OF MEDICAL DRUGS (Cont.)

General Classification	Generic	Trade Name	Psychiatric Side Effects
Miscellaneous Agents (Cont.)	Levodopa (Cont.)	Sinemet	Dyskinesia Agitation Anxiety Confusion Depression Antisocial behavior Suicidal tendencies Increased libido Mood swings

Index

GPSR Compliance

The European Union's (EU) General Product Safety Regulation (GPSR) is a set of rules that requires consumer products to be safe and our obligations to ensure this.

If you have any concerns about our products, you can contact us on ProductSafety@springernature.com

In case Publisher is established outside the EU, the EU authorized representative is:

Springer Nature Customer Service Center GmbH
Europaplatz 3
69115 Heidelberg, Germany

Batch number: 10607212

Printed by Printforce, the Netherlands